# Lecture Notes: Obstetrics and Gynaecology

# Lecture Notes
# Obstetrics and Gynaecology

**Diana Hamilton-Fairley**
MD, FRCOG
Consultant Obstetrician and Gynaecologist
Guy's and St Thomas's Hospital NHS Trust, London

**Second Edition**

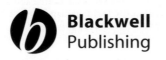

**Blackwell**
Publishing

Blackwell Publishing Inc., 350 Main Street, Malden, Massachusetts 02148-5020, USA
Blackwell Publishing Ltd, 9600 Garsington Road, Oxford OX4 2DQ, UK
Blackwell Publishing Asia Pty Ltd, 550 Swanston Street, Carlton, Victoria 3053, Australia

First published 1999
Reprinted 2000, 2001
Second edition 2004
Reprinted 2006

ISBN-10: 1-4051-2066-5
ISBN-13: 978-1-4051-2066-1

Library of Congress Cataloging-in-Publication Data

Hamilton-Fairley, Diana.
  Lecture notes on obstetrics and gynaecology / Diana Hamilton-Fairley.—2nd ed.
      p.  ;  cm.
  Rev. ed. of: Lecture notes on obstetrics and gynaecology / Geoffrey Chamberlain,
Diana Hamilton-Fairley.
  Includes index.
  ISBN 1-4051-2066-5
  1.Obstetrics.  2. Gynecology.
  [DNLM: 1. Obstetrics.  2. Gynecology. WQ 100 H217L 2004]  I. Title: Obstetrics and
gynaecology.  II. Chamberlain, Geoffrey, 1930—Lecture notes on obstetrics and gynaecology.  III. Title.
  RG526.C43 2004
  618—dc22

                                                                                2004007260

A catalogue record for this title is available from the British Library

Set in 8/12 Stone Serif by SNP Best-set Typesetter Ltd, Hong Kong
Printed and bound by Replika Press Pvt. Ltd, India

Commissioning Editor: Vicki Noyes
Editorial Assistant: Nic Ulyatt
Production Editor: Helen Harvey and Karen Moore
Production Controller: Kate Charman

For further information on Blackwell Publishing, visit our website:
www.blackwellpublishing.com

The publisher's policy is to use permanent paper from mills that operate a sustainable forestry policy,
and which has been manufactured from pulp processed using acid-free and elementary chlorine-free
practices. Furthermore, the publisher ensures that the text paper and cover board used have met
acceptable environmental accreditationstandards.

# Contents

# Preface

Welcome to the second edition of *Lecture Notes: Obstetrics and Gynaecology*. Professor Geoffrey Chamberlain asked me to assist him with the combining of the original well-established separate *Lecture Notes on Obstetrics* and *Lecture Notes on Gynaecology* by joining him as editor of this textbook aimed at undergraduate medical, midwifery and nursing students, junior doctors, nurses and midwives. He told me then that he intended to retire from the editorship for the second edition. I owe him an enormous debt as a teacher, mentor and guide through my career and into the complex area of editing a book with an illustrious list of eminent obstetricians and gynaecologists as its previous editors. He graciously agreed to proof read this edition and I thank him for his helpful contribution to the final version. He continues to work as the Emeritus Professor of History of Medicine at the University of Wales.

In this edition I have asked two of my colleagues at Guy's, King's and St Thomas's Medical School/Guy's and St Thomas's Hospital NHS Trust to expand the sections on Sexually Transmitted Diseases and Breast Disease to reflect the changes in the undergraduate medical curriculum which combines Obstetrics and Gynaecology, Breast Disease and Sexual Health in several UK universities. I would like to thank them both: Dr David Lewis FRCP, MD from Sexual Health and Mr Nicholas Beechey Newman FRCS, MS who wrote the chapter on Breast Disease. I think their two chapters (6 and 18) are a valuable addition to the book and I hope you, the reader, will agree.

Feedback from students, Senior Lecturers and Professors has led to many smaller changes in the book including an expansion on the history taking and examination sections. At the end of each chapter there are five self-assessment questions with the answers/marking schemes given in Answers to self-assessment questions (p. 306). The questions cover the full range that may be found within the examination system in the United Kingdom, both at undergraduate and postgraduate levels, including extended matched questions, scenarios for practicing history taking as in Objective Structured Clinical Examination (OSCE) as well as the more traditional Multiple Choice Questions. I trust they will be of help in the learning and revision process.

Over the decades this series has been translated into many languages, thus reaching an international audience. I hope those using this book all over the world and those who are not doctors in training will find the changes made to this book an addition to their learning even though many of them are based on the changes that have occurred in the British Medical Undergraduate curriculum.

As the editor, I would like this book to aid its readers' understanding of this very important area of health care and that some of you will turn to caring for women and their families as your long-term career. If this book contributes to either or both of these then I am pleased.

Diana Hamilton-Fairley, 2004

# Acknowledgements

I would like to thank the following for their invaluable contribution to this book: Dr David Lewis FRCP, MD Consultant, Department of Genitourinary Medicine, Guy's and St Thomas's Hospital NHS Trust; Mr Nicholas Beechey Newman FRCS, MS Senior Lecturer, Department of Endocrine Surgery, Guy's, King's and St Thomas's Hospital Medical School, King's College London; Professor Geoffrey Chamberlain Emeritus Professor of History of Medicine, University of Wales; and the editorial and publishing staff of Blackwell Publishing.

# Chapter 1

# Basic science

## Female anatomy

The woman's body is built in a different way from that of the male; it is less muscular and therefore has a slighter skeleton to support the muscles. In the abdomen, the non-pelvic organs are similar and subject to the same diseases. Readers are therefore referred to books on general anatomy and this chapter is concerned with female pelvic anatomy. Since much changes in pregnancy we will introduce the pregnancy aspects in this section and Chapter 7.

## Uterus (Box 1.1)

A hollow, muscle-walled organ in the pelvis communicating with each fallopian tube and, through its cervix, the vagina.
Pre-pregnancy: $7 \times 5 \times 3$ cm; weight, 40 g.
Full term: $30 \times 25 \times 20$ cm; weight, 1000 g.

## Structure

Muscle in three layers with vascular anastomosis between them.
**1** Outer: thin, longitudinal, merging with ligaments.
**2** Middle: very thick, spiral muscle fibres with blood vessels between.
**3** Inner: thin, oblique with condensation at each cornu and at the upper and lower end of the cervical canal—the internal and external os.

Increase in size during pregnancy is mostly due to hypertrophy of existing cells rather than increase in number. Changes are stimulated by oestrogen and gradual stretch (maximum effective stretch about term).

## Blood supply (Fig. 1.1)

From the uterine and ovarian arteries, mostly the former. The uterine artery is a branch of the internal iliac artery. It runs in the lower edge of the broad ligament to the junction of the uterine body and cervix before running up the side of the uterus giving off several branches into the myometrium. The ureter lies immediately beneath the uterine artery.

## Cervix (Box 1.2)

Barrel-shaped canal at the bottom of the uterus. (Fig. 1.2) Mostly connective tissue with muscle at upper and lower end (internal and external os). In late pregnancy the ground substance of connective tissue becomes softer with a greater water content and the cervix becomes softer clinically.

## Ligaments

Uterus is supported by ligaments (Fig. 1.3). The principal supports of the uterus are the transverse cervical ligaments (cardinal ligaments), the

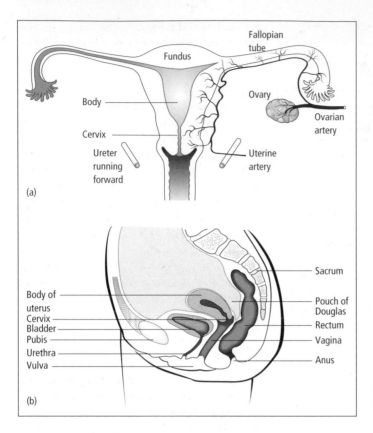

(a)

(b)

**Figure 1.1** Relations of the uterus. (a) Anteroposterior view. (b) Lateral view. See also Box 1.1.

| Box 1.1  Relations of the uterus | |
|---|---|
| Peritoneum | The body and fundus are covered with peritoneum. In front, this is reflected to the upper surface of the bladder. Over the rest of the uterus, the attachment is dense and it cannot be stripped off the uterine muscle |
| Anterior | The uterovesical pouch and bladder |
| Lateral | The broad ligaments with their contents |
| Posterior | The pouch of Douglas. The rectum |

| Box 1.2  Relations of the cervix above the attachment to the vagina | |
|---|---|
| Anterior | Loose connective tissue. Bladder. Pubocervical ligaments |
| Lateral | The ureter 1 cm lateral to the cervix. The uterine artery. Uterine veins. Parametrial lymph glands. Nerve ganglia. The transverse cervical ligament |
| Posterior | Peritoneum of the pouch of Douglas. The uterosacral ligaments |

**Figure 1.2** A longitudinal section of the cervix.

uterosacral ligaments and the round ligament. The round ligament rises from the fundus of the uterus anterior to the fallopian tube and passes into the inguinal canal ending in the labia majora. The broad ligament is made of two layers of peritoneum that run over the fallopian tubes anteriorly to the uterovesical reflection and posteriorly to the rectovaginal reflection. In pregnancy these

are stretched and thickened. They soften because of the progesterone and relaxin effect on collagen.

## Ovary (Box 1.3)

The ovaries have twin functions; both steroid production and gametogenesis. They are a pair of organs on each side of the uterus, in close relation to the fallopian tubes. Each ovary is attached to the back of the broad ligament by a peritoneal fold, the mesovarium, which carries the blood supply, lymphatic drainage and nerve supply of the ovary. The blood supply to the ovaries is principally from the ovarian arteries which arise from the aorta just below the renal arteries.

The ovary is approximately 4 cm long, 3 cm wide and 2 cm thick and weighs about 10 g. A general view of the organs in the pelvis is shown in Fig. 1.1b.

## Structure

The ovary has an outer cortex and inner medulla (Fig. 1.4) and consists of large numbers of primordial oocytes supported by a connective tissue stroma. It is covered by a single layer of cubical,

**Figure 1.3** The ligamentous supports of the uterus. (a) Frontal view. (b) Lateral view. 1, transverse cervical ligament; 2, round ligaments; 3, uterosacral ligaments.

| Box 1.3 Relations of the ovary | |
| --- | --- |
| The ovary lies free in the peritoneal cavity | |
| Anterior | The broad ligament |
| Posterior | The peritoneum of the posterior wall of the pelvis |
| | The common iliac artery and vein |
| | The internal iliac (hypogastric) artery |
| | The ureter |
| Lateral | Peritoneum over the obturator internus muscle |
| | The obturator vessels and nerve |
| | Further out, the acetabulum and hip joint |
| Above | The fallopian tube, which curls over the ovary |
| | Loops of bowel |
| On left | The pelvic colon and its mesentery |
| On right | The appendix if it dips into the pelvis |

**Figure 1.4** Maturation of the oocytes to follicles.

germinal epithelium which is often missing in adult women. Beneath is the fibrous capsule of the ovary, the tunica albuginea, a protective layer derived from fibrous connective tissue.

The cortex of the ovary at menarche contains about 500000 primordial oocytes that may become follicles, cysts about 0.1 mm in diameter. They have a single layer of granulosa cells which produce oestradiol and specially differentiated theca cells which produce androgens.

During each menstrual cycle many primordial follicles are recruited, but usually only one develops fully to become a mature Graafian follicle and expels its oocyte. The granulosa cells multiply and secrete follicular fluid. The oocyte with its granulosa layer projects into the follicle (Fig. 1.4). The stroma cells outside the granulosal cell layer differentiate into:
• the theca interna (a weak androgen secretor);
• the theca externa (no hormone secreting function).

Shortly before ovulation, meiosis is completed in the primary oocyte in response to the luteinizing hormone (LH) surge. The oocyte casts off the first polar body resulting in the number of chromosomes in the remaining nucleus being reduced from 46 to 23. Thus the primary oocyte and the first polar body each contain the haploid number (23) of the chromosomes.

At this stage, the ripe follicle is about 20 mm in diameter. At ovulation it ruptures, releasing the oocyte usually into the fimbriated end of the fallopian tube.

The follicle in the ovary collapses, the granulosa cells become luteal cells while the theca interna forms the theca lutein cells. A corpus luteum develops and projects from the surface of the ovary. It can be recognized by the naked eye by its crinkled outline and yellow appearance. Its cells secrete oestrogen and progesterone. If the ovum is not fertilized, the corpus luteum degenerates in about 10 days. A small amount of bleeding occurs into its cavity, the cells undergo hyaline degeneration and a corpus albicans is formed. If pregnancy does occur, the corpus luteum grows and may reach 3 cm in diameter. It persists for 80–120 days and then gradually degenerates.

## The fallopian tube

The fallopian tube is the oviduct conveying sperm from the uterus to the point of fertilization and ova from the ovary to the uterine cavity. Fertilization usually takes place in the outer part of the tube.

The tube has four parts:
• The *intramural* (cornual) part is 2 cm long and 1 mm in diameter.

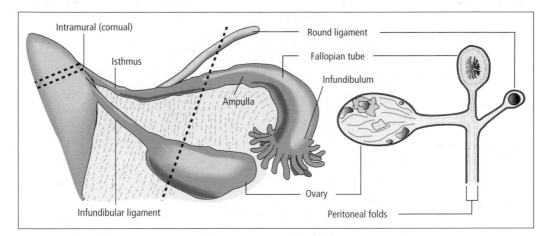

**Figure 1.5** Peritoneal folds to two layers of peritoneum.

- The *isthmus* is thick-walled and is 3 cm long and 0.7 mm in diameter.
- The *ampulla* is wide, thin-walled, being about 5 cm long and 20 mm in diameter (Fig. 1.5).
- The *infundibulum* is the lateral end of the tube. It is trumpet shaped, crowned with the fimbriae that surround the outer opening of the tube. The fimbriae stabilize the abdominal ostium over the ripening follicle in the ovary.

## Structure

The tube has three coats.
- An outer *serous* layer of peritoneum which covers the tube except in its intramural part and over a small area of its attachment to the broad ligament.
- A *muscle* layer with outer longitudinal and inner circular smooth muscle.
- The *mucosa* or endosalpinx which lines the tube that is thrown into numerous longitudinal folds or rugae. The rugae have a core of connective tissue covered with a tall columnar epithelium.

   Three types of cell are found in the mucosa.
- *Ciliated cells*, which beat a current usually in a medial direction.
- *Secretory cells*, which provide the secretion for the rapidly developing blastocyst allowing exchange of oxygen, nutrients and metabolites.

- *Intercillary cells* with long narrow nuclei, squeezed between the other cells. There are rhythmic changes in the epithelium during the menstrual cycle; in the proliferative phase the cells increase in height and activity with increased secretions just after ovulation.

## Vagina (Box 1.4)

The vagina is a fibromuscular canal extending from the vestibule of the vulva to the cervix, around which it is attached to form the fornices.

## Structure

The anterior vaginal wall is about 10 cm long and the posterior wall 15 cm. It is capable of great distension, as in childbirth, after the prolonged

| Box 1.4 Relations of the vagina | |
|---|---|
| Anterior | The bladder and urethra |
| Posterior | Upper—the pouch of Douglas<br>Lower—the rectum, separated by the rectovaginal septum and perineal body |
| Lateral | The cardinal ligaments and the levator ani muscles |

hormonal stimulation of pregnancy. Normally, the anterior and posterior walls are in contact so the cavity is represented by an H-shaped slit.

The walls have:

• an outer connective tissue layer to which the ligaments are attached—it contains blood vessels, lymphatics and nerves;

• a muscular layer consisting of an outer longitudinal layer and an inner circular layer of variable thickness and function;

• the epithelium of stratified squamous epithelium which in adult women contains glycogen and is composed of three layers:

   (a) a basal layer;

   (b) a functional layer;

   (c) a cornified layer.

The epithelium undergoes cyclical changes during the menstrual cycle and characteristic changes during pregnancy. After the menopause it atrophies so that smears taken from postmenopausal women contain a high proportion of basal cells. There are no glandular cells in the vaginal epithelium and so the term vaginal mucosa should not be used.

Vaginal fluid is composed of cervical secretion and transudation through the vaginal epithelium. The vagina allows colonization of lactobacilli which produce lactic acid from the glycogen in the epithelial cells.

## Vulva

The vulva or external genitalia of the female includes the mons, the labia major, the clitoris, the labia minor, the vestibule, the external urethra meatus, the glands of Bartholin and the hymen (Fig. 1.6)

The *mons* is a pad of fat which lies over the pubic symphysis. It is covered with skin in which hair grows profusely from puberty to the menopause.

The *labia major* are two folds of skin which enclose the vaginal opening. They are made up of fatty tissue very sensitive to oestrogen stimulation; the skin of the labia major is covered with hair after puberty.

The *clitoris* contains erectile tissue and is attached to the pubic arch by its crura. Folds of skin running forwards from the labia minor form the prepuce of the clitoris.

The *labia minor* are delicate folds of skin, containing fibrous tissue and numerous blood vessels and erectile tissue. The skin contains sebaceous glands, but no hair follicles, and epithelium which lines the vestibule and vagina.

Mons

Clitoris
Labia major
Urethral orifice
Labia minor
Vestibule
Bartholins gland
Perineum

Anus

**Figure 1.6** The vulva.

The *vestibule* is the area between the labia minor into which opens the vagina, with the external meatus of the urethra in front and the ducts of the Bartholin glands behind.

The *external urethral meatus* is the opening of the urethra covered with squamous epithelium. Skene's ducts from the posterior urethral glands open on to the posterior margin of the meatus.

The *Bartholin glands* are a pair of glands, the ducts of which are lined by columnar epithelium. Each gland is the size of a pea and in structure resembles salivary glands. The secretion is colourless and mucoid and is produced mainly on sexual excitement.

The *hymen* is a circular or crescentic fold of squamous epithelium and connective tissue which partly closes the vaginal entrance in young women. Its shape and size varies. It is often ruptured or stretched by tampon insertion or by intercourse—childbirth destroys it.

## Perineum

The perineum is the area between the vaginal opening and the anus. The perineal body is a pyramidal mass of fibromuscular tissue into which the fibres of the levator ani and the deep transverse perineal muscles are inserted. These are the muscles which are often torn or cut (episiotomy) during childbirth.

## Bony pelvis

The false pelvis is to true pelvis like a saucer on top of a cup. The true pelvis is important in obstetrics, the false pelvis is not. Diameters are shown in Fig. 1.7.

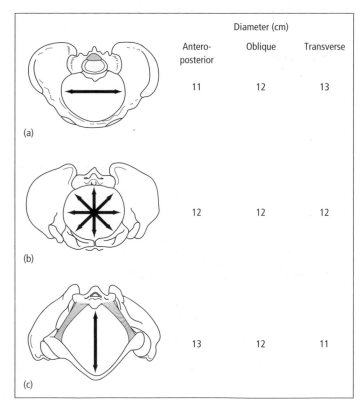

| | Diameter (cm) | | |
|---|---|---|---|
| | Antero-posterior | Oblique | Transverse |
| (a) | 11 | 12 | 13 |
| (b) | 12 | 12 | 12 |
| (c) | 13 | 12 | 11 |

**Figure 1.7** The bony pelvis. (a) Inlet. Longest diameter transverse. Bean shaped. (b) Mid-cavity. All diameters equal. Circle. (c) Outlet. Longest diameter anteroposterior. Diamond shaped.

The longest axis of the pelvis changes through 90° going from top to bottom. Hence the fetus passing through must rotate. There is a long curved posterior wall and a short anterior wall, so the fetus passing through takes a curved course (Fig. 1.8).

The three bones—two ilia and a sacrum—are held together at joints by ligaments, these soften in pregnancy allowing some laxity at these sites.

The coccyx is a fused group of the last vertebrae, hinged on the sacrum by a joint which easily allows bending back in childbirth.

## Pelvic muscles

*Lining lateral wall of pelvis*
• Pyriformis.
• Obturator internus.
*Making pelvic diaphragm*
• Levatores ani comprising:
• pubococcygeus
• iliococcygeus
• ischiococcygeus.
*Beneath pelvic diaphragm*
1 Anterior triangle.
   Deep perineal: compressor urethrae; deep transverse perinei.

Superficial perineal: ischiocavernosus; bulbocavernosus; superficial transverse perinei.
2 Posterior triangle.
   Sphincter ani.

## Essentials of pelvic musculature

1 The pyriformis muscles reduce the useful transverse diameter of upper and mid-cavities, thus thrusting the fetus forward.
2 The pelvic diaphragm and its fascia are like a pair of cupped hands tilted slightly forward (Fig. 1.9). Muscle fibres lace the one hand with the other, being especially thick around the three tubes which broach the diaphragm—the urethra, the vagina and the rectum. These muscle slings pull each of these forward making an extra sphincter.

## Female physiology

### Pituitary hormones

#### Follicular stimulating hormones (FSH)

These are soluble glycoproteins. Production is activated by gonadotrophic releasing hormones

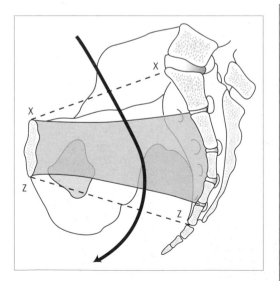

**Figure 1.8** Side view of bony pelvis, showing the plane of the inlet (x–x), the zone of the mid-cavity (toned), and the plane of the outlet (z–z).

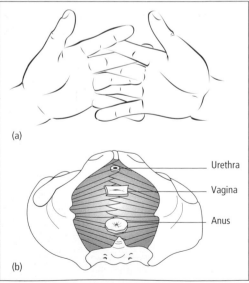

**Figure 1.9** Interlocking hands (a) illustrate the lacing of the muscle fibres in the pelvic diaphragm (b).

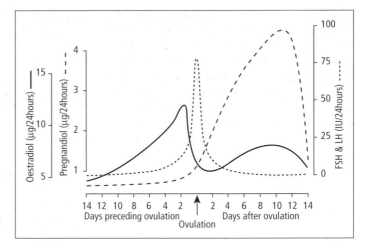

**Figure 1.10** Hormone levels before and after ovulation.

(GnRH) from the hypothalamus. FSH is produced in the anterior lobe of the pituitary and production is increased in the first half of the menstrual cycle. This production is diminished by increasing oestrogen levels (negative feedback) (Fig. 1.10). It leads to recruitment of oocytes and their maturation.

## Luteinizing hormone (LH)

A soluble glycoprotein activated in the pituitary by GnRH. The LH is released from the pituitary in a bolus at mid-cycle initiating ovulation if the

follicle is already primed by oestrogen. Ovulation takes place 36 hours after the LH surge.

## Ovary

In each menstrual cycle over 400 primitive oocytes migrate to the surface of the ovaries under the influence of follicle stimulating hormone (FSH). LH and FSH act in concert to select a single oocyte. When one follicle reaches 20 mm in diameter, the oocyte is squeezed to the surface of the ovary (Fig. 1.11). The remaining follicles atrophy.

The process of ovulation is preceded by:

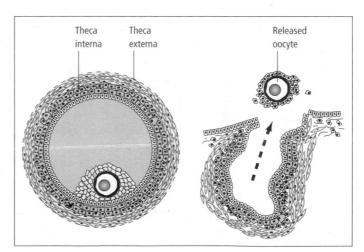

**Figure 1.11** The follicle just before and just after the oocyte is released.

• the release of LH from the pituitary which initiates ovulation and the completion of the first meiotic division;
• a spurt of oestrogen from the tissues of the follicle.

The outward signs and changes associated with ovulation are:
• the cervical mucus becomes less viscid, becoming watery and increasing in amount;
• in some women peritoneal pain is caused by irritation of released blood from the follicle (mittelschmerz);
• the body temperature may increase by about 0.6°C.

## Fertilization

The fimbriated end of the fallopian tube, possibly excited by chemotaxis, closes to embrace the ovary like a hand holding a rugby football. The egg has virtually no transperitoneal passage.

At the time of intercourse millions of sperms are deposited in the vagina. They travel in all directions, some through the cervix, where, in mid-cycle, the molecules of cervical mucus untangle their barbed-wire-like morphology to assume straight lines. A few sperm reach each fallopian tube where they swim counter-current, the first arriving near the oocyte within 30 minutes of intercourse. One sperm only penetrates the zona pellucida by hyaluronidase activity; the tail is shed, the sperm's neck becomes the centrosome and the head is the male pronucleus containing half the genetic potential of the future fetus (Fig. 1.12).

Sperm penetration into the ovum initiates the second meiotic division of the ovum, with a reduction in chromosomes from 46 to 23 and the extrusion of a second polar body. The haploid nuclei of the oocyte and the sperm combine, restoring the diploid state of 46 chromosomes and ferlilization is achieved.

Fertilization usually occurs at the ampullary end of the fallopian tube within 12–24 hours of oocyte production. The fertilized egg then travels along the tube propelled by:

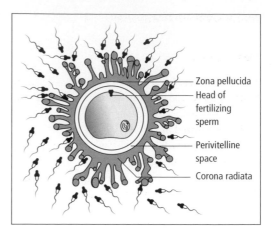

Figure 1.12 Several sperms surround the oocyte, but only one penetrates.

• Muscular peristalsis of the tube.
• Currents in the tube whipped by cilia.

During this time, nutrition and oxygenation are from the fluid secreted by the glandular cells of the fallopian tube lining. Arriving in the uterus 4–5 days later, it is in the cavity for 2–3 days and implants in the thick endometrium in the secretory phase on about day 22 of the cycle. The blastocyst starts to put out pseudopodia so that the surface area available for maternofetal exchange is increased. All transfer is by osmosis and diffusion at this stage.

## Germ cells

There are seven million primordial oocytes in each ovary of the female fetus, which drops to two million at birth and is further reduced to half a million at puberty.

About 400 are initiated during each ovulation cycle; the rest degenerate at a steady rate. At the menopause there are no more follicles available for ovulation and so there is diminution of oestrogen production.

Ovulation is controlled by the ovarian hormones and the gonadotrophins from the pituitary.

## Major ovarian hormones

### Oestrogens

These are mostly produced by the maturing follicle. Levels gradually increase to a peak at the time of ovulation (Fig. 1.13).

The recognized functions of oestrogens are to:
• stimulate growth of the vagina, uterus and oviducts in childhood;
• increase the thickness of the vaginal wall and distal one-third of the urethra by increased stratification of the epithelium;
• reduce vaginal pH by the action of the Doderlein's bacillus on the glycogen to form lactic acid;
• decrease viscosity of cervical mucus to facilitate sperm penetration;
• facilitate the development of primordial follicles;
• inhibit follicle stimulating hormone (FSH) secretion;
• stimulate proliferation of the endometrium;
• increase myometrial contractility;
• stimulate growth of breasts with duct proliferation;
• promote calcification of bone;
• promote female fat distribution;
• promote female hair distribution.

Oestrogen is metabolized by the liver and conjugated with glucuronic acid so that 65% is excreted in urine.

### Progesterone

This hormone is produced by the corpus luteum in large amounts following ovulation and by the placenta in pregnancy. Its functions are to:
• induce endometrial secretory changes;
• increase the growth of the myometrium in pregnancy;
• decrease myometrial activity in pregnancy;
• increase secretory activity in the uterine tubes;
• decrease motility of the uterine tubes;
• increase the glandular activity in the breasts.

Progesterones are metabolized in the liver, 80% becomes pregnanediol.

**Figure 1.13** Pathways of oestrogen metabolism. Oestradiol is a pregnancy oestrogen metabolized by the fetoplacental unit and does not appear here.

## Physiology

### The menstrual cycle

The cyclical interaction of the hormones from the hypothalamus, anterior pituitary and the ovaries is shown in Fig. 1.14.

• The production of oestrogen and later oestrogen and progesterone by the ovaries results in changes in the endometrium.

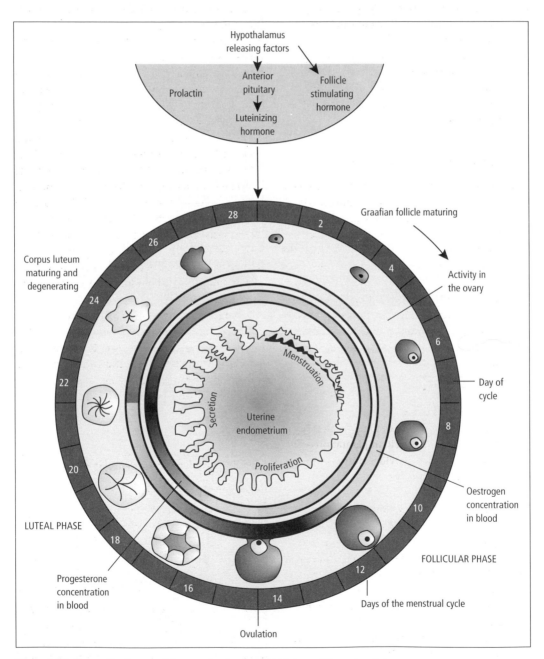

**Figure 1.14** Composite diagram of the menstrual cycle and histology of the endometrium.

• The *endometrium* is the mucous membrane of the uterus, consisting of tubular glands with supporting stroma. There are numerous blood vessels which arise from the spiral arterioles, the terminal branches of the uterine arteries.
• The endometrium rests on the *uterine musculature*; its basal areas are so closely applied they cannot be removed with a curette but can be reached at endometrial ablation.
• The *basal layer* of tubular glands which regenerate following menstruation.
• The *superficial compact layer* is covered with ciliated columnar epithelial cells which extend down into the endometrial glands.

## Changes in the menstrual cycle

At the end of menstruation, the endometrium enters a short resting phase, when it is thin, its glands are straight and the stroma compact and non-vascular. As oestrogen levels rise, the endometrium enters a follicular or proliferative phase with the endometrial glands becoming tortuous; the stroma becomes cellular.

After ovulation, the corpus luteum is formed under the influence of LH; it secretes oestrogen and progesterone. In the luteal phase, the endometrium becomes secretory; it is thick, pale and glycogen appears in the glands which in turn become full of secretions.

### If the ovum is fertilized

The endometrium grows to become the decidua of pregnancy. Stroma cells swell. Implantation occurs on the decidua, which provides nutrition for the rapidly developing blastocyst.

### In the absence of fertilization

About 12–14 days after ovulation, there is an intense spasm of the endometrial arterioles leading to tissue hypoxia and death in the superficial layers. Fissuring of the endometrium follows with cleavage of the endometrium from its spongy layer. It is shed in small areas with accompanying bleeding—the menstrual loss. Following this, regeneration occurs from the remaining basal layer and the cycle recommences.

## The fallopian tubes (Box 1.5)

Their functions are:
• to convey a spermatozoon from the endometrial cavity to the ovum in the outer third of the fallopian tube;
• to transmit the fertilized oocyte into the endometrial cavity;
• to provide nutrients to the developing embryo on its five day passage.

Oestrogen reduces the peristalsis of the tubes; at the time of ovulation there is a reversal of peristalsis to help the sperm to travel more easily up the crypts between the folds of the mucus.

The oocyte is squeezed out of the follicle and sticks to the surface of the ovarian fimbria of the tube. The fimbria embraces the ovary and the oocyte moves directly into the fallopian tube with no transperitoneal journey. Fertilization is by a single sperm penetrating the zona pellucida.

Peristalsis of the muscle of the tube and the action of fine cilia move oviduct fluid and the passive ovum from the peritoneal end of the fallopian tube into the endometrial cavity taking about five days.

During this passage, the fertilized ovum receives nutrition from secretions of the mucosa of the tube. Here gas exchange between the rapidly growing blastocyst and fallopian tube fluid also takes place. These tubal secretions are under the influence of oestrogen priming and increase greatly

| Box 1.5 Relations of the fallopian tubes | |
|---|---|
| Anterior | Top of the bladder |
| | Uterovesical peritoneal pouch |
| Superior | Coils of intestine |
| | On the right, caecum |
| | On the left, pelvic colon |
| Posterior | Ovary |
| | Pouch of Douglas and its contents |
| Lateral | Peritoneum over the obturator muscle |
| | Obturator vessels and nerve |
| Inferior | Structures in the broad ligament |

with progesterone. Mucopolysaccharide concentration and the calcium ions within the tubes also increase.

## The vulva and vagina

The vagina is a tube lined by stratified squamous epithelium which contains no mucous glands and so there are no vaginal secretions. Any lubrication is a combination of secretions from the cervical canal mixed with secretions from vulval glands and a transudate from the vagina.

The labia minor are normally in apposition as are the fatter labia major in normal standing, sitting and lying down positions, only parted when the legs abduct.

## Sexual activity

On sexual stimulation, there is a vascular engorgement of the labia major, minor and the clitoris. The sweat glands of the labia minor increase their secretions and at the same time mucus is secreted from the Bartholin's glands and endocervical glandular epithelium.

Abduction of the thighs opens the labia major and the voluntary musculature of the vagina and vulva helps to dilate the upper vagina whilst gripping the penis in the lower vagina.

The sexual response in women is usually slower than in men, but a plateau of response is more prolonged and it does not disappear so rapidly after orgasm as is often the case in men.

---

**Self-assessment**

**1.1** From the list of words/phrases below fill in the blanks.
The uterine artery is a branch of the (1) _____ artery. The uterus is a hollow, muscle-walled organ in direct communication with the (2)_____ and the vagina. Inferior to the uterine artery lies the (3) _____ The ligaments that support the uterus include the (4) _____ and (5) _____.
(a) external iliac
(b) transverse cervical
(c) pudendal
(d) ureter
(e) pectineal
(f) bladder
(g) fallopian tubes
(h) internal iliac
(i) ovaries
(j) uterosacral

**1.2** Which of the following statements are true?
(a) The granulosa cells secrete androstenedione.
(b) The granulosa cells become luteal cells following the release of the oocyte.
(c) Luteal cells secrete progesterone alone.
(d) The ovary contains around 50 000 oocytes at menarche.
(e) The primordial oocytes are found in the cortex of the ovary.

**1.3** Which of the following statements are true of the menstrual cycle?
(a) The LH surge causes the oocyte to undergo meiosis reducing the chromosome number in the oocyte to 23.
(b) Oestradiol causes the endometrial glands to secrete glycogen.
(c) The endometrium is shed because the spiral arterioles lose their elasticity and start to bleed.
(d) The luteal phase lasts for a fixed duration of 12–14 days.
(e) In the proliferative phase of the cycle the endometrial glands become tortuous.

**Self-assessment** *Continued*

**1.4** Which of the following statements are true?
- (a) Oestradiol exerts a negative feedback on FSH.
- (b) The secretion of FSH and LH is under the control of the thalamus.
- (c) FSH catalyses the conversion of testosterone to oestradiol.
- (d) Testosterone is essential for the production of oestradiol.
- (e) Progesterone concentrations reach their peak at the time of ovulation.

**1.5** Using the words and phrases below label the diagram provided.
- (a) Uterine fundus
- (b) Uterine corpus
- (c) Endometrium
- (d) Isthmus of fallopian tube
- (e) Ampulla of fallopian tube
- (f) Infundibulopelvic ligament
- (g) Internal os of cervix
- (h) External os of cervix
- (i) Fimbriae of fallopian tube
- (j) Round ligament

# Part 1

## The woman

# Chapter 2

# The woman as a patient

## Attitudes of women

The attitudes of women towards their medical attendants has changed in the last 50 years. The subservient doctor-knows-best approach has been modified amongst young and intelligent women who ask more questions. They are more informed about medical matters because of press articles, television, radio and internet. They query the authority of the doctor more, not because they mistrust him or her but to ensure they understand their condition.

In the 1960s there was a more aggressive approach by women asking for more recognition. This had its major opportunity with the onset of oral contraception which for the first time put fertility squarely in the hands of women. Here too was the release from the doctor's benevolent parentalism.

About 70% of women prefer to be looked after by women doctors. This is understandable and if staff ratios allow, this should be attended to.

## Clinical approach

Doctors should remember the sensitive nature of gynaecological and obstetrical problems which are very personal to women. No one wants to visit the gynaecologist but they do if they think it would help. The attitude towards the obstetrician is mollified by the fact that women realize that there are two patients and problems may arise in pregnancy both for the mother and the fetus. Generally, difficulties can be assuaged by allowing more time for such a consultation. Many find it difficult to discuss the intimate sexual details of their lives with doctors and so tact and discretion are needed. Often further points of history come out whilst the examination is being performed or at the next visit.

When examining a female patient, all doctors should have a chaperone, who need not be present during the history but could be introduced at the time of examination. The attitude of the doctor towards the woman is terribly important and can set the whole tone of the relationship. Friendly, but not affectionate, should be the tone of the doctor's behaviour.

## Women's choice

The Patient's Charters issued by the Department of Health have raised expectations about women's choice of doctors. The general practitioners of a given area look after their population of men and women usually with complete confidence on both sides, but provision has been made for the rotation between practices of those who do not wish to accept the management and treatment protocols of a given practice.

When a woman has to be referred to hospital, she may request that she goes to a certain unit. This applies mostly in the big towns, for in rural areas there is usually only one District General Hospital. There again the woman may request to see (or not see) any given consultant for her own reasons. In the out-patients this can usually be arranged but not at an emergency level where consultants work to a rota.

The presence of junior doctors or medical students at teaching hospitals is being highlighted at the moment. Naturally women want privacy, but when it is explained to them that these are the doctors of the future, they usually understand and allow them to be present.

## Ethics

Ethics is the science of morals but probably is better interpreted as the rules of conduct recognized in certain departments of human life. Those in the medical profession owe an ethical duty to do their best for those who seek their care. In latter years the subject has moved more towards the science and people have tried to lay down guidelines.

Generally speaking, the ethics of medicine are covered by the General Medical Council, the British Medical Association and the Ethical Committees of the various Colleges including the Royal College of Obstetricians and Gynaecologists. Details proliferate but a central principal remains that you should do unto others as you would they should do unto you. Always imagine your mother or your daughter as the patient and how you would like them to be treated. This will generally lead to good ethical behaviour.

## The pregnant woman

When a woman becomes pregnant she usually consults her family doctor first. There may be records going back many years and the doctor may know the woman from previous medical encounters. There is already a rapport between the doctor and the woman. While many of the items needed in the antenatal record for the history are already in the practice records, it is wise to keep a pro forma especially for each pregnancy with summaries of detailed notes held elsewhere. A National Maternity Record has now been developed. With team obstetrics becoming common, midwives need to know of certain events in a woman's life. This raises the complication of the inclusion of events of a sensitive nature such as previous terminations of pregnancy or sexually transmitted diseases. Practitioners must seek the permission of the woman as to how much of this goes into the woman's hand-held notes, but for obvious reasons this should be as complete as possible. If the woman wishes to keep confidential essential pieces of information which may affect the clinical management then marks such as an asterisk or euphemisms should be recorded in her notes that will alert your colleagues. For example, if a woman does not wish her HIV status to be recorded then it is acceptable to write that the woman should not have an instrumental delivery or breastfeed. This will clearly indicate to both midwives and doctors that she is HIV positive but will not mean anything to a non-medically trained person who may see her notes.

If the woman attends an antenatal clinic where she is not known, one has to start from the beginning. The history, examination and investigation of the woman are taken at the booking clinic when she attends for the first time in pregnancy (see Chapter 9). Ideally, this should be at 8–10 weeks of gestation but more often in Britain it has slipped to 12–14 weeks, hence invalidating all the help that can be offered to the woman in the first trimester and passing the time when teratogenesis might have been avoided.

## The gynaecological patient

Most women in their lives will consult a doctor about gynaecological symptoms. Initially this will be with a general practitioner. If the condition warrants, the woman may be referred to a hospital gynaecologist. Be it specialist or general practitioner, the same logical processes must be used to make a diagnosis and direct management. (The obstetric assessment is in Chapter 9.)

The gynaecological assessment will be considered under three headings.

- History.
- Examination.
- Investigations.

## History

This is best considered under systematic headings so that no important symptoms are omitted. It is often necessary to ask leading questions.
- The woman herself may not realize the significance of her symptoms.
- She may be reluctant to mention symptoms connected with sexual troubles.

The following is a useful pro forma.

*Personal information*
- Name, age, date of birth.
- Married, single, widowed, divorced, separated.
- Occupation past and present.
- Hours and conditions of work.
- Partner's occupation.
- Type of housing.

*Chief symptom*
- Duration.
- Periodicity.
- Severity and description.

*Any treatment of present complaint so far*
All drugs taken recently must be noted, especially tranquillizers, oral contraceptives, hormones and antibiotics.

*History of past major illness or operations*
- All admissions to hospital with approximate dates.
- A written report obtained from another hospital may be helpful especially with conditions such as infertility, to check what has been done.

*Social history*
- Home conditions (including nature and state of relationships with other people in the residence).
- Conditions of work.
- Occupation.
- Smoking habits.

- Alcohol habits.
- Drugs (cannabis, etc.).

*Family history*
- Health of parents and siblings.
- History of hereditary or familial disease.

*Sexual history*
- Dyspareunia.
- Difficulty with coitus.
- Use of contraception.
- Sexually transmitted diseases.

*Obstetric history*
- Number of pregnancies.
- Dates.
- Mode of termination of each, i.e. full-term birth, premature birth, stillbirth, miscarriage, ectopic pregnancy.
- Abnormalities of:
  (a) pregnancy;
  (b) labour;
  (c) puerperium.
- Birth weights of children and their names.
- Their present state of health.

*Menstruation*
- Age at onset (menarche).
- Approximate duration of each menstrual bleed;

$$K = \frac{\text{days of bleeding}}{\text{length of cycle (dl-dl)}}$$

- Interval from the first day of one to the first day of the next period.
- Estimate of amount and character of loss.
- Any recent change:
  (a) increase;
  (b) decrease;
  (c) clots or flooding.
- Any pain associated with menstruation.
- Date of last period.
- Date of last cervical smear.

*Vaginal discharge*
- Character of discharge:
  (a) mucoid;
  (b) purulent;

(c) colour;

(d) quantity;

(e) bloodstained.

• Discharge may be offensive or may cause:

(a) soreness;

(b) irritation.

*Micturition*

• Frequency, day and night.

• Pain on micturition.

• Urge incontinence (micturition must occur on the urge).

• Stress incontinence (loss occurs on virtually any physical effort).

*Bowels*

• Regularity.

• Use of purgatives.

• Any history of piles, pain or difficulty on defaecation.

• Rectal bleeding.

## Examination

The general appearance of the patient should be observed.

• Height.

• Weight: calculate body mass index (BMI)

$$BMI = \frac{wt(kg)}{ht^2(m^2)}$$

• Does she look anxious or ill?

A systematic examination is made with special attention to the reproductive system.

• The lower eyelid mucous membrane should be inspected for anaemia.

• The breasts should be examined in the over 35-year-old (see Chapter 18).

• Other relevant symptoms, such as breathlessness or cough, call for examination of the heart and lungs.

## Abdominal examination

The patient should be asked to empty her bladder before examining her abdomen and pelvis. The abdomen should be exposed from the costal mar-gin to the pubes and the patient should lie comfortably relaxed. A sheet or light blanket over the pubis is used to prevent unnecessary exposure.

*Inspection*

• Skin quality and fat or wasting.

• Distension or any visible tumour.

• Operation scars, especially a laparoscopy crescent at the umbilicus or lower abdomen curved scar for pelvic surgery.

*Palpation*

This is done lightly at first to test for any localized tenderness or rigidity. Deep palpation is used to confirm the presence of a tumour or enlargement, especially of uterus or ovaries.

*Percussion*

If there is a central tumour it will be dull to percussion with hollow sounds from the flanks. Ascites may produce shifting dullness in the flanks and central resonance.

*Auscultation*

Although this will rarely help, it may give reassurance about intestinal activity, and bowel sounds may be heard. Fetal heart sounds may help make a diagnosis of pregnancy using a handheld Doppler-tone after 12 weeks.

## Pelvic examination

A chaperone should always be present when performing a vaginal examination to act as an advocate for the woman and to potentially protect the doctor (male and female) from accusations of assault or inappropriate behaviour. You should offer a full explanation of the examination you are about to perform. Verbal consent should be obtained from the woman in the presence of a chaperone. Prior to commencing the examination, ensure that you have all the necessary equipment, speculum, swabs, spatulas/cytobrushes, slides that you may require, ready. If you are going to perform a cervical smear ensure that the slide is labelled in pencil (the fixative dissolves ink from biros and pens) with the patient's name, date of birth, hospital number if she has one and the date of the examination before taking the smear.

### The vagina

Vaginal examination can usually be satisfactorily performed by using the index finger alone. This causes less discomfort and muscle spasm. If the vagina is long or voluminous or your fingers are small, a second finger may be needed. The finger(s) should be inserted slowly up to the level of the cervix.

Assessment is by bimanual examination, the other hand being on the abdomen above the pubic symphysis. A three-dimensional image of the pelvis is built up from information obtained from both hands, not just the vaginal one (Fig. 2.1).

### The vulva

The vulva is inspected for:
• swelling;
• inflammation;
• ulceration.

### The urethra

The urethral orifice is inspected for:
• urethritis;
• caruncle.

The patient is asked to cough or strain and any prolapse or stress incontinence of urine is noted.

## Examination with a speculum

This is an essential part of the gynaecological examination. If it must be omitted because the vaginal entrance is too small or because of vaginismus, the examination is incomplete.

The *bivalve speculum* (Cusco's) consists of two limbs jointed at the handle; it is made in various sizes and is useful for general cervical and upper vaginal examination (Fig. 2.2). It is also made in a disposable plastic form. A *Sim's speculum* holding back the posterior wall gives a good view of the cervix and anterior vaginal wall (Fig. 2.3). The woman should be in the left lateral position (see p. 286).

When passing a speculum, it is important to remember that the vagina is directed upwards and backwards; warming a speculum under a warm tap makes it more comfortable.

**Figure 2.2** A bivalve or Cusco speculum used to examine the cervix with the woman in the dorsal position.

**Figure 2.3** A Sim's speculum used to hold back the posterior vaginal wall with the woman in the left lateral position.

**Figure 2.1** A bimanual examination gathers information about the pelvis with both hands.

## Bimanual examination

When a cervical smear or a high vaginal swab is to be taken, it is best to pass the speculum before making a bimanual examination. This examination may be performed in the dorsal or left lateral position, a matter of personal preference among gynaecologists. In either case the patient should be spared unnecessary exposure by covering her with a sheet or light blanket. The gloved index finger may be lightly lubricated and is introduced gently into the vagina.

- The condition of the vaginal walls is noted.
- The cervix is palpated for softening, tears or polypi.
- The uterus is palpated between the two hands noting:
  - (a) size;
  - (b) consistency;
  - (c) shape;
  - (d) mobility;
  - (e) tumours;
  - (f) tenderness on pressure.

The finger in the vagina is now moved into the right lateral fornix, the hand on the abdomen follows to explore for any enlargement or tenderness of the tubes or ovaries. A similar examination is made of the left adnexa. The finger is passed to the posterior fornix to detect swelling in the pouch of Douglas.

## Rectal examination

This can be valuable in certain aspects of gynaecology, but the patient may find it the most uncomfortable part of the whole examination. It permits bimanual examination of the uterus, tubes and ovaries if vaginal examination is impossible or undesirable. It may further be easier to feel a retroverted uterus or a swelling in the pouch of Douglas and allows an easier approach to the parametrium and uterosacral ligaments. The possibility of rectal disease must always be borne in mind.

## Investigations

*Blood*
The haemoglobin level should always be measured before an operation, however minor. It should certainly be done in cases of excessive uterine bleeding (menorrhagia) and as a routine in early pregnancy. Blood disorders may be associated with a bleeding tendency so a platelet count, bleeding time and clotting time may also be done.

In black women, a sickle test should be done, and in women of Mediterranean or Middle East origin, there may be a thalassaemia trait which is diagnosed by electrophoresis.

Serological tests of syphilis and human immunodeficiency virus 1 (HIV 1) antibodies are done after counselling if there is any suspicion of either disease.

Blood urea and other tests for renal function should be done where indicated.

Human chorionic gonadotrophin (hCG) levels may be checked if a pregnancy is suspected. Other hormone levels in the blood may be measured in specific conditions. Their ranges are wide.

*Urine*
The urine should be tested as appropriate for:
- albumin;
- sugar;
- bacilluria by nitrite dipstick;
- microscopy and culture.

*Cytology*
Exfoliative cytology in gynaecology examines cells desquamated from the epithelium of the genital tract. Material may be obtained by scraping the cervix with Ayre's wooden spatula, or a cytobrush. Cytology is principally used in the early detection of premalignant lesions of the cervix and is considered in Chapter 19.

*Colposcopy*
Colposcopy examines the cervix under magnification in the out-patient department. It is used in conjunction with cervical cytology so that biopsies can be accurately taken from suspicious areas and treatment performed (Chapter 19).

*Laparoscopy*
Visual examination of the pelvis and peritoneal cavity is invaluable when investigating pain or fertility potential.

*Hysteroscopy*
Endoscopy of the uterine cavity demands a fluid or gas under pressure to open up the cavity. Then the endometrium can be inspected and biopsied.

*Ultrasound*
Abdominal or vaginal probes may be used. The size of the tumour can be estimated more accurately (Fig. 2.4). The vascularity of the tumour can be measured with Doppler ultrasound and its cystic or malignant nature assessed. Also fibroids can be detected and distinguished from ovarian cysts, often a difficult clinical problem.

Ultrasound is used to monitor the progress of ovulation. A follicle can be found from day 10 of the cycle and its development monitored by a daily scan. When the follicle reaches 20 mm it is close to ovulation and is the best time for the harvesting of oocytes. After ovulation the corpus luteum can be shown in the ovary.

Using ultrasound, a hydatidiform mole can be detected; the vesicles reflect echoes leaving a picture of a series of multiple semicircular reflections, rather like bubble foam/wrap. There is usually no fetus or fetal heartbeat.

In early pregnancy, an embryonic sac may be seen by five weeks with both embryonic tissue and heart beat usually visible by six weeks. An early fetal death can be detected if a sac is present but no fetus. The scan should be repeated a week later and, if an empty sac still found or a fetus but no heart beat, a firm diagnosis made.

Ultrasound can be used in the diagnosis of ectopic pregnancy. Ultrasound may show a cystic area separate from the uterus, but free blood in the pouch of Douglas with an empty uterus and a positive pregnancy test raises high suspicion.

Doppler ultrasound examination can detect deep vein thromboses in the legs or pelvis.

*Magnetic resonance imaging (MRI)*
Pelvic tumours are seen easily while tumour invasion from the endometrium, the cervix or from the ovary can be seen on different cross-sections, enabling staging of these growths to be made without an invasive operation (Fig. 2.5).

Magnetic resonance equipment is currently available in most hospitals in the UK.

*Computerized tomography (CT) scans*
These allow the visualization of many pelvic tumours to assess their position, size and consistency, and is more readily available than MRI.

**Figure 2.4** An ultrasound scan of an ovarian tumour.

**Figure 2.5** An MRI scan of a pelvic tumour. With acknowledgement to Dr Christine Heron, Radiological Department, St George's Hospital.

## X-rays

Straight films of the abdomen can show:

• gas and fluid levels in the obstructed intestine;

• calcium in the urinary tract or dermoid ovarian tumour;

• radiopaque dye instillation shows the outline of the uterine cavity and spill from the fimbriated ends to be seen indicating patency of the tubes at fertility investigations.

## Intravenous urography

The diagnosis of pelvic tumours and renal tract disease may be helped by intravenous urography. Before radical operations in the pelvis the course of the ureters can be checked.

## Barium studies

A barium enema may be helpful in the diagnosis of rectal conditions. A barium meal with follow-through to the ileocaecal region may be useful in cases where symptoms are right-sided.

## Pelvic lymphangiography

By injecting radiopaque contrast material into the lymphatics in the foot, the lymphatic drainage of the lower limb and pelvis is outlined. It is useful to detect secondaries in the lymph glands from malignant disease in the pelvis.

## Ventilation (v)/perfusion (Q) scan

This is used to detect a pulmonary embolism along with serum estimation of D-dimers. Sometimes a spiral CT scan of the chest may be used in pregnancy.

---

### Self-assessment

Ask a friend to role-play a patient and practise taking a history using the following role-plays. The instructions for the candidate are that you should take a history from the role-player in 10 minutes. At the end, the candidate may be expected to give a two-sentence summary of the case. The role-player needs to make up a name for herself and fill in some personal details. The scoring scheme may be purely for communication skills or may include marks for information given. (See Answers to self-assessment questions, p. 306)

**2.1** You are a 22-year-old woman who has come to see the doctor because of painful periods. You have had them since you started your periods at the age of 12. They are becoming worse. The pain is crampy and radiates down the front of your legs. You take Nurofen regularly but it only helps a little bit. The pain starts the day before your period and continues for 3 days. Your periods are regular, bleeding for 5 days in every 26–29 days. You have never been pregnant and are not in a relationship at present. You had a smear last year which was normal. (All other details are up to the imagination of your role-player!)

**2.2** You are a 27-year-old woman who has been trying for a baby for 18 months. You had a child at the age of 22 by a different partner and an ectopic pregnancy 2 years ago. You have never had an infection but, now you come to think about it, you were supposed to take a course of tablets 3 years ago after one of your boyfriends had been to a clinic, but you never bothered. You have been with your current partner, aged 32 for the last 2 years and are planning to get married next year. Your periods are regular and you have no other health problems. Your baby (a boy) was born at term vaginally with no problems. (All other details are up to the imagination of your role-player!)

**2.3** You are a 32-year-old woman who is seeing your GP about future contraception. You have had 3 children and don't really want any more. During your first pregnancy you developed high blood pressure and the baby was delivered at 36 weeks by Caesarean section. Your other two children were born naturally. Your mother has diabetes which was diagnosed in her 50s. Your father is alive and well but has high blood pressure. You do not like taking the pill because you keep forgetting it and it gives you headaches. You are concerned that the other hormonal preparations will make you put on weight which is a problem for your job as an air hostess. You have never had any other illnesses. You smoke 30 cigarettes a day and drink socially. (All other details are up to the imagination of your role-player!)

# Part 2

# The young woman

# Chapter 3

# Puberty and menstrual problems of young women

Puberty defines the period in a girl's life when she undergoes a series of physiological changes which lead to the achievement of sexual maturity and the ability to reproduce.

There are three phases of change:

**1** *Adrenarche*. Increased production of androgens by the adrenal gland which are converted centrally by the liver and ovaries and peripherally in the adipose tissue to oestrogens. This usually starts at the age of 8–10 years and leads to:
- increased sebaceous gland activity;
- sweating;
- hair growth;
- pubic hair which follows axillary hair.

**2** *Sexual characteristics*.
- Usually start at the age of 9–11 years.
- Breast development usually precedes pubic hair growth and takes 5–6 years to reach Tanner's stage 5.
- Pubic hair growth takes only 3 or 4 years and so is often complete before breast development (Fig. 3.1).
- Menarche usually coincides with breast development to Tanner's stage 3.
- Average age of menarche in the UK is 12.9 years. It is earlier in countries nearer the Equator.

**3** *Growth*. The onset of puberty coincides with a rapid increase in growth velocity.
- In girls growth gain is 25–28 cm and in boys 26–30 cm. Boys go through puberty later than girls and therefore start their growth spurt from a higher starting point which accounts for their greater adult height.
- The pituitary gland increases its frequency of pulsed growth hormone (GH) and luteinizing hormone (LH). The mechanism of this is unknown.
- The greatest release of GH and LH is at night during sleep; this may account for the increased need for sleep in adolescents.
- The increase in LH acts on the thecal cells of the ovary to increase androgen production. This starts the maturation of the oocytes in the ovary from primordial phase to the antral phase when they are ready to be recruited for final maturation and release. Once this begins the young girl starts her periods.
- The onset of puberty is weight related; the average weight of a girl starting her periods is 45 kg. Anorexia in teenagers can arrest puberty if they become underweight for their age.

## Germ cells

There are about seven million primordial oocytes or germ cells in each ovary of the female fetus at 15 weeks of intrauterine life. This drops to two million germ cells at birth and is further reduced to half a million at puberty.

About 400 will be recruited during each ovulation cycle during the reproductive life; the rest degenerate at a steady rate. The stromal tissue of the

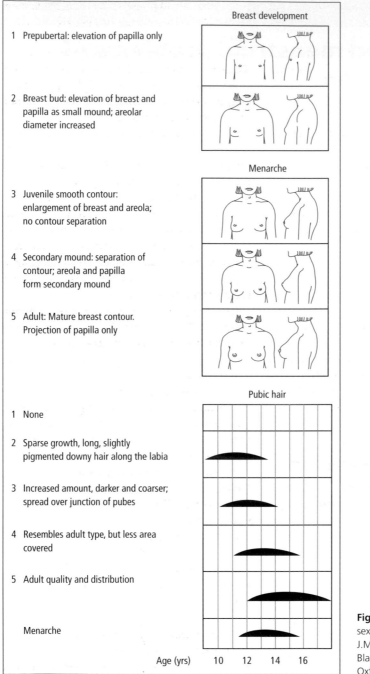

Breast development

1 Prepubertal: elevation of papilla only

2 Breast bud: elevation of breast and papilla as small mound; areolar diameter increased

Menarche

3 Juvenile smooth contour: enlargement of breast and areola; no contour separation

4 Secondary mound: separation of contour; areola and papilla form secondary mound

5 Adult: Mature breast contour. Projection of papilla only

Pubic hair

1 None

2 Sparse growth, long, slightly pigmented downy hair along the labia

3 Increased amount, darker and coarser; spread over junction of pubes

4 Resembles adult type, but less area covered

5 Adult quality and distribution

Menarche

Age (yrs)    10    12    14    16

**Figure 3.1** Tanner's classification of sexual maturity in girls. After Tanner, J.M. (1962) *Growth at Adolescence*. Blackwell Scientific Publications, Oxford.

ovary produces androgenic hormones which may be metabolized in peripheral fat to produce oestrogens.

Ovulation is controlled by the ovarian hormones and the gonadotrophins from the pituitary.

## Menstrual cycle

Three structures are involved with the regulation of ovulation and menstruation.

**1** The anterior pituitary gland.

**2** The ovary.

**3** The uterus.

These are all dealt with in Chapter 1 considering the anatomy and physiology of these organs.

## Amenorrhoea

### Primary amenorrhoea

*Definition*: no periods experienced by the age of 16.

Investigations of this condition may be divided according to whether secondary sexual characteristics are present or not. If absent, girls should be investigated at the age of 16. If present, investigation can wait until the age of 18.

### Causes of primary amenorrhoea

• *Hypothalamic (absence of gonadotrophic releasing hormone, GnRH) or hypogonadatrophic (no LH or follicle stimulating hormone, FSH).*

This may be:

  • Idiopathic.
  • Following radiotherapy.
  • Following surgery.
  • Craniopharyngomas in childhood.
  • Anorexia.
  • Excessive exercise (ballet dancers).
• *Chromosomal.*
• *Congenital.*

### Chromosomal causes

The normal human has 46 chromosomes, 44 autosomes and two sex chromosomes. The number is halved in both gametes, the oocyte and spermato-

zoon; when fertilization occurs the original number is restored in the resulting fertilized ovum (see Chapter 1).

In the normal female the sex chromosomes are XX, in the normal male XY. All oocytes carry the X chromosome, while about half the spermatozoa carry X, the others Y. Thus, the resulting offspring are either XX (female) or XY (male).

Sex chromosome abnormalities mainly arise from non-disjunction (Fig. 3.2). At the division of the primary oocyte while still sited in the ovary, the two chromosomes fail to separate so that a primary oocyte is produced which may have two X chromosomes or none; conversely, the first polar body will contain the converse—none or two. Fertilization by a spermatozoon which may carry X or Y can therefore result in abnormal patterns, XXX, XXY or XO. YO has not been described as this genetic combination is lethal.

The description is a simplification as more complex anomalies may occur, for example mosaics or individuals of mixed chromosomal patterns.

*Turner's syndrome*

• Chromosome pattern XO.
• Incidence about three in 10 000 full-term births.
• Present with primary amenorrhoea for there are either no ovaries or non-functioning streaks of tissue with no oogenesis.
• The vagina and uterus are present.
• Poor breast development.
• Little or no axillary and pubic hair.
• Short stature.
• Webbing of the neck.
• A wide carrying angle in the arms.
• Coarctation of the aorta.
• Congenital malformation of the kidneys may be found.

*Androgen insensitivity syndrome (AIS)*

• Chromosomal pattern XY.
• Due to lack of androgen receptors (deletion on X chromosome).
• Active breast development (hepatic oestrogens).
• Absent or scanty axillary and pubic hair.
• Usually absent uterus with a very short vagina.
• The gonads are testes or undifferentiated

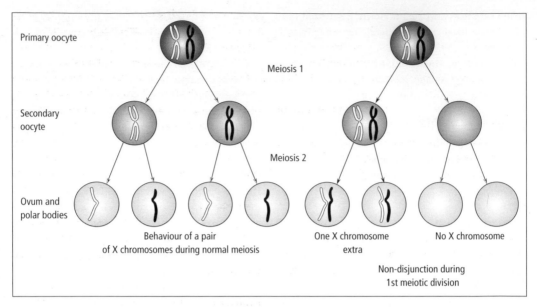

Primary oocyte

Meiosis 1

Secondary
oocyte

Meiosis 2

Ovum and
polar bodies

Behaviour of a pair
of X chromosomes during normal meiosis

One X chromosome
extra

No X chromosome

Non-disjunction during
1st meiotic division

**Figure 3.2** Non-disjunction during meiosis.

gonads and may be intra-abdominal or in the labia major.
• Male serum androgen levels.

*Congenital adrenal hyperplasia (CAH)*
• Chromosomal pattern XX.
• Congenital adrenal hyperplasia is inherited as a Mendelian recessive.
• Female infants are born with ambiguous genitalia.
• Vagina and uterus are present.
• Ovaries are usually polycystic in appearance and anovulatory.
• Defective production of cortisol, most commonly due to 21-hydroxylase deficiency.
• Leads to overproduction of corticotrophic hormone and enlargement of the adrenal cortex.
• Increased adrenal androgen production.
• The clitoris is enlarged and the labia fused.
• Some of these babies are salt losers and become seriously ill in the first week of life.
• Teenagers often develop severe hirsutism and acne.

### Congenital causes

Menstruation not begun by the age of 17 must be distinguished from cryptomenorrhoea—hidden loss caused by obstruction to menstrual flow. This is most often caused by a septum across the vagina just above the hymen at the embryological junction of the Mullerian ducts and the urogenital sinus in the lower third of the vagina. It may be incomplete. A complete septum leads to cryptomenorrhoea (vagina filled with blood) and haematocolpos (uterus filled with blood). The lower part of the vagina may be a solid cord; haematocolpos and haematometra may form above this. On inspection of the vulva a bluish bulge is seen just inside the hymen. There may be cyclical attacks of abdominal pain and a mass may be palpable *per abdomen*, representing a large haematocolpos.

*Treatment*
Under anaesthesia, incise the septum and express the haematocolpos by suprapubic pressure. If infection does not occur, subsequent menstruation and childbearing are normal.

## Investigation of primary amenorrhoea

- A *history* is taken including a family history as AIS may affect other females in the family.
- *Physical examination.* The general examination should begin by recording the girl's height—if by 16 she is less than 147 cm there is a possibility of ovarian agenesis (Turner's syndrome) or (pan)hypopituitarism. If there is a decrease in body weight, calculate Body Mass Index (wt(kg)/ht(m$^2$)). A general examination checks the development of secondary sexual characteristics, hair patterns and density.
- A *pelvic examination* should be performed if the examiner really thinks a positive finding will be there. For most young women with primary amenorrhoea it will not be useful particularly at first consultation. The vulva is inspected to see that the introitus is patent; there may be cryptomenorrhoea, congenital absence of the vagina or a blind vagina as in AIS.
- *Investigations*—a buccal smear and an examination of the polymorphonuclear leucocytes to determine if chromatin positive (probably XX) or chromatin negative (probably XO or XY); in other cases a full chromosome analysis may be needed to exclude mosaicism and AIS.
- *Hormonal investigations* should include LH, FSH, oestradiol and testosterone levels.
- *Ultrasound* will help determine the presence, state and size of the ovaries and any follicular activity. Uterine size can also be seen. It is rarely necessary to perform a laparoscopy to assess the pelvic organs.

## Management

If the girl is normally developed, with normal breast development, the uterus and vagina are normal and she is chromatin positive, the most likely diagnosis is delayed menarche. It is reasonable to await events; menstruation is not established in some individuals before 18 years.

For those with a diagnosable pathological cause, the aim must be to restore normal function as far as possible and, although fertility may not be possible, enable the individual to lead as normal a sexual life as possible.

Cases of Turner's syndrome should receive long-term treatment with cyclical hormones, oestrogen and progestogen (hormone replacement therapy). There is a small risk of uterine carcinoma.

In AIS, the gonads are testes that are often found inside the abdomen or inguinal canal. Since these testes have a 25% risk of becoming malignant (teratoma or dysgerminoma) they should be removed soon after puberty and an artificial vagina may be constructed or dilators used to permit sexual intercourse. Treatment with oestrogen should also be given to augment breast development and prevent osteoporosis.

In cases of congenital absence of the vagina and uterus the ovaries are usually normal. An artificial vagina may be constructed to permit sexual intercourse.

Abnormalities of pituitary secretion should be treated with oestrogen or progesterone until fertility is desired.

## Secondary amenorrhoea

*Definition*: no periods for over 6 months, having once started.

## Causes of secondary amenorrhoea

### Physiological
Amenorrhoea occurs naturally in:
- pregnancy;
- lactation;
- after menopause.

### Pituitary
Total pituitary ablation or destruction by radiotherapy after puberty. Tumours may also destroy it. In Sheehan's syndrome, severe postpartum haemorrhage causes pituitary anoxia with failure of lactation, amenorrhoea and other manifestations of pituitary failure.

Hyperprolactinaemia may be due to a definitive pituitary adenoma or scattered microadenoma causing galactorrhoea, visual disturbances and headaches. It may be a side-effect of some drugs, particularly cimetidine and phenothiazine.

Anorexia nervosa may lead to pituitary damage

and thus to permanent amenorrhoea and sterility. Periods cease before weight loss becomes apparent.

**Thyroid disease**

All thyroid disorders may cause amenorrhoea or excessive bleeding. Correction of the thyroid function may restore normal menstruation.

**Ovary**

Polycystic ovary syndrome (PCOS) is the commonest cause of anovulation in young women, with one in four women having the morphological picture on ultrasound scan. They have stromal hyperplasia of the ovaries, leading to an excess secretion of testosterone and the formation of multiple follicular cysts; it is associated with amenorrhoea, oligomenorrhoea, hirsutism and infertility, secondary to anovulation. Women with PCOS are often hyperinsulinaemic. This predisposes them to obesity and diabetes. Obesity increases the prevalence of anovulation and hirsutism. Anovulation and obesity both predispose women to endometrial hyperplasia/carcinoma because of the effects of unopposed estrogen on the endometrium. Weight control and regular withdrawal bleeds are therefore essential.

Spontaneous premature ovarian failure (POF) in the absence of disease causes premature menopause. The ovary ceases to respond to pituitary gonadotrophins which are usually excreted in excessive amounts or may be normal. This follows a lack of oocytes or their autoimmune destruction in the ovary.

Castration by surgical removal of the ovaries or by exposure to irradiation leads to amenorrhoea.

Extensive destruction of the ovaries by infection or tumours is a rare cause.

**Uterine**

The endometrium can be destroyed by the following.
- Disease:
  (a) tuberculosis;
  (b) severe postpartum infection.
- Formal endometrial ablation (by laser or diathermy).
- Severe curettage usually following pregnancy, miscarriage or therapeutic abortion (Asherman's syndrome).

**General disease**

Amenorrhoea may occur in any debilitating disease, e.g. pulmonary tuberculosis, not necessarily with involvement of the pelvic organs.

Terminal stages of diseases such as Addison's disease and uraemia due to renal disease.

Starvation may lead to amenorrhoea, similar to that seen in anorexia nervosa.

Obesity can also cause amenorrhoea (most commonly associated with PCOS) and in grossly obese young women weight reduction may restore normal menstrual function.

## History

- Family history.
- Hot flushes.
- Drugs such as reserpine, digoxin, phenothiazines and hormones, including oral contraceptives.
- Change in body weight, i.e. obesity or sudden loss of weight.
- Galactorrhoea.
- Headache, visual disturbance (hemianopia).

## Physical examination

- Height measurement.
- Weight.
- Blood pressure.
- Breasts for evidence of pregnancy or milk secretion.
- Pelvic examination to:
  (a) exclude pregnancy (a woman may still conceive in the course of a period of amenorrhoea);
  (b) assess the size and position of the uterus to exclude a pelvic tumour.

## Investigations

- Pregnancy test.
- Computerized tomography (CT) scan or magnetic resonance imaging (MRI) of pituitary area.
- Thyroid stimulating hormone.

- Plasma hormone levels of FSH.
- LH.
- Oestradiol.
- Prolactin.
- Testosterone.
- Progesterone withdrawal test: give a progestogen for 5 days. If the woman bleeds afterwards, she has oestrogen in her circulation and a uterus.

Ultrasound assessment of:

- uterine size;
- pregnancy;
- ovarian size and morphology;
- follicular function.

Examination under anaesthesia if congenital abnormality:

- assess the pelvic organs;
- perform a laparoscopy to inspect the pelvic organs and to take a biopsy of the ovaries.

The differential diagnosis of amenorrhoea is given in Box 3.1.

## Treatment

Treat the cause if one is discovered. If not, management will depend upon whether fertility is desired or not.

Women with low oestrogen levels should be treated with oestrogen and progesterone replacement (the oral contraceptive pill or hormone replacement therapy).

In *anorexia nervosa* the periods may cease before weight loss is evident; treatment should include efforts to restore weight to normal. In *gross obesity*, weight loss may result in normal menstruation.

Teenagers who over-exercise (ballet dancers and gymnasts), should be encouraged to reduce their training schedule.

In *polycystic ovary syndrome*, if the woman is obese, referral to a dietician is recommended to reduce weight. In some women metformin may help to restore ovulation in conjunction with a low-calorie diet. Regular progesterone therapy for 12 days every three months will give a regular withdrawal bleed or the oral contraceptive pill with cyproterone acetate (an antiandrogen) will give a regular period and improve hirsutism and acne.

A *premature menopause* is characterized by low oestrogen levels and high FSH. They should receive cyclical oestrogen and progesterone such as Cyclo-Progynova to prevent osteoporosis.

Where excess of prolactin (over 1000 μu/l) is secreted, perform a CT/MRI scan of the pituitary fossa to exclude a tumour. In the absence of such a space occupying lesion, microadenomata of the

| **Box 3.1  Tests: differential diagnosis of primary and secondary amenorrhoea** | | | | | | | |
|---|---|---|---|---|---|---|---|
| | Chromosomes | FSH | LH | Oestradiol | Testosterone | Prolactin | Progesterone withdrawal |
| *Primary amenorrhoea* | | | | | | | |
| Turner's | XO | ↑ | ↑ | ↓ | = | = | −ve |
| Androgen insensitivity syndrome | XY | ↑ | ↑ | = | ↑ | = | −ve |
| Hypogonadotrophic hypogondism | XX | ↓ | ↓ | ↓ | = | = or ↓ | −ve |
| *Secondary amenorrhoea* | | | | | | | |
| Prolactinoma | XX | ↓ | ↓ | ↓ . | = | ↑ | −ve |
| Polycystic ovary syndrome | XX | = | ↑ or = | = | ↑ | = | +ve |
| Premature ovarian failure | XX | ↑ | ↑ | ↓ | = | = | −ve |

pituitary body are postulated. Treatment of amenorrhoea with prolactin excess is with bromocriptine or the longer acting cabergoline (both are dopamine agonists) in perpetuity. Bromocriptine and cabergoline should be stopped if pregnancy occurs. Periods will return on treatment once prolactin levels are rendered normal.

## Bleeding in infancy

Female infants may have vaginal bleeding during the first week of life. This is rarely significant and probably due to withdrawal of maternally derived oestrogens which had crossed the placenta in pregnancy.

*Precocious puberty* is caused by premature maturation of the ovaries in most cases; very rarely there may be a granulosa cell tumour of the ovary. The breasts grow while pubic and axillary hair develops and endometrial bleeding occurs. Provided a tumour of the ovary can be excluded, the child may be allowed to develop normally but the parents must be warned of the danger of pregnancy.

The differential diagnosis includes:

• a mixed mesodermal tumour;

• adenocarcinoma of the vagina; particularly at risk were adolescent girls whose mothers received stilboestrol during pregnancy but this is now history.

## Menorrhagia under 18 years

*Adolescent bleeding* of a sufficient amount to be considered as menorrhagia is usually dysfunctional, secondary to anovulation. There may be prolonged episodes of painless bleeding and the girl can become anaemic. Examination of the endometrium may show an anovulatory pattern or hyperplasia.

Treatment consists of eliminating any organic cause and correcting anaemia if present. Hormone treatment is usually successful using a progestogen such as norethisterone (15 mg daily) (see Chapter 16). When the treatment is stopped, withdrawal bleeding with shedding of the endometrium analogous with normal menstruation occurs. Treatment should be given cyclically for a further three to six months. An alternative is use of the oral contraceptive pill.

---

### Self-assessment

Read the following clinical scenarios carefully and answer the questions below.

1 A 16-year-old presents with a history of primary amenorrhoea. She is 1.45 m tall and weighs 53 kg (BMI 25.2). On physical examination her breasts are Tanner stage 2, she has a normal vulva and vagina. Her mother reports that she struggles at school and is being teased because she is so short.

2 A 16-year-old girl presents with a history of primary amenorrhoea. She is 1.64 m tall and weighs 47 kg (BMI 17.5). Her breast development is Tanner stage 3 and she has scanty pubic hair, she has a normal vulva and vagina. She represents Greater London in marathon running and is otherwise well.

3 A 17-year-old girl presents with a history of secondary amenorrhoea. She is 1.64 m tall and weighs 56 kg (BMI 21). She started her periods at the age of 14 and they were irregular and light until one year ago when they stopped. On physical examination she has acne on her face and back which she finds distressing. Her legs and arms are hairy and she has hair on her abdomen in an inverted triangle. Her vulva and vagina are normal. Her mother has type 2 diabetes. She is otherwise well.

4 A woman of 24 years old presents to the clinic with secondary amenorrhoea. Her periods started at the age of 12 and were regular until 2 years ago when they became irregular and light. She has noticed a discharge from her breasts and suffers from severe headaches. On physical examination she has a white discharge from her breasts and is otherwise normal.

5 A 15-year-old girl presents to the clinic with primary amenorrhoea. She complains of intermittent abdominal pain and has noticed that her school skirt is becoming tighter. Her weight and height are normal for her age. On examination her breasts are Tanner stage 4 and pubic hair stage 5. Her vulva looks swollen at the introitus and she has a palpable abdominal mass which is tender.

**Self-assessment** *Continued*

Questions

**3.1** From the list below choose the single most likely diagnosis for each of the clinical scenarios above.
  (a) Androgen insensitivity syndrome
  (b) Cryptomenorrhoea
  (c) Pregnancy
  (d) Polycystic ovary syndrome
  (e) Ashermans syndrome
  (f) Turner's syndrome
  (g) Congenital adrenal hyperplasia
  (h) Hyperprolactinaemia
  (i) Constitutional delay of puberty
  (j) Anorexia/exercise related amenorrhoea

**3.2** From the lists below select the most useful first line investigations to establish the diagnosis for each clinical scenario.
  (a) Ultrasound scan
  (b) Ultrasound scan, LH, FSH and testosterone
  (c) Ultrasound scan, LH, FSH, prolactin
  (d) Chromosome analysis
  (e) Pregnancy test
  (f) LH, FSH, oestradiol
  (g) Ultrasound scan, LH, FSH, testosterone, adrenal androgen profile
  (h) Thyroid function tests

**3.3** From the list below select the most appropriate first line treatment for each condition.
  (a) Weight gain
  (b) Removal of gonads/ovaries
  (c) Incision of vaginal septum
  (d) Referral to the antenatal clinic
  (e) Bromocriptine
  (f) Progestogerone therapy every three months
  (g) Creation of a vagina
  (h) Oestrogen replacement therapy
  (i) Prednisolone
  (j) Weight loss

# Chapter 4

# Subfertility

Subfertility is defined as failure to conceive after one year of unprotected coitus at frequent intervals. A woman who has never conceived has primary subfertility, a woman who has conceived before has secondary subfertility, even though this episode did not result in a live birth, e.g. miscarriage or ectopic pregnancy.

## Causes of infertility (Box 4.1)

### Both partners

• Mechanical difficulty in coitus with inadequate penetration, often associated with lack of ability in the male to maintain an erection.
• Periods of separation so that there is no intercourse at the most fertile time.

### Male

• Impotence.
• Premature ejaculation.
• Azoospermia/oligospermia ($<20 \times 10^6$/ml).

---

**Box 4.1 Factors in infertility**

| | |
|---|---|
| Ovulation disorder | 30% |
| Tubal factor | 30% |
| Male factor | 30% |
| Unexplained infertility | 10% |

---

• Poor sperm motility.
• >10% abnormal forms.

### Female

• Fallopian tubes—infection may close or partly obstruct.
• Ovarian dysfunction (Box 4.2):
  (a) ovulation may not occur;
  (b) ovulation is irregular with anovulatory cycles;
  (c) polycystic ovary syndrome;
  (d) hyperprolactinaemia;

---

**Box 4.2 Causes of anovulation**

**Primary ovarian dysfunction**

| | |
|---|---|
| Genetic, e.g. Turner's syndrome | 1% |
| Autoimmune | |

**Secondary ovarian dysfunction**

*Disorders of gonadotrophin regulation*

| | |
|---|---|
| Hyperprolactinaemia | 15% |
| *Functional* | |
| Weight loss | 10% |
| Exercise | |

*Gonadotrophin deficiency*

| | |
|---|---|
| Pituitary tumour | |
| Pituitary infarction | 4% |
| Pituitary ablation | |
| *Polycystic ovary syndrome* | 70% |

---

(e) perimenopausal;

(f) premature ovarian failure.

• Intact hymen—a woman may complain of subfertility when her marriage has not been consummated.

• Vagina—congenital malformation.

• Uterus—congenital malformation, or tuberculous endometritis.

## Investigation of the infertile couple

### History from the female

• Age, occupation, length of time with partner, use of contraception or avoidance of pregnancy, previous sexual activity.

• Previous pregnancies, including abortions, miscarriages, ectopic.

• Menstrual history: age at onset, cycle and duration of flow, dysmenorrhoea, ovulation pain, recent change in the cycle.

• Vaginal discharge: character, amount, whether associated with irritation or soreness.

• Previous illnesses, especially pelvic inflammatory disease (PID), diabetes, renal disease.

• Operations, especially in the abdomen or pelvis.

• Coitus frequency, difficulties, relation to fertile days.

• Previous investigation or treatment of infertility.

### Examination of the female

• General examination—physical development, evidence of endocrine disorder.

• Abdominal examination—scars, tenderness, guarding, masses.

• Vaginal examination—state of introitus, size and mobility of the uterus, uterine enlargement, enlargement of the ovaries.

### History from the male

• Age, occupation, including absence from home, length of time with partner and duration of infertility.

• Sexual performance—frequency, ability to ejaculate in upper vagina.

• Previous relationships, fathering of any pregnancies.

• History of mumps with orchitis, injury to genitalia or operations for hernia or varicocoele, any recent debilitating illness.

### Examination of the male

• General build and appearance.

• Examination of genitalia, hypospadias.

• Palpation of testicles, size, consistency. Relate size to standard models (Fig. 4.1).

### Investigations

#### Seminal analysis (Box 4.3)

Best performed on a masturbation specimen which should be examined within two hours of collec-

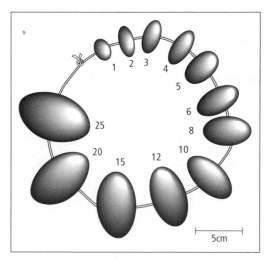

**Figure 4.1** Models of testicular size to allow a standardization of the examined testes size with an objective comparison.

| Box 4.3  Normal seminal analysis | |
| --- | --- |
| Volume | 2–5 ml |
| Liquefaction time | Within 30 minutes |
| Count | 20–150 million/ml |
| Motility | >50% motility at 1.5 hours |
| Sperm morphology | >10% normal forms |

tion. It should not be from semen ejaculated at intercourse using a condom as most modern sheaths are lubricated with spermicidal cream.

The motility of sperms is important—direct, straight moving sperms being the more likely to effect fertilization.

There should be at least 20 million sperms per millilitre with a total count of not less than 100 million. Fertility reduces progressively with numbers below this. Abnormal forms should not exceed 10%. Reliance should not be placed on a single sperm count.

In cases of severe oligospermia/azoospermia the cause should be sought. It may be due to a chromosomal abnormality such as Klinefelter's syndrome (XXY). It may be due to primary hypogonadism, when the level of gonadotrophic hormone will be high, or secondary hypogonadism, where gonadotrophic hormone will be low; in the latter case there may be excess of prolactin secretion, usually due to a pituitary tumour and possibly responsive to bromocriptine. Other causes of azoospermia may be related to congenital absence of the vasa deferentia or to obstruction in the epididymis.

## Basal temperature charts

The woman may keep charts of her basal temperature for a period of three months. This is best taken first thing in the morning before leaving bed. In theory, the raised progesterone levels elevate the basal body temperature by 0.3–0.5°C within 12 hours of ovulation. The graphic chart produced bears some relation to ovulation when it is regular. However, the correlation of temperature to ovulation is less easily seen when ovulation is irregular. Other extraneous causes of temperature fluctuation (e.g. 'flu) intrude on this test as do unusual life rhythms (e.g. nurses on night duty). These charts are very difficult to use prospectively and have largely been abandoned.

## Ovulation predictor tests

A daily test using a few drops of urine which detects the LH surge by giving a colour change on a

stick in the presence of a high LH. When it is positive the woman knows that she is going to ovulate within 36 hours. It is helpful in women with a regular cycle but in women who have PCOS and an irregular cycle it is rarely helpful since they can have a raised LH in the follicular phase without a mature follicle.

## Tests for tubal patency

Hysterosalpingography using a radiopaque dye shows blockage of the tubes and indicates the site of the obstruction; it can also demonstrate a congenital malformation of the cavity of the uterus which will not be apparent at laparoscopy. A new contrast medium containing microbubbles may be injected transcervically and its passage along the fallopian tube detected with ultrasound (HyCoSy®).

Tubal patency may be tested under direct vision at laparoscopy. A solution of methylene blue is injected through a tightly fitting cannula in the cervical canal. The passage of the dye may be observed. When the tubes are normally patent the dye pours out of the fimbriated end of the tube into the pouch of Douglas. Tubal obstruction may be recognized as can the presence of adhesions; a hydrosalpinx may be seen to fill with dye which does not spill.

## Hormone tests

Serum progesterone levels in the mid second half of the cycle (days 21–23 of a 28 day cycle) are ten times as high as those of the rest of the cycle (30 ng/ml compared with 3–6 ng/ml) if ovulation has occurred. Luteinizing hormone (LH), follicle stimulating hormone (FSH), testosterone (if polycystic ovary syndrome is suspected) should be taken between days 3–8 of the cycle.

Prolactin levels should be measured to exclude microadenomata of the pituitary gland; levels above 1000 μu/l are significant and should lead to computerized tomography (CT) scan of the pituitary fossa.

## Ultrasound

An ultrasound scan of the pelvis, especially with a vaginal probe, gives excellent views of the ovaries and uterus if pathology in either is suspected (e.g. polycystic ovary syndrome).

## Treatment of subfertility

A couple seeking medical advice for subfertility are obviously anxious and concerned. They should always be offered help even if the period of subfertility is relatively short. In most couples, investigations should be done after one year of trying.

About 25–30% of women seeking advice for subfertility become pregnant during investigation and treatment. There are various lines of treatment which may prove successful depending on the condition found.

## Correction of coital difficulties

An intact hymen should be removed or dilated. A vaginal septum may have to be removed but usually they cause little difficulty. The woman should be taught to pass vaginal dilators and this helps to give her confidence. The use of a lubricant at coitus also helps.

In the male, the commonest problems with fertility are premature ejaculation and inadequate erection. Both of these are discussed in Chapter 6.

## Lesions of the uterine body

Removal of small uterine polypi (see p. 223) at curettage is often successful. Myomectomy should be performed if the fibroids are blocking the fallopian tubes or are submucous (see p. 231). Laparoscopy or laparotomy may reveal other conditions such as endometriosis or peritubal adhesions which require relevant therapy.

## Lesions of the tubes

Various operations may be undertaken to restore patency and function in cases where the tubes have been damaged by infection (most commonly with chlamydia).

- *Salpingostomy* where the fimbrial end is opened and held open by turning out a cuff (commonly done laparoscopically).
- *Tubal reimplantation* where the isthmus is blocked. The medial tubal end is freed and is reimplanted into the uterine cavity.
- *Salpingolysis* where peritubal adhesions are divided (usually at laparoscopy).
- *Reanastomosis* if the tube is blocked in midsegment; the obstructed area is resected and the open ends reanastomosed often using microsurgery.

Results of many of these operations are disappointing because:

- *patency* can easily be restored but the tube may be too rigid to allow peristalsis;
- *infection* may have caused the tube to be fixed to other organs by adhesions and so the fimbrial end cannot freely manoeuvre and thus harvest the oocytes;
- after surgery there may be *too short a length of tube* so that passage of the fertilized oocyte is so rapid that the endometrium is not yet ready to receive it.

In consequence, the success rates of tuboplasty after infection range from 2 to 10%. The best results come after reanastomosis of sterilization procedures when most surgeons will report a 40–60% success rate, which can be improved to about 75% by the use of microsurgery. Despite these poor results there are some women who will be prepared to submit to such an operation even though the hope of a successful pregnancy is slight. For the majority of women with tubal disease, *in vitro* fertilization (IVF) gives the best chance of a successful pregnancy (see p. 43).

In cases of non-ovulation, further investigation is indicated.

If there is a high level of prolactin on more than one occasion a CT scan should be done to exclude a pituitary tumour. Excess of prolactin is treated with bromocriptine or cabergoline. As prolactin levels return to normal, menstruation restarts and normal fertility is restored.

Cases of primary or secondary ovarian failure show high levels of FSH and low levels of oestrogen. Induction of ovulation is impossible for there are no more oocytes, but the patient should be offered oestrogen replacement therapy.

Cases of ovulation failure with low FSH and LH levels may be treated by the use of gonadotrophins. Human menopausal gonadotrophin (hMG) contains both gonadotrophins or FSH can be given alone. Treatment with these must be monitored carefully with ultrasound to prevent hyperstimulation, secondary to multiple ovulation and thence to multiple pregnancy.

In practice, 75 iu of FSH are given daily from about days 2–3 of cycle. The dose is increased weekly, depending on the ultrasound examination of the ovary which shows the number and size of follicles coming towards ovulation. When the response is satisfactory, an injection of human chorionic gonadotrophin (hCG) is given which acts in a similar manner to the LH surge. Once a satisfactory dosage pattern has been established in one cycle, this can be repeated in other cycles in up to six treatment courses or until a pregnancy is achieved.

Cases of anovulation with polycystic ovary syndrome may be treated with clomiphene citrate. The dose is 50 mg for five days commencing on the third day of menstruation and mid-luteal progesterone levels on day 21 are measured to confirm ovulation. Provided ovulation occurs treatment should be repeated for six months or until the woman is pregnant. If the first dose is unsuccessful it is increased maximally to 150 mg daily. There is a rise of multiple follicular development from this hyperstimulation and therefore multiple pregnancies are more common (5–10%).

## Treatment of male infertility

If it has been established that male factors are associated with infertility, treatment can proceed. This is best done in two phases:
- less invasive treatments;
- more specific therapies.

### Phase one

The first phase should last about three months. Two specimens of semen should be examined to establish levels in the sperm count. Certain aspects of the man's way of life may need to be altered:
- over-exertion;
- excessive smoking;
- excess alcohol consumption;
- poorly controlled diabetes;
- hypertension;
- being overweight.

If the scrotal temperature is raised, it is wise to wear boxer shorts to allow the testes to hang in a cooler atmosphere.

The timing of intercourse may need discussion so that, around the time of ovulation, the couple have intercourse. A few days of abstinence before this may boost the sperm count if there is a deficiency; otherwise timing is irrelevant.

Any varicocoele causing a raised temperature of the scrotum and the efferent ducts from the testes is managed by ligation. Three-quarters of men improve their sperm count after this if a varicocoele has been a feature.

### Phase two

Specific treatments will depend upon the results of investigations. A low sperm count with low FSH and testosterone level may indicate treatment with stimulating hormones (very rare).

In the absence of hormone deficiency, endocrine therapy is less easily justified. Hyperprolactinaemia is rare in males, but if it is present then bromocriptine should be used.

Impaired fertility is associated sometimes with an increased incidence of chronic prostatitis. If present, long-term, low-dose antibiotic treatment may remove this potential cause (erythromycin 250 mg twice a day for a month).

Sperm washing has been described with variable results. Ejaculated sperm is washed in phosphate buffered saline and resuspended for insemination into the uterus (intrauterine insemination, IUI). His partner is usually treated with clomiphene or FSH to increase the number of mature oocytes to 2 or 3 to increase the chance of conception. The risk of a multiple pregnancy is around 10% and ovarian hyperstimulation syndrome (OHSS) 1%.

Generally speaking, the management of male factors of infertility is disappointing and the success rate usually ranges between 20 and 40%. The introduction of assisted conception techniques has altered this considerably.

## Assisted conception

Artificial fertilization methods have increased in use greatly in the last decade with probably over 10 000 children in the world born as a result. Artificial fertilization has received considerable media cover but should be considered as only one part of infertility management, particularly for those who cannot transmit sperms or eggs along the fallopian tubes due to their damage or absence (Box 4.4) or abnormal sperm.

Patients selected for programmes are usually under 40 years of age and in a stable relationship. They should be free of medical or psychological disease and the woman should have a normal uterus.

### Technique

For the process to take place, it is essential that oocytes be recovered. Most women now have ovarian cycles stimulated by gonadotrophins following treatment with a gonadotrophic releasing hormone (GnRH) analogue to stop the woman's own hormone production. hCG is given to stimulate ovulation. This can be monitored by daily ultrasound scanning when follicle size can be measured; the follicle should measure about 20 mm in diameter for oocyte recovery.

| Box 4.4 Indications for *in vitro* fertilization (IVF) | |
|---|---|
| **Cause of infertility** | **%** |
| Disease or absence of the tubes | 50–70 |
| Endometriosis | 7–15 |
| Sperm abnormalities or low count | 5–20 |
| Sperm antibodies | 1–5 |
| Idiopathic infertility | 3–15 |
| Failed donor insemination (DI) | 1–5 |

Oocytes are aspirated through the posterior fornix of the vagina or bladder guided by ultrasonic scanning. Usually several (3–15) oocytes are recovered at the same procedure.

The oocytes are mixed on a warmed flat dish in special media with semen obtained from the husband by masturbation. Fertilization takes place *in vitro* and under specially controlled conditions of temperature and atmospheric gases. The eggs are allowed to develop to the four–eight cell stage, and introduced to the woman's uterus through the cervix, using a fine cannula in as atraumatic a fashion as possible. A maximum of two or three fertilized ova are inserted 2 days after egg collection.

Luteal support with progesterone or hCG is given in the days following embryo replacement until 8–10 weeks of pregnancy or when menstruation begins if conception has not occurred.

### Results

Conception rates at established IVF units are about 20–30% per cycle. Success should be judged by a live birth and not just by the implantation of a fertilized egg—a biochemical pregnancy shown by a rise in hCG levels. The average take home baby rate in the UK is 20%.

### Gamete intra-fallopian tube transfer (GIFT)

If the tubes are present and patent but conventional methods have failed, one may use gamete intra-fallopian tube transfer (GIFT). The oocytes are recovered at laparoscopy under general anaesthesia. Prepared motile sperm from the male semen is then passed through the laparoscope into the fallopian tube and one or two of the oocytes are put into the same tube. The whole procedure takes about half an hour and there is no extracorporeal phase. Success rates are slightly lower than IVF. It is less commonly offered as a treatment these days.

### Zygote intra-fallopian transfer (ZIFT)

Zygote intra-fallopian transfer (ZIFT) puts fertilized

ova back into the fallopian tube two days after fertilization instead of replacement into the uterine cavity as in GIFT. This technique is very rarely used.

### *In utero* insemination (IUI)

Washed semen are injected into the uterine cavity to meet an oocyte by travelling up the tube as happens naturally.

### Direct injection of sperm into oocyte (intracytoplasmic sperm injection—ICSI)

Micromanipulation is performed at special centres placing an individual sperm under the zona and into the oocyte. This has a similar success rate to IVF. Sperm may also be extracted from the epididymis or testis in cases of azoospermia.

### Artificial insemination

In cases where the male is infertile, insemination with donor semen (donor insemination, DI) may be considered; this is best done by a doctor. Careful counselling of the couple about the implications is essential. Success rates are 15–40% per ovulation.

### Donors

Facilities should be available for accumulating a sperm bank with samples from young donors preferably of proven fertility. A sufficient variety of donors must allow the matching of height, hair colour and race by the doctor in charge of DI. Each donor's sample can only be used to help six couples.

### Samples

Samples are produced by masturbation and are usually divided into tubes or straws of about 0.5 ml each, so that the average donor will produce enough to fill six to ten tubes at any ejaculation. These are stored in liquid nitrogen under careful conditions and checked every two years.

### DI and HIV

Until recently, fresh semen was used for DI; this was marginally better at achieving pregnancy than using frozen semen. One of the major fears of artificial insemination has become the theoretical risk of contamination from HIV. In consequence, all donor units now check their donors for HIV antibodies at the time they produce their sample. The samples are then frozen and the donor is rechecked three months later in case he was incubating AIDS at the time he produced the sample. If the second test is negative then the sample can be used for insemination. The percentage of pregnancies achieved is 10–20% less than with fresh semen.

### Technique

The woman is positioned comfortably and a speculum inserted to expose the cervix. Insemination is usually performed into the cervical canal with recently defrosted semen; not more than 0.5 ml of semen is used because it would be painful to distend the canal with a greater volume than this.

### Disclosure of donor

Changes in society are occurring that demand greater freedom of information. One of these may be that, in future, a child from a pregnancy which started with DI may wish to know the identity of the donor. If this becomes law, the donor must give his consent before giving the first semen sample. Short of this, confidentiality must be kept and the clinic must keep information about donors and recipients separately, but be capable of linking.

### Adoption

In cases of intractable infertility, adoption may be considered although there is a great shortage of babies for adoption in the Western world.

### Surrogate mothers

Increasingly, society is accepting the use of *surrogate parenthood*. If a woman has no uterus or has had it surgically removed, she still can make oocytes. Gametes, fertilized by her partner, can be cultured in the uterus of another woman, perhaps a relative such as a mother or a sister. This baby is genetically the same as the parents and only lodges for 38 weeks in the body of another.

Other variations include donated oocytes or sperm if such gonadal material is unavailable naturally. In the UK, the baby is legally the child of the woman who bears him or her, i.e. the surrogate mother and legal issues have arisen in the past when the surrogate mother changes her mind and wishes to keep the baby after birth.

---

### Self-assessment

**4.1** Which of the following statements are true?
(a) On semen analysis more than 10% normal forms is considered normal.
(b) The commonest cause of anovulatory subfertility is hyperprolactinaemia.
(c) Women with premature ovarian failure (POF) can be successfully treated with follicle stimulating hormone (FSH).
(d) Male subfertility due to oligospermia can be successfully treated with intracytoplasmic sperm injection (ICSI).
(e) The risk of multiple pregnancy in ovulation induction is around 30%.
(f) The commonest cause of anovulatory subfertility is polycystic ovary syndrome.
(g) Progesterone levels should be tested in the mid-follicular phase.
(h) A sperm count of 10 million per ml would be considered normal.
(i) Tubal patency can be checked using ultrasound.
(j) Progesterone levels should be tested in the mid-luteal phase.

**4.2** Which of the following are associated with causing tubal damage leading to tubal subfertility?
(a) *Trichomonas vaginalis*.
(b) Gonorrhoea.
(c) Previous ectopic pregnancy.
(d) Use of the oral contraceptive pill.
(e) Chlamydia.

**4.3** Match the diagnosis (a–e) to the first line treatment (1–10) that could be offered to give the best chance of a successful pregnancy.
(a) Bilateral tubal blockage.
(b) Polycystic ovary syndrome.
(c) Hyperprolactinaemia.
(d) Oligospermia due to Klinefelter's syndrome.
(e) Turner's syndrome.

(1) Egg donation.
(2) Bromocriptine.
(3) Follicle stimulating hormone (FSH).
(4) Weight gain.
(5) *In vitro* fertilization.
(6) Weight loss.
(7) Intracytoplasmic sperm injection.
(8) Clomiphene.
(9) Tubal surgery.
(10) Donor insemination.

# Chapter 5

# Pregnancy prevention

Contraception is the use of temporary techniques to prevent pregnancy while allowing intercourse to continue. The ideal contraceptive should be safe, harmless and not interfere with the sexual enjoyment of either party.

Distinguish between family planning and population control.
• *Family planning*, a personal matter demanding a low failure rate.
• *Population control*, where the need for cheapness and ease of use may make a less exacting standard of efficacy acceptable.

The failure rate of any method of contraception is judged by the Pearl Index (PI): the number of women having regular intercourse who become pregnant within a year out of 100 couples using the method.

$$PI = \frac{\text{number of pregnancies}}{\text{number of couples using the method}} \times 100$$

## Contraception

### Trends

Contraception has been available in the UK for several centuries, mostly in the form of barrier methods in the earlier days. In the 1960s, the hormonal method and intrauterine devices (IUDs) became popular. In the 1970s, free family planning was available from the National Health Service. This led to an increase in availability and uptake of all methods in all groups of age, sex or marital status. In the 1970s doubts were raised about the risks of hormonal contraception which, by the 1980s, had been resolved somewhat only to be followed by the fears of HIV which led to the wider use of the condom for safer sex. At the same time, the long-lasting IUDs came on the market and offered less intrusion upon sexual life. In the mid-1990s long-lasting injectables also became more widely used. Table 5.1 shows the World Health Organization (WHO) data in 2001 of various usages in different regions.

Sterilization, a permanent method, also has increased in popularity since the late 1970s so that about a quarter of couples choose this as their method.

## Counselling

Family planning and birth control need discussion of more than just the mechanics of the methods. They are part of reproductive life linked with emotional and sexual life. There is sometimes embarrassment surrounding family planning and so this matter is not discussed openly. For example, contraceptive advertising is not accepted on the London Underground, but is at Heathrow Airport. It is for professionals to try and help break these barriers by discussing the matter in a clear and simple fashion.

**Table 5.1** World wide usage of contraceptives by percentage. Data from the World Health Organization, 2001.

| | Oral contraceptives | Intrauterine device | Condom | Other methods | Sterilization | |
|---|---|---|---|---|---|---|
| | | | | | Male | Female |
| More developed regions | 17.3 | 7.6 | 15.0 | 2.7 | 7.0 | 10.4 |
| Less developed regions | 5.9 | 16.3 | 3 | 3.9 | 3.6 | 22 |
| World | 7.8 | 14.9 | 5 | 3.6 | 4.1 | 20.1 |

**Box 5.1  Check list of contraceptive counselling**

When discussing any methods of contraception consider:
• suitability
• side-effects
• risks
• benefits
• how it works
• after sales service
• professional care needed

The use of contraception is influenced by many factors other than just the regulation of reproduction. These include:
• cultural background;
• religion;
• partnership status;
• personal health;
• personal habits.

The influence of peer comments is probably even greater than those of professionals. If a woman has met someone who had a bad time on the pill, this will be remembered more than advice given by the family planner. When counselling, the professionals should listen quite as much as they should advise. There are not enough data available on the use of methods to be absolute. The failure rate is not the only thing that influences people. When counselling, the items in Box 5.1 should all be included. The provision of contraception is one of the most intimate areas of an individual's life and requires high skills in communication and information giving.

# Methods used by the female

## Hormonal
• The pill—combined oral contraceptive (oestrogen and progestogen).
• The emergency pill—high dose progestogen.
• The mini-pill—progestogen-only pills.
• Injectable hormones—progestogens.
• Implantable hormones—progestogens.

## Intrauterine contraceptive devices (IUCDs)
• Copper bearing devices.
• Progestogen bearing devices.

## Barriers
• Diaphragm or Dutch cap.
• Cervical cap.
• Vault pessary.
• Vaginal sheath.

## Chemical spermicides
• Soluble pessaries.
• Creams, foams and jellies.
• Medicated sponges.
• Douching.

## Hormones: oral contraceptives

### Combined pill
The pill is used by about a third of women in the UK who use contraception. There is a wide range of oral contraceptives (Table 5.2). Most are a mixture of oestrogen and a progestogen taken for all of the 21 days of the packet.

**Table 5.2** Some examples of oral contraceptives in current use in the UK.

| Pill type | Preparation | Oestrogen ($\mu$g) | Progestogen (mg) | |
|---|---|---|---|---|
| *Combined* | | | | |
| Ethinyloestradiol/norethisterone | Loestrin 20 | 20 | 1 | |
| | Loestrin 30 | 30 | 1.5 | |
| | Brevinor | 35 | 0.5 | |
| | Norimin | 35 | 1 | |
| Ethinyloestradiol/levonorgestrel | Microgynon 30 | 30 | 0.15 | |
| | Eugynon 30 | 30 | 0.25 | |
| | Ovran | 50 | 2.25 | |
| Ethinyloestradiol/desogestrel | Marvelon | 30 | 0.15 | |
| Ethinyloestradiol/gestodene | Femodene | 30 | 0.075 | |
| Ethinyloestradiol/norgestimate | Cilest | 35 | 0.25 | |
| Ethinyloestradiol/norethisterone | Norinyl-1 | 50 | 1 | |
| | Ortho-Novin 1/50 | 50 | 1 | |
| *Biphasic* | BiNovum | 35 | 0.5 | (7 tabs) |
| | | 35 | 1 | (14 tabs) |
| *Triphasic* | TriNovum | 35 | 0.5 | (7 tabs) |
| | | 35 | 0.75 | (7 tabs) |
| | | 35 | 1 | (7 tabs) |
| Ethinyloestradiol/levonorgestrel | Trinordiol | 30 | 0.05 | (6 tabs) |
| | | 40 | 0.075 | (5 tabs) |
| | | 30 | 0.125 | (10 tabs) |
| Ethinyloestradiol/gestodene | Tri-Minulet | 30 | 0.05 | (6 tabs) |
| | | 40 | 0.07 | (5 tabs) |
| | | 30 | 0.1 | (10 tabs) |
| *Progestogen ONLY* | | | | |
| Norethisterone | Noriday | — | 0.35 | norethisterone |
| | Femulen | — | 0.5 | ethynodiol diacetate |
| Levonorgestrel | Microval | — | 0.03 | |
| | Neogest | — | 0.075 | norgestrel |

The pill:
• inhibits ovulation by interfering with gonado-trophin releasing hormones;
• modifies the endometrium preventing implantation;
• makes the cervical secretion more viscid and less permeable to spermatozoa.

*Advantages*
• The pill is the most effective method of reversible birth control provided the instructions are followed and it is taken regularly.
• The method is not related to the act of intercourse.

• Women who suffer from dysmenorrhoea or heavy periods often find their periods less painful and the flow diminished.
• Menstruation occurs at regular intervals of four weeks.
• Haemoglobin levels are maintained so that anaemia is less common.
• Acne and hirsutism may improve.

*Metabolic effects*
In different women there may be as much as a 10-fold variation in tissue levels of the hormones and therefore of their effects because of:

- difference in absorption;
- difference in liver metabolism of steroids;
- difference in fat layers of body as fat absorbs steroids avidly.
  
  Glucose tolerance may be impaired.

  There may be an increase in:
- low density lipoproteins;
- cholesterol;
- serum iron;
- serum copper;
- circulating blood coagulation factors VII, IX;
- fibrinogen.

*Side-effects*
- There may be fluid retention and weight gain.
- Break-through bleeding may occur in the first cycle and later if the amount of oestrogen is too low.
- Thromboembolism may occur, mainly with high oestrogen dosage and a very small increased risk in users of desogestrel/gestodene preparations.
- Skin pigmentation like the chloasma of pregnancy may develop.
- Migraine may be aggravated.
- Depression occurs in a few.
- There is a little evidence that the pill is carcinogenic to the cervix or the breast. Much of this relates to the higher-dose oestrogens and progestogens used in oral contraceptives (OCs) 40 years ago.
- There is a lower incidence of cancer of the ovary (by 40%) and endometrium (by 50%).

*Contraindications*
- The most serious hazards are:
  (a) thromboembolism;
  (b) coronary thrombosis;
  (c) cerebrovascular accident.
- The pill should be avoided in women:
  (a) with a history or family history of thrombophlebitis, severe heart disease or cerebrovascular accidents;
  (b) over 40 if they are obese and smoke heavily;
  (c) with liver damage including recent infective hepatitis or glandular fever;
  (d) with a history of breast cancer;
  (e) with excess weight, more than 50% of ideal;
  (f) with moderate hypertension;
  (g) with true sickle cell disease—genotype SS or SC (but not sickle trait, genotype AS).

Women taking the pill who undergo surgery face an increased risk of thrombosis and embolism during the post-operative period. The pill should ideally be stopped four weeks before elective surgery and immediately in the case of illness or accidents leading to long immobilization.

*Drug interactions*
Certain drugs may interfere with the absorption, metabolism or efficacy of oral contraceptives.
- Phenytoin.
- Barbiturates.
- Anti-tuberculous drugs (e.g. rifampicin).
- Antibiotics (e.g. griseofulvin and tetracycline).

The dose of hypoglycaemic agents may need increasing while the effect of corticosteroids may be enhanced. Epileptic women may need double the normal oral contraceptive dose to inhibit break-through bleeding and achieve maximum safety if they are on sodium valproate or clonazepam.

*Prescribing the pill*
A careful *history* should be taken with reference to conditions such as heavy smoking which may increase the risk of the pill.

*Examination* should include a record of blood pressure and body weight. The breasts, heart and abdomen should be examined. A pelvic examination should be made to exclude pelvic pathology.

The choice of oral contraception often depends on the doctor's preference; the list of available pills is extensive (Table 5.2). In general:
- 20 µg pills are best kept for the very slim;
- 50 µg pills are only used as emergency contraception or for women with epilepsy.

Watch for interacting drugs that are also being taken. The choice lies between a 30 or 35 µg pill to be taken either continuously or as one of the biphasic or triphasic pills.

The first pill is taken on the first day of menstruation. Successors are either taken for 21 days with seven pill-free days during which a withdrawal bleed occurs or continuously depending on the brand. Good instructions come with each packet and should be read.

There may be some side-effects such as early morning nausea, breast tenderness and slight bleeding during the first cycle. The *tricyclic regime* suits some women; here a 35 µg pill with varying doses of progestogen is given for 21 days, then 7 pill free days when bleeding should occur. This may help sufferers from migraine or epilepsy.

The combined pill should not be given during lactation, the progestogen-only pill being preferred then. The pill may be started on the second day after a miscarriage or termination of pregnancy.

The method should be carefully explained and discussed. The woman is advised to report adverse effects immediately. Regular examination with tests for blood pressure, glycosuria and excessive weight gain is essential.

*Forgotten pills*

If a pill is missed, advise the woman to take the missed one as soon as it is realized. If it is within 12 hours of the usual time, contraception is probably secure. If longer than this, the pill may not work. Additional contraception (i.e. condom) or abstinence is advised for seven days. If the missed OC is within the last seven days of the pack, go straight into the next cycle's pack—there will probably be no period but contraceptive effect will be maintained. If the missed pill is within the first seven days of a pack the couple should be advised to use additional barrier contraception for at least two weeks.

**Emergency pill (post-coital contraception)**

Oestrogen taken in large doses after unprotected coitus and before implantation may prevent pregnancy. Combined preparations containing 50 µg of ethinyloestradiol and 250 µg of levonorgestrel (Ovran or Norinyl-1) may be used in double dose. Two tablets are given immediately and repeated after 12 hours. High dose levonorgestrel alone is now the recommended emergency contraceptive. The main side-effects are nausea and vomiting.

Treatment should be given within 72 hours of a single incident of unprotected intercourse. The next period can be early or be late; the woman should have a pregnancy test if she does not menstruate.

An alternative, which is being evaluated and may be more effective, is the antiprogesterone mifepristone.

**Progestogen-only pill**

Progestogens are used for oral contraception; they probably act not by inhibiting ovulation but by their effect on the cervical mucus and the endometrium. They also reduce tubal motility so increasing the risk of ectopic pregnancy.

The progestogen-only pill is taken continuously at the same time of day from the first day of menstruation. If the pill is delayed more than three hours, additional precautions or abstinence are needed until the pill has been taken continuously for 14 days.

There is a failure rate of 1–4 per 100 women/years. There may be irregular bleeding or amenorrhoea and the risk of thrombosis is less than that for the combined pill. They are useful in older women and in women with serious medical disorders, e.g. sickle cell disease.

**Injectable contraceptives**

Those most commonly used consist of a progestogen given either by intramuscular injection or as subcutaneous implants. They are not the first choice for contraception but are widely used in less developed countries and in the UK for women when other methods are unacceptable or contraindicated.

Depo-medroxy-progesterone acetate (Depo-Provera) is given in a dose of 150 mg repeated every 12 weeks or 90 days. Norethisterone enanthate (Noristerat) is given in doses of 200 mg every eight weeks.

Side-effects include weight gain, irregular bleeding and amenorrhoea.

Silastic capsules injected subcutaneously under local anaesthesia are now available in the UK. Levonorgestrel implants (Norplant) offer up to five years of protection and can be removed when the return of fertility is required. Alternatively, at five years they can be replaced.

## Intrauterine devices

Intrauterine devices have existed for centuries. In the past devices were made of plastic, one of the better known being the Lippes loop, which is rarely seen in the Western world now. These have been superseded in UK practice by devices incorporating copper; some also have a silver core or have extra copper on the horizontal arms. In the UK the following devices were available in October 2002, one of which is shown in Fig. 5.1.

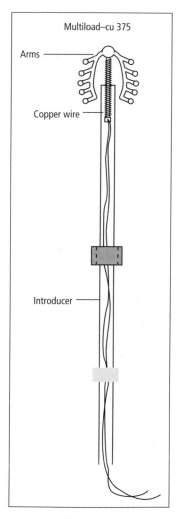

**Figure 5.1** One type of intrauterine contraceptive device in current use.

1 Copper devices (copper inhibits sperm motility)
  • Multiload.
  • Cu 250.
  • Cu 250 short. ⎫ Copper wire on stem.
  • Cu 375. ⎭
  • Gyne T 380 (copper wire or stem and arms).
2 Copper devices with silver core
  • Nova-T.
3 Progestogen devices
  • Mirena (levonorgestrel 20 μg/day)

*Advantages*

An IUD gives permanent protection and requires no attention at the time of intercourse. Provided that there are no complications, a device can remain in the uterus for up to five years; in the last decade of reproductive life, this time may be extended as potential fertility is less.

*Disadvantages*

A skilled doctor or nurse is required to insert an IUD. When first inserted there may be pain and bleeding. The menstrual flow may be increased and the periods prolonged for a few months. There is risk of flaring up pre-existing tubal infection.

*Complications*

• The device may pass unnoticed, especially during menstruation.
• Pelvic infection may occur.
• Increased risk of rejection in nulliparous women.
• Perforation of the uterus may occur with the coil moving into the peritoneal cavity. This is usually at the time of insertion particularly with an acutely anteflexed or retroflexed uterus. If it occurs with a copper device it should be removed, either by laparoscopy or by laparotomy.
• There is no evidence that IUDs are carcinogenic.
• The thread may disappear. The continued presence of the device can be checked by ultrasound. Removal is usually easy in the outpatients department.
• While the rate of intrauterine pregnancy is reduced, that of ectopics is not. Hence, there is a relative increase in ectopic pregnancy after IUD insertion.

• The progestogen intrauterine system (IUS) reduces menstrual flow and often dysmenorrhoea. It has a lower incidence of pelvic inflammatory disease.

*Contraindications*
An IUD should not be inserted in the presence of:
• pelvic infection;
• large or submucosal uterine fibroids;
• genital malignancy;
• abnormal bleeding; ⎫
• menorrhagia. ⎭ except Mirena

*Method of insertion*
The device is supplied in a sterile pack with full instructions for insertion. This should be done with aseptic and antiseptic precautions (Fig. 5.2).
• The best time is at the end of menstruation.
• The cervix is exposed and may be steadied with a single-toothed forceps.
• A uterine sound measures cavity length.
• The device is loaded into the introducer and inserted.
• The introducer is withdrawn and the nylon threads cut leaving 1.5–2.0 cm in the upper vagina.
• The woman should be taught to identify the threads.

A vasovagal attack may occur at the time of insertion, following cervical stimulation. This usually responds on stopping the insertion and lowering the woman's head. Formal resuscitation is very rarely needed, but facilities should be available at the family planning clinic for the rare occasion.

*Post-coital contraception*
An IUD may be used for post-coital contraception to prevent implantation if inserted within five days of unprotected intercourse. The woman must be seen again to ensure menstruation has occurred. This is an emergency measure, but if normal menstruation occurs the device may be left for permanent contraception.

*Pregnancy*
The pregnancy rate with copper devices is reported as 1.4 per 100 women/years. Should pregnancy occur the possibility of ectopic pregnancy must be excluded.
• If the tail of the device is visible the device should be removed by pulling gently on the thread.
• If the tail of the device is not found the position of the device must be checked by ultrasound.
• The device may be left in the uterus throughout pregnancy.

**Barrier contraception**
The most effective is the *vaginal diaphragm* or Dutch cap which consists of a watch spring or coiled spring edged with a dome of latex. They are made in various sizes and for maximum safety must be used with a spermicide jelly or cream.
• The correct size must be selected before examination (Fig. 5.3).
• The woman should be taught how to insert and remove it.
• Always use it with a spermicide.
• Leave it in for eight hours after intercourse.
• A check of the fit and, if needs refitting, after six months, and after childbirth.

If there is prolapse or a retroverted uterus, an alternative is the *cervical cap* made of rubber or plastic. This is harder to get in place and easier to displace at intercourse.

The *vaginal sheath* is a plastic bag which lines the vagina. It retains its place by a spring ring in the fornices. The woman can insert it at leisure. It has

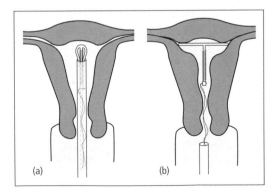

**Figure 5.2** Method of insertion. (a) The T-shaped IUD is straightened inside a plastic tube and inserted through the cervix. (b) When pushed from the hollow tube it resumes its old shape.

**Figure 5.3** The diaphragm fits snugly to the walls of the vagina occluding the cervix from the rest of the vagina.

mixed popularity among women and their partners.

**Chemical contraceptives**

These are mainly spermicides. They may be bought over the counter and do not need professional advice. Creams, gels, soluble pessaries and foaming preparations exist. The failure rate is relatively high if used alone.

A disposable plastic sponge impregnated with spermicide (nonoxinol-9) can be placed high in the vagina. It is less effective than the diaphragm with a PI of about 9 per 100 women/years.

**Douching**

Douching immediately after intercourse with warm water or a weak solution of vinegar (one teaspoon to a pint) is a time honoured but ineffective method. It does not affect those sperms which have already passed up the cervical canal.

## Methods used by the male

## The sheath

The sheath, condom or French letter is one of the commonest methods of contraception. It requires no medical intervention and can be bought in many non-medical places. For maximum safety the woman should insert a chemical contraceptive in case the sheath bursts or slips off. Another advantage is that it reduces the spread of sexually transmitted infections, including HIV.

## Coitus interruptus

This is the oldest and a widely practised method: the male withdraws before ejaculation. It is not always reliable for human beings are frail. It may prevent complete satisfaction to both partners. In *coitus reservatus* the man enters the vagina but does not ejaculate. This is even more unreliable for who wants to stop?

## Methods used by both partners

## The safe period or natural family planning

In theory ovulation occurs only once in each menstrual cycle, so there are days when a woman can expect to be infertile. These can be calculated in various ways.
• The calendar method based on working out the fertile period from previous cycles (Fig. 5.4).
• The basal temperature method depends on the rise of basal temperature which follows ovulation.

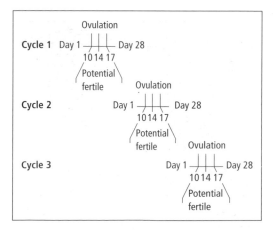

**Figure 5.4** The fertile time to avoid when using the calendar method of contraception.

Intercourse is stopped for three days before and after ovulation.

• Teaching the woman to note the changes in cervical mucus which occur at ovulation and mark the peak of fertility. Instead of sticky glue-like mucus, it becomes thin and runny. Motivation is important as is adequate instruction.

• Ovulation predictor tests, but these are expensive.

The disadvantage of the safe period is that it is not really safe if menstruation is irregular, after childbirth or abortion or in women approaching the menopause.

## Sterilization

Sterilization is an operation aimed at the permanent occlusion of tubes carrying the gametes.

### Counselling for sterilization

Sterilization is an important step in the life of any man or woman. It should be considered as irrevocable for, while reversal is possible for both males and females, success cannot be guaranteed even in the most expert hands. Counselling is important and consent must be given in writing. The consent of the spouse is no longer necessary legally, but it is desirable that the couple should be seen together and the full implications of the procedure explained.

A girl under 16 cannot consent to sterilization, nor can her parents insist on it. The same applies to individuals who are mentally retarded to a degree that they cannot understand the meaning and consequences of the operation. At present such operations can only be performed with the consent of a High Court judge.

### Female sterilization

The most practical place to block the female genital tract is at the fallopian tubes. These are deep inside the peritoneal cavity, so their approach is a bigger procedure than operating on the male. The use of the laparoscope has reduced much of the need for large incisions in the majority of cases, but

it is still an intraperitoneal operation requiring a general anaesthetic and the availability of full surgical skills.

### Laparotomy sterilization

The woman should plan to stay in hospital for 2–3 days depending on how fit she is. The simplest operation was described by Pomeroy; it is not often performed now. A more common technique is the Irving method, where each tube is divided and separated. The medial end is implanted in a tunnel in the wall of the uterus.

The operation of formal surgical division is commonly performed these days whilst doing an elective Caesarean section when the abdomen is open. The failure rate is about 2–4 per 1000 operations.

A lesser abdominal operation (Mini-Lap) can be performed by an experienced surgeon. A 5 cm transverse suprapubic incision is extended to the rectus sheath and the surgeon then separates the rectus muscles. This allows a bivalve speculum to be introduced through the incision into the peritoneal cavity. Through this, each fallopian tube in turn can be sought, drawn up and operated upon. It is divided and the two ends overlapped so that the ends are separated. This operation is often done in developing countries where laparoscopy is not readily available. The failure rate for this operation is about 1–2 per 1000 operations (Fig. 5.5).

Two clamps mid section excised

Ends are overlapped and tied

**Figure 5.5** Division and overlapping of tubes at mini-laparotomy.

## Laparoscopic sterilization

This operation is performed through a small incision but is potentially just as hazardous as a larger operation. It should only be performed by those who are skilled in general gynaecological surgery because the abdomen may have to be opened at any time to deal with complications. These are, however, uncommon and usually the laparoscopic sterilization can be done as a day case.

The tube is then blocked by one of three methods.

**1** A *mechanical clip* (Hulka–Clemens, Filshie) may be applied to each tube. This may be a spring-loaded clip or a plastic one with a grip (Fig. 5.6).

**2** A *silastic ring* (Falope ring) may be applied to the medial narrow part of each tube through the laparoscope (Fig. 5.7). A knuckle of tube is drawn up and over it is slipped a silastic ring which constricts the neck of the knuckle. This causes necrosis of the tube at the bound point, which then fibroses, blocking the lumen and then pulls apart leaving the tube with a gap.

**3** *Unipolar or bipolar diathermy* used to cauterize the fallopian tube in two places about 1 cm apart in the isthmal area. There is a risk of heat damage. For this reason, it is less commonly used in the Western world.

Failure rates of laparoscopic sterilizations are about 2–3 per 1000 operations.

## Other methods

Transuterine methods of sterilization without anaesthesia are being attempted using a hysteroscope and passing catheters through the uterine cavity into the fallopian tubes. A rapidly setting plastic resin is injected; alternatively, electrical cautery or cryosurgery by narrow cooling probes has been used by the same route. None of these methods has yet been shown to produce reliable results.

## Causes of failure

Despite these operations, a woman may still get pregnant in 2–3 per 1000 cases in the UK.

• The woman may already have a fertilized oocyte in the proximal tube or even the uterus at the time of the operation. Hence try to operate in the first two weeks of the cycle.

• All women undergoing sterilization should have a pregnancy test before the procedure.

• The occluding clip or ring may be correctly placed but spring off or break after the operator has left the abdomen. Unless a good knuckle of tube is brought through the elastic ring, it may not be pinching it securely. The clip may re-open under pressure of the tissues although this is less common with the beaked Filshie clip. Very rarely steril-

**Figure 5.7** A silastic ring and its method of application. (a) The springy forceps grasp the tube. (b) Retracting the forceps draws the tube through the plastic ring. (c) Passing the forceps back releases the tube and the tube is constricted at its neck by the ring. (d) The loop becomes hypoxic, dies and the ends separate when the ring drops off.

**Figure 5.6** Clip sterilization. (a) A Filshie clip and (b) its method of application.

ization clips have broken. Thus they have no oc-clusive effect on the fallopian tube and have been removed subsequently from the abdomen in pieces.

• Although the tube is blocked by the clip and the short length of fibrosis it causes, the two ends of the tube may not separate. A small fistula can form between the contiguous ends bypassing the occluding device or burrowing through the short length of fibrous tissue. This would allow sperm to pass up readily although fertilized eggs might pass down less commonly; in consequence an ectopic pregnancy may result.

• The occluding device may be put on the wrong structure. Laparoscopic sterilization should be done only when the surgeon has good vision. Occasionally, however, with less than perfect sight, a clip is put on the round ligament just in front of the fallopian tube.

A hysterosalpingogram is occasionally per-formed 16 weeks after the operation to ensure tubal blockage. It is unwise to do it before as the pressure of the injected dye may disrupt healing tissues and produce a fistula between the blocked parts of the tube.

## Male sterilization

Blockage is performed by division of each vas def-erens in the groin, a lesser surgical operation than for the female, and done under local anaesthesia (Fig. 5.8). Unguarded intercourse should await two semen specimens showing no sperm, often as long as 16 weeks after the surgery.

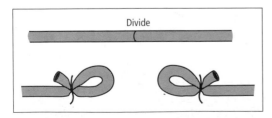

**Figure 5.8** Male sterilization. Divided ends of the vas deferens are turned back and ligated to ensure that the open ends are not just separated but point in opposite directions.

Complications are few:
• Haematoma of scrotum.
• Infection.
• Failure of blockage.
• Long-term generation of sperm antibodies and non-specific antibodies in later life.

## Termination of pregnancy

Pregnancy may be terminated by intervention with instruments or by drugs. If done incorrectly, there is a high risk of trauma and death of the mother. It is illegal in some societies, but many sovereign states have now passed laws which allow a termination to be performed by doctors under certain constraints.

Religious and cultural factors dictate whether termination is allowed in a country. Generally, termination of pregnancy (TOP) is unacceptable to the Roman Catholic Church, to Moslems and some other major world religions. In actuality, women seek termination of unwanted pregnancies world-wide, irrespective of the official religion or laws of a country.

In some countries, TOP is used as a part of the contraceptive programme; in Communist Eastern Europe, up to a third of women used termination as their primary means of contraception. In most of the Western world, this is not so, for it is appreciat-ed that TOP has many more complications than the more conventional methods of contraception.

Four factors have recently rendered TOP safer in Western society.
• Better training of doctors in the subject.
• Safer general anaesthesia or wider use of local anaesthetic agents.
• Asepsis and antisepsis have reduced infection.
• Liberalization of abortion laws encourage early medical advice.

### Position in the UK

Major changes in TOP were associated with the 1967 Abortion Act (which does not apply in Northern Ireland) and the subsequent 1991 amendment. Before then, a few TOPs had been car-ried out under an *obiter dictum* or case law which said that a physician may recommend a pregnancy be terminated if he thought that the continuation of pregnancy would harm the mother's physical or mental health. Since the 1967 Abortion Act, the position has been codified into statute law. This was modified in 1991 so that now there are five indications which must be certified in advance by two doctors who should have seen and examined the woman. These are reproduced in Box 5.2, taken from the Abortion Act Certificate A.

In addition, in an emergency, one doctor alone may recommend TOP to save the woman's life or health. This indication is very rarely used.

In England and Wales, the various indications are used in the following proportions (2002):

|   | % |
|---|---|
| A | 0 |
| B | 1 |
| C | 94 (from 85% in 1995) |
| D | 4 |
| E | 1 |
| Emergency | <0.01 |

Assessment of the data by age is shown in Fig. 5.9 along with the proportion of births reported in these age groups. There is a shift to the younger women in the distribution of terminations.

Ninety per cent of TOPs in Britain take place before the 12th week of pregnancy and only 2.5% are performed after the 20th week even though the law at present allows this up to the 24th completed week. A legal TOP must be notified by the operating surgeon to the appropriate Department of Health in England, Scotland or Wales.

## Methods

Any woman presenting with a request for a TOP should be assessed carefully. Her GP may know the circumstances of the family well, but the hospital doctor will not. The alternative to abortion is continuation of the pregnancy and its sequelae must be considered:

- adoption;
- placing child with foster parents;
- the mother's parents taking the child.

Often none of these are acceptable and the woman wishes to go on with the abortion. The GP usually sends her on to a gynaecologist for a second opinion and action, having signed the first half of the Abortion Act Certificate A.

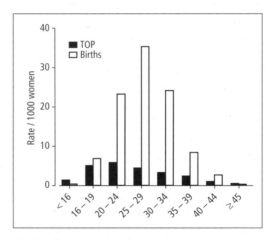

**Figure 5.9** Terminations of pregnancy (TOP) by age compared with births.

---

**Box 5.2  Extracts from the Abortion Act Certificate A 1991**

A  The continuance of the pregnancy would involve risk to the life of the pregnant woman greater than if the pregnancy were terminated

B  The termination is necessary to prevent grave permanent injury to the physical or mental health of the pregnant woman

C  The pregnancy has NOT exceeded its 24th week and that the continuance of the pregnancy would involve risk, greater than if the pregnancy were terminated, of injury to the physical or mental health of the pregnant woman

D  The pregnancy has NOT exceeded its 24th week and that the continuance of the pregnancy would involve risk, greater than if the pregnancy were terminated, of injury to the physical or mental health of any existing child(ren) of the family of the pregnant woman

E  There is a substantial risk that if the child were born it would suffer from such physical or mental abnormalities as to be seriously handicapped

In the hospital, if in agreement with the GP, the specialist signs the second part. Time should be allowed for the woman to reconsider; if she wishes to go ahead she is checked for fitness for operation under anaesthesia and tested for chlamydia. The future method of contraception is discussed to avoid a repeat unwanted pregnancy. Many women are day case admissions, especially those seen in the earlier weeks of gestation (before 14 weeks). TOP must be performed in a National Health Hospital or clinic specifically licensed for the purpose.

## Early abortion

### Surgical termination

For pregnancies up to 12 weeks' gestation, TOP is often by a vacuum aspiration of the uterine cavity. A hollow plastic catheter is passed through the cervix which has been gently dilated, usually after prostaglandin ripening. A vacuum suction then removes the uterine contents and a gentle curettage ensures the uterus is empty. This technique has few complications and a high success rate.

### Medical termination

The use of antiprogesterone steroids like mifepristone has spread from Europe to the UK, but not widely in the USA because of the views of their politicians. An increasing number of women at less than 9 weeks' gestation elect for this day case TOP which is very effective in producing total abortions in 96%—a figure comparable with the success rate of aspiration TOP. Women opt for this since it avoids anaesthesia and surgery; they consider it more natural and it gives them control.

Used in the outpatients, a single oral dose of mifepristone is given followed 36–48 hours later by 200–600μg oral misoprostol or 0.5mg gemeprost vaginal pessary. While the measured blood loss in both medical and surgical methods is the same, women report a longer period of blood loss after medical TOP.

Mifepristone is also most useful at 16–18 weeks' gestation when 200mg is given 24 hours before prostaglandins ($PGE_{2\alpha}$) and works swiftly.

Mifepristone can also be injected into ectopic gestational sacs in ectopic pregnancy (Chapter 8) and can be used for post-coital emergency contraception.

### Complications of early termination of pregnancy

• *Haemorrhage*—separation of the sac and forming placenta causes blood loss. Syntometrine is often needed intravenously to help the myometrium clamp down.
• *Perforation*—if the uterus is perforated, laparoscopy with examination and repair of the uterus may be required.
• *Infection*—TOP is an invasive procedure, passing instruments through the potentially septic area of the vagina into the sterile area of the uterus. The operator cleans the upper vagina with antiseptic before starting and antibiotics may be given before the operation if vaginal infection is suspected.

If infection occurs, particularly with chlamydia, it must be treated promptly with antibiotics or a tubal infection may follow leading to future infertility.
• *Incomplete termination*—this leads to retention of products of conception. Bleeding occurs and re-evacuation of the uterus is necessary.
• *Psychological complications*—many women have a natural grief reaction after early TOP; if the abortion was voluntary, that reaction passes in a few weeks or months. Should the woman have been coerced into termination, the reaction can continue for much longer; up to 25% of women in this latter group may require psychotherapy.

### Future pregnancies

Early TOP usually has no effect on future pregnancies. If the cervix is properly dilated (usually not more than 8mm), there should be no cervical incompetence following early TOP; this is more commonly found after 10–12mm dilatation, particularly if no prostaglandin was given preoperatively to ripen the cervix.

## Mid-trimester abortion

After 14 weeks of gestation, pregnancy termination becomes more difficult.

## Morcellation and extraction

In the hands of an expert and experienced gynaecologist, under anaesthesia the cervix can be dilated to well beyond 10 mm. Crushing instruments are introduced into the uterus to break up the fetus which is then extracted piecemeal. This is an unpleasant and potentially hazardous way to abort, but in expert hands it does mean the whole procedure is over in a few minutes with the mother asleep and unaware of the abortion. She often goes home later the same day.

## Prostaglandins

The uterus can be made to contract by giving prostaglandins ($PGE_{2\alpha}$) *per vaginam*, intra-amniotically, extra-amniotically or intravenously. Under sterile conditions, an amniocentesis can be performed drawing 20 ml of amniotic fluid. In its place, 40 mg of $PGE_{2\alpha}$ is injected in the amniotic cavity. Alternatively, $PGE_{2\alpha}$ gel/tablet is inserted into the vagina causing the uterus to contract.

A mini-labour follows and delivery usually takes place in 10–20 hours. This is painful and so should be well covered with analgesia, even an epidural. Evacuation of the placenta is needed in many cases.

## Hysterotomy

If prostaglandins are not available, pregnancies after about 14 weeks require a surgical termination and a mini-Caesarean section is performed. There is no lower segment and so the uterine incision has to be vertical. This is rarely done in the UK now but often in the USA.

## Complications

• *Bleeding*—this is uncommon after prostaglandin TOP, because the uterus has been contracting through the mini-labour. However, the placenta is often retained in terminations between 14 and 22 weeks of pregnancy and often requires removal under general anaesthesia.

Bleeding is not a major problem after hysterotomy for it is a surgical procedure at which haemostasis is achieved at the time of the operation.

• *Infection*—infection is not common after mid-trimester abortion procedures and should be prevented as it is in any labour or surgical operation by good asepsis and antisepsis.

• *Psychological problems*—these are commoner after mid-trimester abortion. The woman has been pregnant for a longer period and the fetus is more developed. This is an area of great sensitivity which the attendants must be very careful in handling. Some people wish to bury the fetus with a religious service; these natural reactions should be assisted.

• *Future pregnancies*—following mid-trimester TOP, the cervix has been dilated and cervical incompetence can follow.

A vertical hysterotomy scar on the uterus might cause a problem, for it is more liable to rupture in a subsequent pregnancy than a lower segment transverse incision.

## Later terminations

Until 1991, TOP was only permitted in England, Wales and Scotland before 28 weeks, the time of presumed viability in law. With modern neonatal developments, the law has reduced this to 24 weeks. Clauses C and D limit terminations to below 24 weeks, but the other clauses (risk of death, grave permanent injury to the mother or fetal abnormalities) are not time limited. Sometimes ultrasound may only show a fetal abnormality at 26–28 weeks or cordocentesis done for karyotyping studies may give results as late as 28–29 weeks.

Late termination is difficult to accept for the woman and to all who have to care for the woman, but it is a logical extension of the law's previous position with more up to date diagnostic tests on the fetus. Such terminations are usually done with mifepristone and prostaglandins.

**Self-assessment**

**5.1** OSCE role-play question (10 minutes).

**Candidate's instructions:** A 14 year-old girl comes to your practice requesting contraception. You are the GP who is going to counsel her. She has no medical illnesses and her weight is normal.

**Role-player's instructions:** You are a 14-year-old girl who is fully developed. Your periods started when you were 11. You have been going out with a 16-year-old boy in your school for the last three months. Your relationship has developed to the point that you are thinking about having sex with him. Your parents do not know about the relationship and you do not want to tell them. You get on reasonably well with your father but he is never at home as he is a long distance lorry driver. You constantly fight with your mother who does not understand you at all and would be horrified that you had a boyfriend. She disapproves of your friends and will not let you go out late at weekends. You tend to defy her and take the consequences in the morning. You know that she would be furious if you got pregnant so you want to be sensible and take precautions so this can't happen. Your friend has told you to go to the GP and get the pill. She has reassured you that s/he cannot tell your parents without your permission. You haven't told your boyfriend because you do not want him to know that you are ready for sex, you just want to be protected in case. You have no medical problems, you smoke three cigarettes a day and are of normal weight. You have never taken any illegal substances. The rest is up to the imagination of the role-player.

**5.2** OSCE role-play question (10 minutes).

**Candidate's instructions:** A woman of 35 comes to your clinic requesting sterilization. She is fit and well and of normal weight. You are the doctor who will counsel her.

**Role-player's instructions:** You are a woman of 35. You have 3 children and do not want any more. You have been married for 12 years and your children are 10, 7 and 3 years old, all fit and well. You and your husband have discussed this and have decided that you should have the operation. You have been on the pill for the last three years but you know you should stop taking it as you smoke 40 cigarettes a day. Your periods were regular but quite heavy before you had your youngest daughter. You have no other medical problems and all the children were normal deliveries at term. You do not want to use barrier methods because they are messy and unreliable. You are not keen on a coil because you have heard they cause heavy periods and infection. You are worried about putting on weight after the operation and have heard that the mini-pill and the injections are also bad for your weight. All other details are up to the role-player.

**5.3** Which of the following statements are true about the combined oral contraceptive pill (COCP)?
(a) COCP should be started on the seventh day of a woman's period.
(b) If the woman misses the first two pills in her packet she should use additional protection for at least two weeks.
(c) COCP should be taken at the same time of day to ensure protection from unwanted pregnancy.
(d) A past medical history of thrombosis is an absolute contraindication for prescribing the COCP.
(e) Women on antiepileptic medication should be prescribed a pill with a low estrogen content.

**Self-assessment** *Continued*

**5.4** Which of the following are absolute contraindications to the use of an intrauterine contraceptive device.

(a) Past history of pelvic inflammatory disease.

(b) Past history of sickle cell disease.

(c) Past history of termination of pregnancy.

(d) Past history of an abnormal cervical smear.

(e) Past history of heart valve replacement.

**5.5** Which of the following are recognized methods of emergency contraception.

(a) High dose estrogen given in two doses 12 hours apart.

(b) High dose estrogen and progestogen given in two doses 12 hours apart.

(c) High dose progestogen given in two doses 12 hours apart.

(d) Endometrial curettage.

(e) Insertion of an intrauterine device (IUD) within five days of unprotected intercourse.

# Chapter 6

# Benign diseases, genital tract infections and sexual problems

## Introduction

This chapter will address benign conditions and infections affecting the lower genital tract. In reading the chapter, it is useful to remember that all infections may be sexually transmitted (STIs) and therefore it is essential to consider this possibility in all women who are, or have recently been, sexually active. It is important to have knowledge of these diseases which are the most widespread infectious diseases in the UK and many other parts of the world. Some of the STIs have significant long-term sequelae including infertility, ectopic pregnancy, chronic pelvic pain as well as the possibility of mother-to-child transmission during pregnancy or at delivery and postpartum (if breast-feeding).

The increase in the reported incidence of STIs in the UK and other countries reflects a number of factors, including worsening of access to overburdened sexual health services, a more liberal attitude to sexual intercourse, the younger age of starting sexual activity, a lack of political will to deal with STI-related issues, and less than ideal sex education in some schools and homes. In addition, the introduction of more sensitive DNA amplification-based techniques has resulted in more diagnoses of some conditions, e.g. *Chlamydia trachomatis*. The UK has a well-established network of genitourinary medicine (GUM) clinics which provide primary care access to patients at risk of STIs. These clinics provide quarterly statistical returns on their workload; a statutory requirement in the UK (KC60). In addition, these clinics have health advisers who oversee partner notification (contact tracing) of all patients diagnosed with important STIs. They also possess expertise in risk assessment for HIV infection and provide pre- and post-test counselling for those wishing to know their HIV status.

In an attempt to deal with the alarming increase in STI diagnoses and the increasing waiting times in GUM clinics, the UK Government recently released a National Strategy for Sexual Health and HIV which aims to increase the amount of STI testing and treatment undertaken in general practice and community reproductive and sexual health (family planning) services. However, it should be noted that, despite the importance of sexual ill-health among younger members of our society, the UK Government has not chosen to make sexual health a National Service Framework. This political move would ensure a marked improvement in the quality of sexual health services in the UK.

Any health care worker who takes on the responsibility of treating an STI (presumed or confirmed) must ensure that sexual partners are treated as well. There is little or no point in treating the index case when they will simply be reinfected by an untreated partner. Even if they are no longer at risk of reacquiring the STI from their expartner, it is important that the source is treated from the public health view point.

## Taking a sexual history

**1** History of presenting condition.
- Describe the current symptoms.

**2** Sexual contact history.
- Cover sexual contacts for the past three months (six months if secondary syphilis or acute hepatitis B are likely).
- Gender of partner(s) and whether regular or non-regular partner.
- Sexual orientation of patient.
- Type of sexual intercourse: vaginal, oral, anal, fingers, sex toys.
- Use of condoms and other contraceptive methods.

**3** History of past STIs.
- Ask about past chlamydial, gonococcal and syphilis infection.
- Warts and herpes may recur spontaneously.
- Fully document previous treatment for positive treponemal serology.
- Document previous HIV test result (with year).

**4** Recent antibiotic and drug history.
- Relevant for gonorrhoea in terms of possible resistance.
- Document allergies.

**5** Hepatitis B immunization.
- Hepatitis B immunization is recommended for those using IV drugs, sex workers and those who are partners of Hepatitis B carriers.

**6** HIV risk assessment.
- Necessary only for period since last negative HIV test.
- Number of sexual partners with whom patient practised unprotected vaginal or anal intercourse.
- Has the patient had unprotected sexual intercourse with men in *or* from high HIV-risk countries.
- IV drug abuse with sharing of needles.
- Blood transfusion at time when blood supplies were not checked for HIV antibodies.

## Benign conditions

### The vulva and vagina

### Pruritus vulvae

Pruritus vulvae is a common symptom—an irritation of the vulva sufficient to lead to scratching.

*Causes*
*Irritating vaginal discharges* of *Trichomonas vaginalis* or monilia. Since many infections are common to the vulva and vagina, these are considered collectively in later sections. Other causes are:
- *Parasites* such as scabies and crab lice.
- *Fungi* such as athlete's foot affects the feet, the groin and the vulva.
- *Sensitivity to drugs* or chemicals including:
  (a) soap and disinfectants;
  (b) detergents used for washing underwear;
  (c) contraceptives made of rubber;
  (d) commercial spermicides;
  (e) ointments containing benzocaine and amethocaine.
- *Iron deficiency anaemia* associated with glossitis.
- *Gross vitamin deficiencies*, A and B group, especially in elderly women.
- *Glycosuria* due to any cause, but principally diabetes. Glycosuria probably causes irritation because the vulva becomes infected with a fungus. A random fasting blood glucose should be measured.

*Degenerative conditions* of the vulva occur mainly in postmenopausal women and are associated with irritation and soreness. There are two main varieties.
- *Vulval dystrophy*—an important, but uncommon condition specific to the vulva. It presents as a thickening and hypertrophy of the vulval skin often spreading into the groin and around the anus. The hypertrophic keratin layer causes white patches (which used to be called leukoplakia). It may be precancerous and tends to recur in time after surgical removal of the vulva. Diagnosis is by biopsy; this shows thickening and increase in depth of the keratin layer, while the basal papillae are hypertrophied and dip deeply into the dermis.

• *Lichen sclerosus et atrophicus* is an atrophic condition usually seen in postmenopausal women and pre-pubertal girls. It differs from vulval dystrophy in that it is atrophic and does not spread beyond the skin of the vulva itself. Biopsy shows a general thinning of all the layers of the skin; the keratin layer is deficient and the basal papillae are flattened. There is hyaline change in the dermis which is infiltrated with lymphocytes.

Careful investigation reveals a cause for pruritus vulvae in over 90% of cases. True pruritus must be distinguished from soreness of the vulva, also a common symptom, and often caused by vaginitis, oestrogen deficiency states and postmenopausal atrophy.

*Investigations*
These should include:
• a careful *history*, including the use of any substance which might lead to allergy;
• *examination* to determine characteristics and limits of physical signs;
• *bacteriological examination* of vaginal secretions and scrapings from the skin;
• a full *blood count*;
• a fasting blood glucose if relevant;
• *biopsy* of the skin of the vulva.

*Treatment*
Women tend to be very sensitive and shy about pruritus and often delay in seeking advice. Self-medication often makes the condition worse.

No treatment should be attempted without full examination and investigation. Blind treatment may mean that a serious condition, such as an early carcinoma or diabetes, is overlooked. With full investigation, the cause can be found in almost every case. The help of a dermatologist may be sought in difficult cases. The treatment is that of the cause, e.g. diabetes or anaemia.

Fungal infections should be treated with imidazole drugs and vaginal applications should be supplemented with antifungal creams for vulvitis.

Dystrophy and lichen sclerosis may respond to ointments containing hydrocortisone. In cases which do not improve, simple vulvectomy may be undertaken but the condition often returns.

Care should be taken in using local analgesics, especially benzocaine and amethocaine, as acute sensitivity may develop.

## Non-STI conditions of the vulva

• *Infections, boils and carbuncles* may affect the vulva, especially in women with glycosuria and diabetes.
• *Swellings of Bartholin's gland.* Cysts of Bartholin's duct and a Bartholin's abscess are common. Both present as swellings in the fourchette. An acute abscess is painful and tender like a boil; an abscess may rupture spontaneously, but tends to recur. Treatment of both cysts and abscesses is by marsupialization which permits adequate drainage and in many cases the function of the gland is retained. The pus in an abscess should always be cultured and a search made for gonococci in the urethra and cervix, since some Bartholin's abscesses are due to gonorrhoea.
• *Vaginal and uterine causes.* A patient complaining of a lump in the vulva may be suffering from:
  • prolapse;
  • a large polyp;
  • inversion of the uterus;
  • a vaginal cyst.

## Conditions of the urethra

*Urethral caruncle* occurs mostly in postmenopausal women. It presents as a bright red, exquisitely tender swelling at the posterior margin of the urethral meatus. Symptoms include dysuria, bleeding and dyspareunia. Treatment is to excise the caruncle with diathermy.

*Prolapse of the urethra*, which may be acute or chronic, involves the whole circumference of the urethra and not just the posterior margin of the meatus. It may give similar symptoms to a caruncle. If symptoms are severe, the prolapsed urethra must be excised and repaired.

## Conditions of the vagina and cervix

Infections of the vagina may or may not be sexually-transmitted infections (STIs), whereas infections of the cervix are usually caused by one of two STI pathogens, *Neisseria gonorrhoeae* and *Chlamydia trachomatis*.

Natural protection of the genital tract is provided by:
• squamous epithelium thickened by oestrogens;
• low pH(4) from lactic acid derived from intra-epithelial glycogen breakdown;
• mucus from the cervix, Bartholin's gland and Skene's glands rich in bactericidal lysozymes.

This protection is diminished by a number of causes.
• Pre-pubertal and postmenopausal low oestrogen levels resulting in a thinner epithelium, a higher pH and less mucus production.
• Antibiotics which destroy the commensal flora, in particular lactobacilli (Doderlein's bacilli).
• Chemical douches which wash away the natural protective secretions.
• Foreign bodies in the vagina such as pessaries or tampons.
• Abortion and menstruation which render the pH more alkaline and remove the protective discharge in the cervical cavity.
• Debilitation.

*Symptoms*

VAGINAL DISCHARGE
• Details of the onset, e.g. postcoital, postantibiotics.
• The volume—does it soil the clothing or require sanitary towels to be used?
• The colour and consistency:
  (a) white and thick—candidiasis;
  (b) yellow, green and frothy—trichomoniasis;
  (c) mucus—cervical origin.

*Itchiness* or pruritus is commonly associated with candidiasis and trichomoniasis.

SORENESS
• Comes with secondary bacterial invasion or herpes simplex.

CERVICITIS
• Postcoital or intermenstrual bleeding.
• May be associated with pelvic pain or deep dyspareunia.

ULCERATION
• Associated with viral infections (herpes) or exposure to chemicals, e.g. detergent which causes inflammation.

OFFENSIVE DISCHARGE
• Often associated with anaerobic bacterial activity caused by foreign bodies and carcinoma.

*Examination*
Inspect the vulva for:
• reddening;
• oedema;
• excoriation from scratching;
• ulceration.

Inspect the external urethral meatus for prolapse or caruncle.

Vaginal examination to check for:
• patchy, reddening associated with trichomoniasis;
• white plaques associated with candidiasis;
• punctate vesicle type ulceration associated with herpes simplex.

Examine the cervix for:
• reddening;
• mucopurulent cervical discharge;
• contact bleeding.

Palpate the urethra for thickening and tenderness. Check the Bartholin's glands are not enlarged or tender.

*Investigations*
Swabs should be taken from the cervical canal, lower urethra, posterior fornix and from any overt lesions on the walls of the lower genital tract. Instant microscopy in saline can sometimes demonstrate the presence of *Trichomonas vaginalis* and candida. All the swabs should be sent to the laboratory in Stuart's medium as speedily as possible for culture.

*Treatment*

The principles of therapy for infection are:
• to avoid indiscriminate treatment;
• to ensure that there is no sexually transmitted disease or carcinoma present;
• to avoid excessive treatment, which may lead to a chemical vaginitis.

### Foreign bodies in the vagina

This usually presents with a foul discharge caused by the anaerobic organism. This is commonest in:
• children—beads or toys, etc;
• mentally subnormal—beads or coins, etc;
• those in custody—vagina used to hide objects (e.g. drugs), which are then forgotten.

Treatment requires the removal of foreign bodies. Lactic acid pessaries restore pH and encourage regrowth of lactobacilli.

### Toxic shock syndrome

Caused by a *Staphylococcus aureus* septicaemia toxaemia. Associated with:
• obstructed drainage of menses by tampons;
• abrasion of the cervical surface by tampons;
• retrograde flow of menses into the peritoneal cavity.

*Symptoms*

Shivering, diarrhoea, erythematous rash and fainting. Occurs mostly on second and third days at the peak of menstrual flow.

*Physical signs*
• Hypotension.
• Fever.
• Tenderness of vagina and cervix.

*Treatment*
• Removal of tampon.
• Intravenous fluid resuscitation.
• Systemic antibiotics, e.g. Magnapen.

## Microbiology and therapy of common genital tract infections

### Bacterial vaginosis

This condition is due to an imbalance in the vaginal microflora, although the exact mechanisms which result in this change remain uncertain. There is a decrease in the number of acid-producing lactobacilli and an increase in other vaginal organisms, including *Gardnerella vaginalis, Mycoplasma* species, *Mobiluncus* species and other anaerobes. It appears to be more common in certain ethnic groups, e.g. African Caribbeans, and also in those who are sexually active.

*Symptoms and signs*

Typically there is a creamy vaginal discharge, often with an offensive fish-like smell. Sometimes, it is the smell alone which brings the patient to the doctor. The symptoms tend to be worse around the period and the smell may be exacerbated after unprotected sexual intercourse due to the alkalinity of semen. In more severe cases, there may be vulval soreness and itching.

*Investigations*

The diagnosis of bacterial vaginosis (BV) should be made by Gram staining a specimen taken from the lateral wall of the vagina. It is no longer recommended to culture for *Gardnerella vaginalis* as this organism is a normal commensal in the vagina of some asymptomatic women. Features consistent with BV include a reduction in numbers (or absence) of lactobacilli, the presence of mixed flora consistent with an increase in anaerobes and *Mobiliuncus* species and the presence of more than 20% 'clue cells'. Clue cells are vaginal epithelial cells with an adherent mixture of Gram negative and positive organisms (Fig. 6.1).

*Treatment*
• Metronidazole 400 mg two times a day for five days.
• 2% Clindamycin cream at night for seven nights.
• No indication to treat the male partner as this is not an STI.

**Figure 6.1** Gram-stained slide showing 'clue cell' in bacterial vaginosis. With acknowledgement to Professor Catherine Ison, Sexually Transmitted Bacteria Reference Laboratory, London.

### Candidiasis (thrush)

This is caused by a dimorphic fungus which exists in both yeast and mycelial forms. It thrives in sugar-rich environment and is commonly found in:

- pregnancy;
- diabetes mellitus;
- oral contraceptive or oestrogen therapy;
- following exposure to broad-spectrum antibiotics which kill off the competing commensal organisms.

*Symptoms*
- Vulval itching.
- Superficial dyspareunia.
- Vaginal discharge of various appearances, including thick 'cottage cheese' and watery 'milky' types.
- May be asymptomatic and found incidentally on speculum examination or cervical cytology.
- As this is not an STI, there is no need to treat the male partner.
- Men in contact with candidal proteins may develop a blotchy red rash on their glans penis.
- Diabetic men may develop extensive candidal balanitis, which may be the presenting feature of their diabetes.

*Treatment*
- It is important to treat intravaginally with a pessary or cream as well as topically on the vulva.
- A number of suitable imidazole agents exist, e.g. clotrimazole 500 mg pessary as a single dose with two weeks of topical 1% clotrimazole cream to the vulva twice daily for two weeks.
- Oral fluconazole 150 mg as a single dose or itraconazole 200 mg twice daily for one day may be used when topical therapy is not suitable.
- Male candidal-associated balanitis responds well to a combination of 1% hydrocortisone and an antifungal, e.g. Canestan HC or Daktacort, given twice a day for one to two weeks.

## Sexually transmitted diseases

### Trichomoniasis

This is an STI in which the male is transiently colonized from the reservoir in the female vagina. This occurs because the adhesion proteins of this protozoon organism are expressed preferentially in acid pH, typically found in the vagina whereas the male urethral pH is approximately 7.4. In addition, trichomonads are repeatedly washed out of the urethra when men micturate. The organism can colonize the male prostate, and the female equivalent (Skene's glands).

*Symptoms and signs*
The woman has an intensely irritating vaginal discharge with inflammation of the vulva, vagina and cervix. The cervical appearance may manifest as a 'strawberry cervix'. The vaginal discharge is greenish-yellow, frothy and offensive with a fish-like smell. Men typically have no symptoms but, when present, the symptoms include urethral discomfort, dysuria and occasional urethral discharge.

*Investigations*
Same day diagnosis may be made with the use of a saline wet-mount in which a drop of vaginal fluid from the posterior fornix is placed in a drop of saline on which a coverslip is floated. The trichomonads have a characteristic motility due to

their five flagella. Culture is more sensitive although the gold standard is DNA amplification, currently unavailable in many clinical settings. It is important to screen for other common STIs.

*Treatment and follow-up*
• This is an STI, so sexual partner(s) *must* be treated with antimicrobials.
• Metronidazole 2 g single dose or 400 mg twice a day for five days.
• Tinidazole 2 g single dose.
• Various complicated regimens exist for metronidazole resistant trichomoniasis and referral to an STI specialist is recommended.
• Partner notification (contact tracing) should be initiated at diagnosis.
• Patients should return for a test of cure when they have been off antibiotics for at least seven days.

## Chlamydial infection

*Chlamydia trachomatis* is the most common bacterial STI in the UK and the predominant organism responsible for pelvic inflammatory disease (PID) and ectopic pregnancy. It is a potent mediator of chronic inflammation and causes fine adhesions in the pelvis surrounding the tubes and ovaries. There may be adhesions between the liver capsule and diaphragm (Fitz-Hugh Curtis syndrome). There has been a recent increase in

*Chlamydia* cases in men and women in the UK (see Fig. 6.2).

*Symptoms and signs*
Many women are asymptomatic although male partners may complain of either dysuria or a urethral discharge, which is mucopurulent in nature, and may occasionally present with epididymoorchitis. If symptoms/signs are present in women, they may include any of the following: vaginal discharge, mucopurulent cervical discharge, cervicitis, deep dyspareunia, pelvic pain, cervical excitation and other symptoms of PID.

*Investigations*
• Chlamydia trachomatis is difficult to grow and requires a specialist laboratory.
• DNA amplification techniques, which have increased sensitivity over other diagnostic methods, are the diagnostic methods of choice (e.g. SDA, PCR, TMA).
• DNA amplification tests can be performed on non-invasive specimens such as urines or vulval swabs. These tests will detect both dead and live organisms but will not provide data on antimicrobial susceptibility.
• Enzyme linked immunoassay (ELISA) techniques are still used in many laboratories.
• Fluorescent-labelled monoclonal antibodies can be used to detect chlamydial organisms on an endocervical smear.

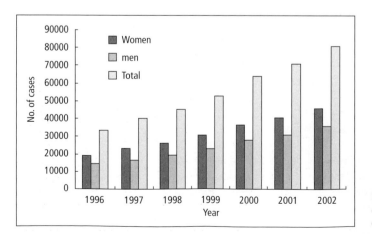

**Figure 6.2** Uncomplicated chlamydial infection in England and Wales (1996–2002). (Source, PHLS.)

• It is important to screen for other common STIs.

*Treatment and follow-up*
• This is an STI, so sexual partner(s) *must* be treated.
• Azithromycin 1 g single dose.
• Doxycycline 100 mg twice a day for 10 days.
• Tests of cure are not necessary with the above regimens although are recommended with erythromycin-containing regimens.
• Longer regimens are used to treat PID and epididymo-orchitis.
• Partner notification (contact tracing) should be initiated at diagnosis.

## Gonorrhoea

The STI is caused by *Neisseria gonorrhoeae*, a Gram negative diplococcus which is often found within neutrophils in genital specimens. There has been a recent increase in gonorrhoea cases in men and women in the UK (see Fig. 6.3).

*Symptoms and signs*
Primary sites of infection in women include the endocervix, urethra, oropharynx, anorectum and Bartholin's gland. In men, the urethra, oropharynx and anorectum are the sites of primary infection. Usually there are no symptoms of infection in women, although they may present with vaginal

discharge, dysuria, lower abdominal pain, deep dyspareunia or signs of ascending infection suggestive of PID. Men with urethral gonorrhoea usually have evidence of a dysuria and a purulent urethral discharge. Sore throat or anorectal discharge may occur with oropharyngeal or anorectal infection, although these infections are usually asymptomatic.

*Investigations*
• GUM clinics can provide same day diagnosis of gonorrhoea by Gram-staining endocervical and urethral smears (sensitivity 25–40%).
• The best site to sample for gonorrhoea is the endocervical canal which will be culture positive in 90% of genital cases.
• There will be an increased diagnostic yield if the urethra and anal canal are also cultured. About 2% of female genital gonorrhoea is only detected if the anal canal is sampled in addition to the urethra and endocervix; it is thought that most cases of anorectal colonization result from self-inoculation of this anatomical area via spread of vaginal discharge rather than through unprotected anal intercourse.
• The organism is extremely fastidious and so the swabs should be either spread directly onto appropriate culture medium (as happens in some GUM clinics) or be sent to the laboratory as soon as possible. Stuart's transport medium may increase the yield if a delay is envisaged in the transport process.

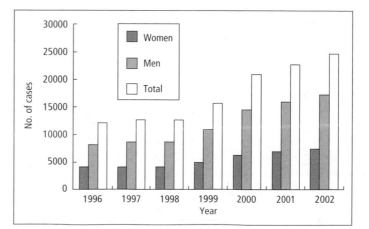

**Figure 6.3** Uncomplicated gonorrhoea in England and Wales (1996–2002). (Source, PHLS.)

• Once isolated, the gonococci can be screened for antimicrobial susceptibility.
• DNA amplification tests are now available for the diagnosis of gonorrhoea using non-invasive specimens such as urine or vulval swabs. These tests will detect both dead and live organisms but will not provide data on antimicrobial susceptibility.
• It is important to screen for other common STIs.

*Treatment and follow-up*
• Amoxycillin 2 g oral and Probenecid 1 g oral, both as a single dose.
• Ciprofloxacin 500 mg oral single dose.
• Ceftriaxone 250 mg i.m. single dose.
• Cefotaxime 500 mg i.m. single dose.
Longer courses are recommended for the treatment of upper genital tract complications.
• Penicillin resistance may be chromosomally-mediated or plasmid mediated through the production of beta-lactamase (penicillinase).
• High-level ciprofloxacin resistance is increasing worldwide.
• No documented resistance to third generation cephalosporins has yet been reported.
• Partner notification (contact tracing) should be initiated at diagnosis.
• Patients should return for a test of cure when they have been off antibiotics for at least three days.

## Herpes simplex infection

Genital herpes is caused by herpes simplex virus (HSV) types 1 and 2 which enter the host through mucocutaneous surfaces. The viruses are able to establish latency and subsequent reactivation may give rise to repeated episodes of the disease. Factors involved in reactivation include local trauma, menstruation, HSV 2 viral type and stress.

*Symptoms and signs*
The first attack is often characterized by extensive genital ulceration together with local regional lymphadenopathy and systemic symptoms. The ulceration may last up to three weeks if untreated and first attacks are more severe in vulval and perianal locations in comparison with penile infection. The

lesions present as vesicles which burst to leave a superficial tender ulcer with an erythematous halo and a greyish-white exudate. Complications include dissemination to distant sites (e.g. finger, thighs), meningitis, sacral radiculomyelopathy and urinary difficulties or retention. Recurrent infections are shorter and less severe than primary infections. Prodromal neuralgia-type pain radiating down the thigh or buttocks is common.

*Investigations*
• Culture of HSV using a swab of vesicular fluid (best) or ulcer base which is sent to the laboratory in viral transport medium.
• Amplification of HSV target DNA by the polymerase chain reaction (PCR).
• Serology is not helpful in individual diagnosis but may have a role in the management of partners of patients with known HSV type 2 recurrent genital lesions.

*Treatment and partner notification*
• Primary episodes should be treated with aciclovir 200 mg five times a day for five days (double dose in HIV positive patients).
• Recurrent episodes generally do not need treating.
• If more than six recurrent episodes occur per year, consider maintenance therapy with aciclovir 400 mg twice a day for 6 month minimum.
• The value of partner notification (contact tracing) for first attack HSV episodes is debated as these may occur after many years since infection.

## Genital warts

Genital warts, also known as condylomata acuminata, are caused by various genotypes of the human papillomaviruses (HPV). Some HPV types (e.g. 16 and 18) are associated with oncogenicity or intraepithelial neoplasia.

*Symptoms and signs*
In females, genital warts typically occur on the vulva at the vaginal introitus, posterior fourchette, on the labia, around the clitoris and in the perineal and perianal regions. In men, warts occur at the

frenulum, around the coronal sulcus, on the inner aspect of the prepuce, on the penile shaft, within the meatus and at the perianal margin. Proctoscopy may reveal internal warts as far as the squamocolumnar junction between the anus and the rectum. The lesions feel hard to the touch and are often raised with an irregular surface. The application of 5% acetic acid may help in the diagnosis of uncertain lesions but the technique is non-specific and not suitable for widespread use.

*Investigations*
- The diagnosis is a clinical one.
- It is important to screen for other common STIs.

*Treatment*
- Self-application of podophyllotoxin may be undertaken in which the reagent is applied to the warts twice a day for three days followed by a four day rest. This cycle may be repeated three more times before the patient is reviewed by a clinician.
- Cryotherapy.
- Imiquimod topical therapy three nights per week for four weeks, followed by clinical review.
- Trichloroacetic acid (caustic agent to be handled with care).
- Electrocautery.
- Surgery (curettage, scissor excision).

*General advice*
- Warts may recur within the first year after therapy in up to one-third of cases.
- Condoms should be used with new sexual partners.
- Long-term partners are likely to be already infected with the same HPV genotypes as the patient, so instructions on condom use may not be helpful in this situation.
- Partner notification (contact tracing) should be initiated at diagnosis.
- It is important to ensure that cervical smears are being undertaken in line with the recommendations for national screening programmes (see Chapter 19).

## Syphilis

This disease, caused by *Treponema pallidum*, was a major cause of morbidity and mortality in the pre-antibiotic era. It remains an important disease in resource-poor settings and has recently re-emerged as an important STI in gay men, many of whom are HIV positive. There continue to be outbreaks of syphilis among women in the USA and, more recently, this has occurred in the UK. There exist epidemiological links to crack cocaine use, social deprivation and ethnic minorities in these cases.

*Symptoms and signs*
Syphilis can present in the primary stage (9–90 days), secondary stage (six weeks to six months) or tertiary stage which include gummatous lesions, neurosyphilis and cardiovascular syphilis (10–40 years). Alternatively, latent syphilis may be detected in patients during opportunistic serological screening at GUM or antenatal clinics. Patients are only infectious during the first two years of the infection, i.e. primary, secondary or early latent stages, which will be the focus of this chapter. Congenital syphilis may occur in infants born to those women who are infected and book late for their antenatal care, or in whom infection is acquired after their initial booking blood tests are performed. The outcome for the fetus varies depending on the gestational stage at which infection is acquired.

The primary stage is manifest by a typically painless ulcer at the site of inoculation, often associated with regional lymphadenitis. Characteristically the ulcer is indurated with a serous exudate, although ulcers in women tend to have more subtle clinical appearances. In women, the ulcer is usually on the vulva but may be intravaginal, on the cervix or in the perineal or perianal regions. In men, the ulcer may be in the coronal sulcus, on the penile shaft or on the glans penis. Gay and bisexual men may present with primary lesions at the anal margin, or on the tonsils, lips or nipples.

Secondary syphilis manifests with a widespread maculopapular rash, which may affect the palms and soles, as well as with generalized lymphadenopathy, mouth ulcers, condylomata lata in moist areas and alopecia.

*Investigations*
In centres equipped with a dark ground micro-

scope, examination may be made of lesional material placed in a drop of saline under a floating coverslip. Suitable material includes ulcer exudate, samples from open skin lesions and condylomata lata, as well as sterile aspiration of lymph nodes. Pathogenic *Treponema* species have a characteristic appearance and motility.

Serology remains the mainstay of diagnosis but is unable to distinguish between the different pathogenic treponemes, which include *Treponema pertenue* (yaws) and *Treponema carateum* (pinta). In the primary stage, treponemal serology is generally positive in 70–80% of occasions but should be positive in 100% of cases in the secondary phase. It is important to re-test serology at three months in patients with genital ulceration to ensure that syphilis is excluded. Most laboratories now screen with a treponemal-specific ELISA method detecting IgG, and confirm this with the *Treponema pallidum* particle agglutination test (TPPA). Alternative treponemal tests include the fluorescent treponemal antibody test (FTA). Activity of the disease is measured with non-treponemal tests, which detect anticardiolipin antibodies, such as the rapid particle reaginic test (RPR) or the Venereal Diseases Research Laboratory test (VDRL). Measurement of activity is useful as it provides a marker to monitor therapeutic response as evidenced by a fall in RPR/VDRL titre. Once infected with syphilis, the specific treponemal tests generally remain positive, so the only way to detect a subsequent re-infection is by testing with the RPR or VDRL.

It is important to screen for other common STIs.

*Treatment and follow-up for early syphilis (>2 years duration)*
• Benzathine penicillin 2.4 Megaunits i.m. as a single dose.
• Doxycycline 200 mg twice a day for two weeks.
• Penicillin allergic pregnant women should be treated with erythromycin 500 mg four times a day for 2 weeks. Due to lower efficacy and poor placental transfer of this drug, it is recommended that babies are retreated at birth with benzylpenicillin and the mother retreated with doxycycline after breast-feeding has ceased.

• Warn patients about the Jarisch–Herxheimer reaction which may need cover with paracetamol and bed rest for 24 hours.
• Partner notification (contact tracing) should be initiated at diagnosis.
• RPR/VDRL serial measurements should be performed at one, three, six and 12 months post-treatment.

## Human immunodeficiency virus infection (HIV)

HIV is a human retrovirus that causes the acquired immunodeficiency syndrome (AIDS). Through the action of reverse transcriptase, the RNA virus is able to make a double stranded DNA copy of its genetic material that can be inserted into human DNA and establish latent infection. The virus is reproduced whenever the infected cell multiplies. The virus uses the CD4 receptor and a number of co-receptors (CCR5, CXCR4) to enter susceptible cells which can include lymphocytes, macrophages and microglial cells. Infection can lead to:
• asymptomatic infection;
• symptomatic HIV infection;
• AIDS.
The presence of antibodies is used in diagnosis of the disease but they are not protective. Presently, there is no effective vaccine against the virus.

Transmission occurs through infected body fluids being in contact with the body fluids of the recipient in the presence of a break in the integrity of the exposed mucosal surface (Fig. 6.4). Another

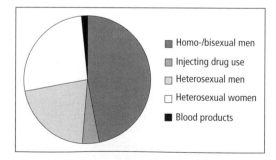

**Figure 6.4** Estimate of prevalent HIV infections among adults in the UK at the end of 2001 adjusted for underreporting and failure to access services. (Source, PHLS.)

major route of infection is blood-borne, either through sharing needles for IV drug use or through transfusion of whole blood and concentrated blood products. Blood products are currently tested for HIV antibodies and so new infections rarely occur through this route now. At the start of the HIV epidemic in the developed countries, most cases of HIV were detected in gay/bisexual men, haemophiliacs and drug addicts. At the current time in the UK, the greatest increases in newly diagnosed cases are occurring in heterosexual men and women, the majority of whom are thought to have acquired their infection overseas.

The fetus can be infected *in utero* from the mother, although it is thought that the majority of transmission occurs at birth and through breast-feeding. The current policy in the UK of prescribing antiretrovirals in the second and third trimester, performing Caesarian section and avoiding breast-feeding has dramatically reduced the risk of mother-to-child HIV transmission (Fig. 6.5). Essential to the success of this policy is encouragement for all pregnant women to undergo HIV testing at antenatal booking. It should be pointed out that, in resource poor countries, a balance has to be made between the risk of preventing HIV transmission through stopping breast-feeding and the risk of gastroenteritis through imperfect bottle feeding.

*Symptoms and signs*
• Seroconversion illness is rarely seen in practice but presents with a glandular fever-type illness which may be associated with a rash. Neurological manifestations such as Guillain-Barre syndrome and encephalitis have been described.
• Asymptomatic infections by definition are only detected by screening.
• Symptomatic HIV infection may present with non-specific weight loss, fatigue, lymphadenopathy, diarrhoea and night sweats. Clues may come from recurrent vulvo-vaginal or oral candidiasis, recurrent and extensive genital warts, shingles, worsening eczema and psoriasis, or oral hairy leukoplakia on the tongue.
• AIDS is determined by the onset of certain opportunistic infections or AIDS-related malignancies. Examples include tuberculosis, *Pneumocystis carinii* pneumonia, cryptococcal infection, cryptosporidiosis, Kaposi's sarcoma and lymphoma.

*Investigations*
• Detection of anti-HIV antibodies in the serum by ELISA.
• Confirmation is obtained using different ELISAs (usually 2 more).
• Western blots can be performed to investigate discrepant results in reference centres.
• Plasma viral load gives an estimation of the amount of HIV virus replication.
• The immune status of the patient is measured by sequential CD4 counts.
• It is important to screen for other common STIs.

*When to treat HIV infection?*
• The best time to start treatment may vary

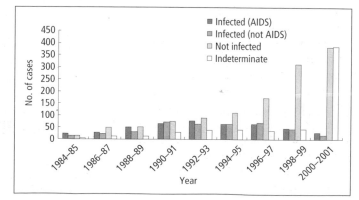

**Figure 6.5** Children born to HIV infected mothers (1984–2001). Indeterminate category includes infants under 18 months when last tested for HIV antibody and without evidence of HIV infection (includes 95 children lost to follow up). (Source, PHLS.)

between countries and has varied over time within countries.

- In the UK, treatment is recommended for all patients with a CD4 count of less than $200 \times 10^6/l$, regardless of the presence or absence of symptoms.
- In the UK, treatment should be considered in patients with a CD4 count between $200–350 \times 10^6/l$ if they are significantly symptomatic due to HIV infection or their CD4 count is falling rapidly.
- In the UK, although not clearly of benefit on clinical grounds, some patients undergoing HIV seroconversion may elect to go on short course (one year) of HIV therapy in an attempt to preserve immunological memory.

*HIV treatment options*

- There now exist many drugs with which to treat HIV infection.
- It is now accepted that patients should take three active HIV drugs as highly active antiretroviral therapy (HAART).
- In patients on salvage therapy, more than three drugs with diminished activity may be used (mega-HAART).
- Adherence is crucial to the success of therapy and resistance rapidly ensues if patients do not adhere meticulously to their regimens.
- Monitoring of HIV RNA viral load shows whether the HAART is working and patients should remain undetectable (<50 copies/ml) on their regimens if adherent until resistance ensues.
- Antiretroviral resistance can be readily measured using genotypic assays but must be done whilst patients are on the drugs in question.
- Most patients have wild-type virus archived in sanctuary sites and this virus will replicate and replace resistance virus once drug pressure is removed as resistant virus strains tend to be less fit.
- Classes of drugs include nucleoside analogues (NRTIs), nucleotide analogues (NtRTIs), non-nucleoside analogues (NNRTIs), protease inhibitors (PIs) and fusion inhibitors.
- NRTIs include AZT, 3TC, ddI, d4T, ddC, abacavir.
- NtRTIs include tenofovir.
- PIs include nelfinavir, saquinavir, lopinavir, ritonavir, indinavir, amprenavir, atazanavir.

- T20 is the first of a new class of fusion inhibitors which needs to be given by subcutaneous injection (salvage therapy at present).
- Regimens are chosen on the basis of side-effect profile, patient's daily schedule, pill and dosage burden, previous HIV drug therapy, CD4 count and presence of AIDS-defining illnesses.
- Some HIV drugs are available in combination tablets to help with adherence, e.g. Combivir (AZT + 3TC).
- Some PIs require boosting with low dose ritonavir to achieve sufficient drug levels in body fluids, e.g. lopinavir and saquinavir.
- There have been trials assessing the efficacy of interleukin-2 (IL-2) therapy as an immunotherapeutic agent but the results have not been promising.

*HIV prevention and partner notification*

- Partner notification (contact tracing) should be initiated at diagnosis.
- The importance of using condoms for sexual intercourse must be explained to all HIV seropositive patients in order to prevent new infections.
- The patient should avoid acquiring drug resistant HIV virus from other sexual partners as this will limit the success of future therapeutic drug interventions.
- IV drug users should be provided with sterile needles through needle exchange programmes.
- Blood and blood products as well as organ donations need to be screened for HIV prior to use.
- Health care workers should take precautions to ensure they do not become infected through sharps injuries or contact with potentially infectious body fluids of patients.
- Surgical instruments should be autoclaved satisfactorily and inspected for possible contamination before use in theatres.
- There is no effective HIV vaccine available at the present time although several trials are ongoing with potential vaccine candidates.

## Sexual problems

Many students do not like considering patients' sexual problems, for they feel they have hardly sorted out their own sexual lives and are therefore ill-equipped to help others. A more open discussion of this subject helps the student to be at ease when discussing sexuality later with patients. It helps the students to become more aware of their attitudes and how these may influence the future doctor/patient relationship.

Patients often consult their doctors about sexual problems and expect them to have the knowledge and skills to help them. It is necessary for a doctor to know the interrelation of sexually related matters and their treatments to general diseases such as heart disease and hypertension.

The facts of human sexuality have not always been known but, by proper analysis, assessment and randomized controlled trials of various therapies, more is becoming comprehensible.

## History and examination

As with the rest of medicine, a systematic approach to sexual problems can help make a diagnosis. A full general and gynaecological history should be taken including details of past gynaecological events, the type of contraception used and obstetric history.

The sexual problem should be discussed allowing the woman or man to use their own phrases, preferably in their own time. If they wander, pointed questions drawn from the following material may be needed to bring them back to the point.

### Questions

- Duration and frequency of intercourse.
- Factors making the problem better.
- Factors making the problem worse.
- Problem happens with other partners.
- Other associated factors such as alcohol, work or drugs.
- Other life events at the time of onset.
- The relationship of the partners.
- History of previous sex knowledge.
- Family background to sex education in childhood.
- Past sexual relationships.
- Possible child abuse.

- Present sexual history.
- Details of usual sex activities, e.g. position and foreplay.
- Sexual fantasies.

Examination is usually unrewarding.
- In the male—obvious abnormalities of the penis and testes should be excluded.
- In the female—the ease of allowing a pelvic examination may be helpful in assessing the degree of the problem. Any structural abnormalities of the vulva, vagina, cervix or uterus should be excluded. The examination can be used positively as an opportunity to educate about genital anatomy. The use of a mirror to help a woman identify her clitoris can be helpful.

It is important to detect general physical abnormalities which might make intercourse difficult or painful before exploring the possibility of psychosexual problems. The patient's comfort or discomfort with their own body and specifically genitalia can give useful information.

## The male

Although this is not strictly a part of gynaecology, anyone dealing with sexual problems must have a knowledge of the male partner and his problems.

### Failure to ejaculate

The inability to produce semen is not always associated with the sex drive itself or the ability to have an erection.

*Causes*
- Sympathectomy.
- Psychosexual features:
  (a) past humiliating sexual rejection;
  (b) fear of a pregnancy in partner;
  (c) past maternal domination;
  (d) repressive sexual teaching as a child;
  (e) doubts about sexual orientation.

*Treatment*
Sympathectomy aspects can be treated with drugs.
- Thioridazine or
- Indoramin.

The psychological aspects may require long-term psychotherapy, because many cases are due to the man avoiding depositing semen in his partner's vagina; this produces further anxieties.

Lesser degrees can be dealt with by sympathetic handling by the woman and extravaginal sexual techniques. The encouragement of the use of erotic material can help if there is loss of control at the point of ejaculation.

## Premature ejaculation

Ejaculation occurs with minimal stimulation or before or shortly after penetration and before either party wishes it.

Ejaculation is under sympathetic control mediated by adrenoreceptors. It probably means that the mediated system enhances this whilst the serotonin balance is inhibitory. These equilibria may be over-ridden by behavioural patterns.

*Causes*
Behavioural patterns are associated with:
• inexperience;
• adolescent conditioning to rapid response;
• rejection by other women.

*Treatment*
Men can be treated individually or with their partners. Sympathetic handling by the woman is important. Male confidence must be generated as he learns to recognize the point of ejaculatory inevitability and to control stimulation to delay ejaculation until the time of his choosing. A squeeze technique applied by the woman to the penis at the moment before ejaculatory inevitability can produce delay in ejaculation.

If a programme is embarked on over the course of weeks or months, this produces good results.

Drugs are occasionally helpful if there is poor response to the psychological approach:
• Clomipramine or
• 5-hydroxytryptamine (5HT) reuptake inhibitors may be helpful.

## Erectile dysfunction

Impotence in the male may be primary or secondary. The former is nearly always psychological due to problems in the family background/upbringing while secondary impotence may be physical or psychological.

*Causes*

STRUCTURAL
• After major pelvic operations.
• Pudendal vein thrombosis.
• Hypospadias.
• Peyronie's disease (fibrosis of the dorsum of the penis).

ENDOCRINE DISEASE
• Diabetes.
• Hypogonadism.
• Hypothyroidism.
• Pituitary tumour.
• Cushing's syndrome.

MEDICAL PROBLEMS
• Peripheral vascular disease.
• Hypertension.
• Cerebral vascular accident.
• Multiple sclerosis.
• Spinal cord injury.
• Increasing age.

DRUGS
• Alcohol.
• Antihypertensives.
• Antidepressants.
• Antipsychotics.
• Hormones.

PSYCHOLOGICAL FEATURES
• Stress.
• Performance pressure.
• Parental influence.
• Ignorance of sexual matters.
• Poor self image.
• Guilt.
• Anger.
• Relationship problems.

It is important to differentiate the psychogenic from the organic causes. The former are associated with:
- rapid onset;
- a recent depression;
- life or family stress;
- normal erections:
  - (a) on waking;
  - (b) masturbation;
  - (c) in response to erotic material;
  - (d) with a different partner.

*Treatment*
Psychological treatment starts with reassurance and education leading on to non-demand, touching exercises based on Masters and Johnson's sensate focus programme.

Erection can be produced by pharmacological means.
- Papaverine injected into the corpus cavernosum works by smooth muscle relaxation.
- Other injectable drugs are phentolamine and prostaglandin $E_1$. These work particularly for men with spinal cord injuries.
- To avoid the problems of injection of the penis, intraurethral prostaglandins or oral Viagra are both being tried in several countries. Preliminary results would seem favourable to producing an erection without serious side-effects.
- Some anti-hypertensives may be changed for others which have less effect on the erectile function.

## The female

## Superficial dyspareunia

Vaginal pain during intercourse may be due to a variety of causes. Physical causes of superficial dyspareunia include:
- infection of the vulva or vagina;
- dermatological disease of the vulva or vagina;
- postmenopausal atrophy;
- painful perineal scar from episiotomy;
- an undilated hymen—this is very rare and mostly related to women who maintain virginity into the late 30s.

*Treatment*
Dealt with according to the cause. Surgical reconstruction may be required for badly healed episiotomy or a rigid undilated hymen.

## Deep dyspareunia

This is felt higher up in the vagina and in the pelvis. It often lasts for some hours after intercourse and can be reproduced at vaginal examination by pressing over relevant parts of the female pelvis.

*Causes*
- Chronic pelvic infection.
- Endometriosis.
- Pelvic tumours.
- Fixed uterine retroversion trapping ovaries behind, e.g. in endometriosis.
- Pelvic congestion.
- Bladder or bowel pathology.
- Failure of arousal response. Superficially this is due to failure of lubrication and deeply due to failure of vaginal ballooning during coitus.

*Treatment*
That of the basic cause; results depend on the responsiveness to the treatment of physical problems.

Results where no pathology is demonstrated are variable. In these women, dyspareunia may be due to intra- or interpersonal conflicts. The use of lubricants and delay of penetration until the woman is fully aroused can be helpful.

## Vaginismus

Spasm of the superficial and deep pelvic muscles prevents the introduction of the penis and is apparent at a pelvic examination.

*Causes*
There may be an organic cause but usually it is a psychological result of apprehension and fear. Previous attempts at forced entry may lead to this.

*Treatment*

A sympathetic approach to examination can help, but no force should be used. Attempts should stop before pain is caused and the woman should feel in control at all times.

Occasionally examination under anaesthesia may be required to exclude structural causes and thus be able to reassure the woman that she is anatomically normal. Usually this is not necessary as she is likely to respond to gradual desensitization techniques. To this end, the use of graduated vaginal trainers is often helpful. Fingers or tampons are sometimes preferred. Referral to a trained sex therapist may be needed.

## Anorgasmia

This is not uncommon in the female. It is nearly always psychological, but in a small percentage it is physical.

*Causes*

A failure to:

- receive stimulation—psychological in origin;
- respond to stimulation—due to family upbringing/background;
- performance pressure from partner or self;
- doubts about sexual orientation.
  Other causes:
- fear of pregnancy;
- dyspareunia;
- debilitating disease;
- chronic constipation.

*Treatment*

Mechanical and organic causes are treated appropriately. Psychological causes require the attention of a sex therapist who would discuss the problem fully with the individual or the couple.

Too easily the woman is labelled as frigid and then accepts this as a part of life. Fifty per cent of women are not orgasmic during penetrative sex, but are orgasmic with clitoral stimulation. Understanding this can help remove pressure from both partners to achieve coital orgasm on every occasion.

Treatment usually involves helping the woman

to achieve orgasm through masturbation and learning to lose control. The use of erotic material or a vibrator can help. Progress to coital orgasm is then made. Use of vibrators may also help with coital orgasmic problems.

## Rape

Rape is unlawful sexual intercourse with a woman against her will; only the slightest penetration of the vulva by the penis is required. Issues of whether the hymen is intact or if semen has been deposited in the vagina are irrelevant.

Rape is unfortunately all too common and the woman may report it to the police, sometimes a day or so later. A doctor may then be called to examine the victim of alleged rape. The practitioner should ensure that he or she has the authority and consent for the examination and has the equipment for taking the appropriate specimens properly.

A history of what happened is taken and careful notes made. Examination is made of the general demeanour of the woman and of her clothing. Bruises and scratches around the lower abdomen, thighs and vulva should be noted, preferably in a diagrammatic form. The vulva should be examined in detail for bruising or tears.

If any suspicion of semen in the vagina is found, a careful specimen should be taken, placed in appropriate containers and labelled fully in the presence of a woman police constable (WPC) and the complainant. This should then be handed to the WPC for transport to forensic laboratories and a receipt should be received or the chain of evidence may be questioned in any subsequent legal enquiry.

Other swabs and blood may be taken to exclude sexually transmitted diseases. While these often have no legal standing, they may be important in the medical management of the woman's future.

Many police forces have a rape investigation team who are able to satisfy both the law and the psychological needs of the woman who is in this situation. A knowledge of the procedures involved is helpful to all practitioners.

## Criminal abortion

One of the results of the laws about therapeutic termination of pregnancy in England, Wales and Scotland has been the massive reduction in criminal abortions. Not a single death has been reported in the 20 years covered by the Confidential Enquiries into Maternal Deaths (1982–2001). This is a very satisfactory situation in the UK but criminal abortion still goes on throughout the world. It is estimated that of the half a million women who die every year of maternity causes, about a quarter of these do so from incompetently performed illegal abortions.

If a doctor is asked to examine a woman who may have undergone a criminal abortion, he or she first must obtain her consent if she is conscious.

### History
This should be taken but may be only partly truthful.

### Examination
The woman may be pyrexial with dull pain in the lower abdomen. Pelvic examination may show the cervix to be soft and the os dilated. Blood or pregnancy tissue may be passing through it. There may be signs of the bite of a volsellum (toothed forceps) on the anterior lip of the cervix. She may have an offensive discharge coming through the cervix. Damage to the genital tract may occur, e.g. the posterior fornix is commonly perforated by incompetent abortionists who force their instruments into the cul-de-sac of the vagina and penetrate it, breaching the peritoneal cavity.

### Treatment
The woman should be admitted to hospital. Antibiotics should be given urgently, a broad spectrum used at first until the results of high vaginal swabs are known. Consider the diagnosis of gas gangrene and if relevant give antigas gangrene serum. If the woman is still bleeding from the uterus, a curettage may remove septic products from the cavity and hasten healing. If the bleeding still persists or is very heavy, hysterectomy may be required for infection may have entered the substance of the uterus. Check the haemoglobin level; a blood transfusion may be required for toxic anaemia. Watch for anuria which commonly follows gross toxic infection.

Whilst confidentiality to the patient is the first concern of the doctor, if the woman becomes seriously ill or approaches death, legal authorities may be involved. Take advice about this from the legal department of the hospital or the doctor's defence society. Keep careful notes. Be prepared to take, or act as witness to a dying declaration.

**Self-assessment**

**6.1** Which of the following statements are true of sexually transmitted infections (STIs)?
  (a) Gonorrhoea in women is best diagnosed by cultures of material from the posterior vaginal fornix.
  (b) Syphilis is adequately treated in penicillin-allergic pregnant women by erythromycin.
  (c) Contact tracing partners of women with first attack genital herpes is helpful.
  (d) Bacterial vaginosis should be diagnosed by culture of a high vaginal swab (HVS) for *Gardnerella vaginalis*.
  (e) *Chlamydia trachomatis* is routinely diagnosed by culture of endocervical swabs.

**6.2** Which of the following statements are true about HIV infection?
  (a) It is caused by a DNA virus that binds to the CD4 receptor.
  (b) Seroconversion commonly presents with a glandular fever illness.
  (c) In the UK, all patients with a CD4 count below $200 \times 10^6$/l should be encouraged to start anti-HIV drugs.
  (d) Antiretroviral resistance testing will show resistance patterns to both current and previous anti-HIV drugs.
  (e) Tenofovir is a new nucleotide reverse transcription inhibitor.

**6.3** Ask a friend to role-play a patient and practise taking a sexual history using the following role-play. The instructions for the candidate are that you should take the history from the role-player in eight minutes. At the end, the candidate may be expected to give a four-minute summary of the case and outline appropriate investigations for this lady. The role-player needs to make up a name for herself and fill in some personal details. The scoring system will award marks for communication skills, history-taking and appropriate investigations (maximum 12 marks).

  **Role-player's instructions:** You are a 35-year-old married woman with two healthy children, aged five and seven. You have come to the doctor because of vulval itching. You last had sexual intercourse (unprotected, only divulge if asked) with your husband three nights ago and have been together for over 10 years. Recently, your husband went to Thailand on a business trip. Two weeks previously, whilst he was away, you had sex with a male friend and the condom broke (only divulge this if asked). Your last smear test was normal one year ago and you have never had an STI before. You are very worried.

**6.4** Which of the following statements are true?
  (a) Female vulvovaginal candidiasis has an offensive smell and presents with vulval itching.
  (b) Condylomata lata do not respond well to podophyllotoxin.
  (c) Women who have been raped once have a higher chance than average women of being raped again.
  (d) The forensic examination and STI screening are best done at the same time by the same doctor.
  (e) Trichomoniasis is best detected by culture of *Trichomonas vaginalis*.

**6.5** Which of the following are true?
  (a) Examination of patients with psychosexual problems is rarely rewarding.
  (b) Ejaculation is under parasympathetic control.
  (c) Psychosexual problems are best managed by seeing both partners together.
  (d) Vaginismus only occurs with penile entry into the vagina.
  (e) Anorgasmia is more common in men than women.

# Part 3

# The reproductive years

# Chapter 7

# The mother and fetus in pregnancy

For most women, childbearing is a major event in their lives. The basic changes of pregnancy are covered in this chapter; the rest of pregnancy and childbirth are discussed in Chapters 8–14 and a short chapter, Chapter 15, covers those aspects the obstetrician should know about the newborn child.

## Maternal changes in pregnancy

During pregnancy, oestrogen increases vascularity and progesterone permits muscular relaxation and softening of the connective tissue sheath of the vagina by an increase in fluid. Over 38 weeks the tube becomes much more stretchable so that, by full term, the vagina and vulva permit the passage of an infant with a head diameter of approximately 10 cm. The perineum with the squamous epithelium in the region of the fourchette does not always stretch so readily and so may tear on occasions.

Pregnancy causes alterations not just in the mother's pelvis and abdomen but the whole body. Adaptations in the function of various systems occur to minimize the stresses imposed and are interlinked smoothly so the function of the whole organism does not deteriorate.

## Uterus

By term, a litre of blood can be in the uterine vasculature. Branches increase in size, number and diameter from each side of the uterus. The placental site gets preferential blood supply. Penetrating branches pass through the myometrium, under the surface of the decidua. They become spiral arteries and penetrate the decidua. In early pregnancy their exits into the placental bed pool are narrow, but trophoblast invasion by 16 weeks normally widens them into deltas so reducing resistance and improving flow. If invasion is incomplete, flow is restricted so that:
• in late pregnancy, the fetus gets fewer nutrients for growth;
• in labour, the fetus gets less $O_2$ and so fetal distress follows more readily.

The uterus grows through hypertrophy of the myometrial cells rather than by an increase in numbers of myometrial cells. From 28 weeks the lower third of the uterus thins and becomes less vascular forming the lower segment of the uterus (hence lower segment Caesarean section).

## Metabolism

Increased to provide for:
• Growth of fetus and placenta.
• Increased growth of the uterus.
• Increased growth of support systems.
• Preparation for lactation.

*Weight increase* (Table 7.1)

Usually 10–14 kg (22–30 lb) in whole pregnancy. For example:

0–14 weeks: 2 kg (4.5 lb)—may be a loss because of vomiting;

13–28 weeks: 5 kg (11 lb);

28–40 weeks: 5 kg (11 lb)—may be a loss in last 2–3 weeks because of diminution of amniotic fluid.

The rest is extracellular fluid, fat and protein storage—6 kg.

A sharp increase in the mother's weight gain in late pregnancy may indicate increased water retention, a facet of pre-eclampsia. Weight loss, if persistent, may reflect poor fetal progress although there is little precision in this and many obstetricians do not use weight as a measure of well-being.

*Protein*

The fetus needs little protein in early pregnancy so the woman is in negative balance.

Two-thirds of the fetal protein is acquired in the last 12 weeks (a half in last 4 weeks). Also maternal uterus and breasts use much protein in growing tissues and storage occurs for lactation. Approximately 12 g of nitrogen a day are needed for the development of these and the fetus.

*Carbohydrate*

Pregnancy is diabetogenic and calorie need is slightly increased.

*Fat*

The fetus accumulates fat late, from 2% of the fetal body weight at 32 weeks to 12% at term. Fetal neolipogenesis accounts for most of the baby's fat

**Table 7.1** Breakdown of approximate weight increase during pregnancy.

| Fetus | 3.5 kg | 7 lb |
|---|---|---|
| Placenta | 0.5 | 1 |
| Amniotic fluid | 1.5 | 2 |
| Uterus | 1.0 | 2 |
| Blood increase | 1.5 | 3 |
| Breasts | 1.0 | 2 |
| Total | 9.0 kg | 17 lb |

with low transfer rate of precursors across the placenta. The mother has a higher circulating lipid and lipoprotein level.

*Calcium*

The fetus utilizes calcium late, taking from the long bones of the mother. If the stores are insufficient the fetus still utilizes calcium leading to maternal osteomalacia. Maternal serum calcium levels stay steady.

*Iron*

Iron is mostly passed to the fetus in the last weeks of pregnancy. It is stored in the liver. The mother may have poor iron stores because of:

• too little in diet, therefore give supplements;

• too poor absorption.

## Cardiovascular system

*Load*

Pregnancy is an increased load so more work is required by the heart.

• Growing fetal tissues which have high $O_2$ consumption rates.

• Hypertrophied uterus and breasts require more $O_2$.

• Increased muscular effort by mother to cope with weight gain of 10–14 kg (22–30 lb).

• In last weeks of pregnancy, the placental bed may act like an arteriovenous fistula. More work is required to overcome this shunt.

*Cardiac output*

Increased needs are met by increasing cardiac output.

Cardiac output = stroke volume × pulse rate.

In pregnancy, pulse rate is raised but most increase in output comes from larger stroke volume with enlarged heart chambers and muscle hypertrophy.

Output increases rapidly in the first trimester by up to 40% and steadies for the rest of pregnancy (Fig. 7.1).

During labour, cardiac output can increase by a further 2 l/min in association with uterine contractions.

**Figure 7.1** Cardiac output in pregnancy in normal women. The lines on the graph represent the mean ± 2 SD of the mean.

Systolic and diastolic pressure is much lower in early and mid-pregnancy, rising in the last trimester. Peripheral resistance is decreased and, since cardiac output is raised, pulse pressure is increased.

*Blood volume*
Return of blood to the heart is maintained by an increased blood volume. Plasma volume increases more than red cells so that relative haemodilution occurs. This used to be called physiological anaemia, but this is a bad term, for no pathological process can be physiological.

*Heart changes*
Pregnancy is a hyperkinetic state. The heart is:
• Enlarged.
• Pushed up.
• Unfolded upon aorta.
These changes produce electrocardiogram (ECG) and X-ray changes which are normal for pregnancy, but may appear pathological if interpreted without knowledge of pregnancy.

There are also sometimes extra murmurs, normal hypervolaemic sounds such as the systolic ejection murmur and that over the internal mammary arteries supplying the breasts.

## Respiratory system

Pressure of the growing uterus forces the diaphragm up and lower ribs out but vital capacity is not reduced in late pregnancy.

Raised progesterone levels increase respiratory rate.

## Urinary tract

*Renal function*
• Renal plasma flow increases by 30–50%.
• Glomerular filtration rate increases by 30–50%.
• Tubular re-absorption increases by 30–50%.
• Patchy glomerular leak happens occasionally (e.g. glucose).

*Lower urinary tract*
• Bladder more irritated as growing uterus pushes on it.
• Ureters:
  (a) Longer, wider, lower tone because of progesterone effects.
  (b) Stasis in ureter and pelvis of kidney may lead to infection.

## Alimentary tract

• Teeth more susceptible to spreading caries and gingivitis because of increased cortisone levels.
• Nausea and vomiting.
• Hypomotility of gut may lead to constipation.
• Hypochlorhydria—regurgitation of alkaline chyle into stomach.
• Slow emptying of gall bladder.
• Increased gastro-oesophageal reflux.

## Early fetal development

Fetal development is well documented in most mammalian species including the human.

Since many women cannot time the precise act of coitus at which fertilization occurred, it is conventional to date pregnancy in weeks from the 1st day of the last normal menstrual period (LNMP). The difference in the clinical timing of pregnancy and biological age (from conception) is readily understood on realizing that no-one becomes pregnant in the first half of a menstrual cycle. The first 14 days of pregnancy do not exist using the 1st day of the LNMP as a method of timing (Fig. 7.2).

The following milestones are particularly important.

*Four weeks (from LNMP) or 14 days biological life*
- Sac 2–3 mm.
- Ectoderm
- Mesoderm ⎫ formed.
- Endoderm ⎭
- Yolk sac formed.

*Six weeks (from LNMP)*
- Sac 20–25 mm; embryo 10 mm—can be seen on ultrasound.

- A cylinder with head and tail end formed.
- Pulsation of heart tube.
- Body stalk (umbilical cord) formed.
- Villi appear in cytotrophoblast.

*Eight weeks (from LNMP)*
- Sac 30–50 mm; fetus 20 mm (Figs 7.3 and 7.4).
- Sex glands differentiated.
- Limbs well formed, toes and fingers present.
- Centres of ossification present.

*Twelve weeks (from LNMP)*
- Sac 100 mm; fetus 90 mm.
- Primary development of all organ systems.
- Nails on fingers and toes.

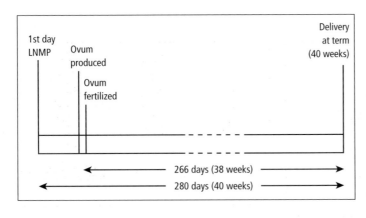

**Figure 7.2** The differences between the actual length of gestation and the calculated length of pregnancy from the LNMP.

**Figure 7.3** Different stages of fetal growth. The fetus at 8, 10 and 12 weeks are shown two-thirds of actual size.

**Figure 7.4** Different stages of fetal growth. (a) Ultrasound showing a sac at 7 weeks. (b) Ultrasound showing a sac and fetus at 12 weeks.

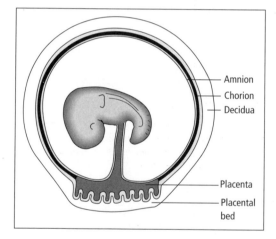

**Figure 7.5** Formation of placenta in relation to fetus and fetal membranes.

**Figure 7.6** Development of blood vessels in the villi. (a) Mesoderm appears *in situ* in the core of a villus of proliferating trophoblast cells. (b) Blood vessels form and join up with those in the mesoderm layer. (c) Capillaries from arterial side circulate blood back to veins.

## Early placental development

The placenta (Fig. 7.5) is formed from:
- chorion
- decidua basalis  } covered by amnion.

Villi are buds from chorionic plate. At first they are made of cytotrophoblast tissue only. Mesoderm appears *in situ* in the centre of the core of each villus (Fig. 7.6).

In this mesodermal core, angioblastic strands are formed. The cells on the edge of these become the endothelium of blood vessels and the central cells, the red blood cells. The vessels of the villus join the vessels formed in the mesoderm. By 22 days, the fetal heart pumps blood and a functioning circulation starts.

By eight weeks, the villi are 200 μm in diameter with a well-organized circulatory system and a double layer of epithelium (cytotrophoblast covered by a cellular syncytiotrophoblast).

Further demands of fetal metabolism require swifter exchanges at the placenta. These come as a result of:

1 Greater surface area—longer and branching villi.
2 Thinning of epithelium so that syncytiotrophoblast is in direct contact with blood capillary.
3 Nuclei in syncytiotrophoblast migrate from areas over capillaries where exchange actually occurs.
4 Localized dome-like swellings occur on the villi protruding into the intervillous space. These areas are especially thin-walled and are probably the site of much of the gas exchange.

Villi are like fronds of seaweed under water as the maternal blood circulates around them (Fig. 7.7). As the placenta grows, fetal size is proportional to the surface area available for exchange at first. The number of stem villi does not increase after the 12th week. Hence the number of lobules is now fixed. The rest of growth is by proliferation and by growth of peripheral villi.

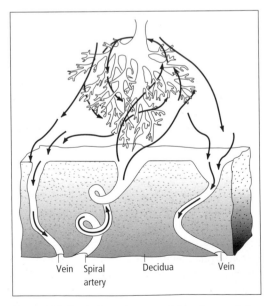

**Figure 7.7** Circulation of maternal blood around fine exchange villi.

## Fetal physiology

The major functions will be reviewed particularly where they differ from adult physiological patterns.

## Cardiovascular system

The heart is beating by 22 days and can be detected with vaginal ultrasound at 5 weeks (from LNMP).

There are bypasses in the system since the lungs are not used; less than 10% of blood goes through them (Fig. 7.8). These bypasses include:
• foramen ovale between the right and left atria so that the majority of oxygenated blood passes straight to the left side of the heart.
• ductus arteriosus from the pulmonary artery to the aorta so that only a small amount of blood from the right side of the heart goes into the lungs and the rest can use the bypass into the aorta.

Umbilical blood flow increases with fetal weight. This increase is disproportionate, but with enhanced $O_2$ carrying capacity of the fetal blood, the total $O_2$ transport is increased. Flow is about 100 ml/kg/min, as measured experimentally, but may be greater *in vivo*.

*Fetal haemoglobin*
HbA (adult haemoglobin) differs from HbF (fetal haemoglobin) by a 25% alteration of amino acid radicals in chains. At any given $Po_2$, the $O_2$ dissociation curve of HbF is to the left of HbA so it has greater $O_2$ affinity (Fig. 7.9). The fetus has higher Hb concentration than the adult (18 g/dl in the blood compared with 13 g/dl) allowing further $O_2$ uptake at the placenta and greater release to tissues. Production of HbF diminishes before birth and has usually ceased by the age of one year (Fig. 7.10).

## Respiratory system

Within 1–2 minutes this has to adjust from an intrauterine to an independent state. Vascular loops occur in the lungs by 18 weeks. Alveoli develop by 22 weeks.

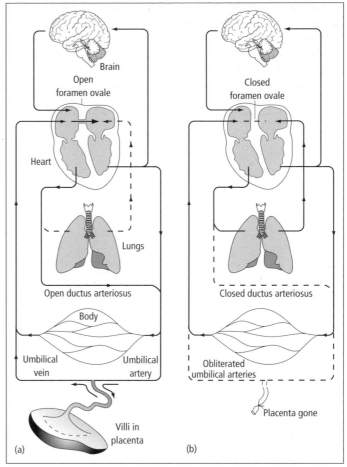

**Figure 7.8** (a) The fetal circulation. (b) The neonatal circulation. Note closure of bypasses after birth.

Surface tension of alveolar epithelium is decreased by surfactant lipoproteins, which are not present in the immature fetus. Hence if they are born prematurely it is difficult to open up their lungs and respiratory distress syndrome occurs. Production of surfactant increases after 34 weeks.

Before birth, the alveoli are closed and the trachea is filled with lung fluid. This is different from amniotic fluid and is secreted from glandular cells in the periphery of the bronchiolar system. Small spontaneous chest movements occur, but if the fetus is made hypoxic, larger efforts are made; then (and only then) is amniotic fluid drawn into the trachea. Most non-stressed infants are born with a respiratory tract filled with lung fluid, not amniotic fluid.

Fetal development is mostly by growth (Fig. 7.11); most congenital defects that are going to occur will have been formed by 10 weeks. The critical periods in the development of the human embryo are shown in Fig. 7.12.

Growing from one cell to six billion demands organization of cells into functioning systems so that all can metabolize under optimal conditions. The rate of growth is greatest in the first weeks. Cellular increase is under the control of maternal and fetal hormones; at first, oestrogens are most influential, then later insulin-like growth factors. In very early pregnancy oestrogens regulate the supply of nutrients in uterine fluid. Later they regulate the course of the blood supply to the placental bed.

After mid-pregnancy, growth is also determined by placental transfer. This could be impaired by:

**1** A low environment supply from the mother of:
- oxygen—only has effect in last weeks, e.g. living at high altitudes;
- nutrients—shows with extremes of specific deprivation or general starvation.

**2** Reduced blood flow to the placental bed. This follows lack of normal invasion of the arcuate arteries by trophoblasts at 16–18 weeks. This can be estimated by Doppler ultrasound.

**3** Poor exchange across the syncytiotrophoblast membrane; if this should be reduced a smaller baby results.

Overall growth is determined by:

**1** Genetic factors inherited from both parents.

**2** Placental transfer of nutrients dependent on:
- placental bed flow rates;
- placental membrane transfer.

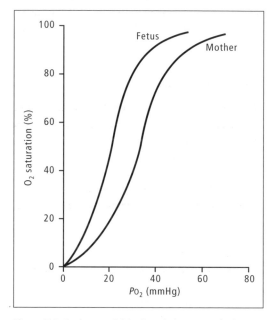

Figure 7.9 Oxyhaemoglobin dissociation curves for human maternal and fetal blood at pH 7.4 and 37°C.

Figure 7.11 The weight gain of the fetus and newborn child. The growth potential falls off in the last few weeks of pregnancy. Note that, after the immediate weight drop, neonatal growth continues at the same incremental rate as it did in the uterus.

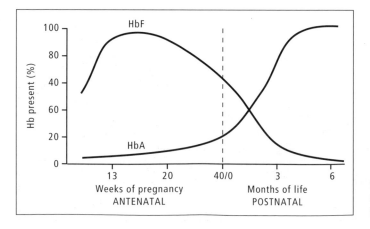

Figure 7.10 Proportion of HbF and HbA present at different stages of fetal and postnatal life.

## Changes that occur in the fetus at birth

- Closure of the ductus arteriosus
- Closure of the foramen ovale
} Occurs with the first breath so that 100% of deoxygenated blood passes through the lungs.

- Obliteration of the umbilical arteries and veins (Fig. 7.8b).

## Placental physiology

### Exchange

The placenta is the fetal exchange station. Compare Fig. 7.13a and Fig. 7.13b. Figure 7.13a is an adult with organs of homeostasis (kidney, skin and lung) communicating with the outside environment—the air in the case of humans. Figure 7.13b shows the fetal situation where these same homeostatic organs only communicate with the amniotic sac—a closed cavity. All exchange must take place via the placenta to the mother and thence (using her kidneys, skin and lungs) to the outside. The placenta is called the lung of the fetus but is also its liver and kidneys. Transfer of nutrients, waste products, etc., occur predominantly by diffusion but active transport mechanisms exist for larger molecules.

### Placental hormones

The placenta has a second set of functions, that of an endocrine organ making hormones that regulate the following:
1 Rate of growth of fetus.
2 Activity of uterus to:
   - prevent premature expulsion of fetus;
   - encourage labour contractions at correct time.
3 Activity of other organs:
   - breasts;
   - ligaments of pelvis in pregnancy.

The hormones made by the placenta are detailed below.
- *Chorionic gonadotrophin*
  - Made in: cytotrophoblast.
  - Function: prolongs corpus luteum (early); may control progesterone metabolism (late).

**Figure 7.12** Critical periods of various areas of the human embryo. Abnormalities are likely to follow if appropriate teratogens act on tissues at these sensitive times.

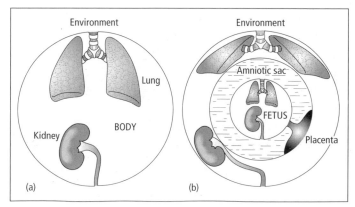

**Figure 7.13** (a) Non-pregnant woman. (b) The fetal environment in the pregnant woman.

- *Oestrogens*
  - Made in: all tissues of placenta.
  - Function: stimulate uterine growth and development.
- *Progesterone*
  - Made in: cytotrophoblast.
  - Function: damps down intrinsic uterine action in pregnancy.
- *Human placental lactogen*
  - Made in: syncytiotrophoblast.
  - Function: alters glucose and insulin metabolism; may initiate lactation.

Placental tissues age. Maximum efficiency is at 37–38 weeks; many functions deteriorate after this.

Beware extrapolations between transfer and endocrine functions of the placenta. Correlations may not be valid.

## The fetus and placenta at term

### The fetus

The anatomical features of the fetus which most concern the obstetrician are those found in the mature fetus after 36 weeks' gestation. The most important area is that which is largest, hardest and most difficult to deliver—the head.

*The head*
Certain measurements should be remembered (Fig. 7.14). These diameters engage in the maternal pelvic brim at different degrees of flexion of the fetal head on the neck.

The intracranial arrangement of meninges is important (Fig. 7.15) because, under stress, it can be damaged to produce intracranial haemorrhage.

*The body*
The rest of the fetus will usually pass where the head leads. The bisacromial diameter of the shoulders is about 10 cm.

## Placenta

A discoid with 15–20 lobules packed together.
- *Fetal surface.* Covered with amnion (not chorion which fuses with the placental edge). Fetal vessels

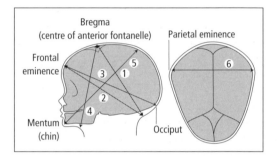

**Figure 7.14** The important diameters of the fetal head of a 3-kg baby:
**1** Suboccipitobregmatic, 10 cm: vertex presentation
**2** Suboccipitofrontal, 11 cm: various flexions of cephalic presentations
**3** Occipitofrontal, 12 cm
**4** Submentobregmatic, 10 cm: face presentation
**5** Mentovertical, 13 cm: brow presentation
**6** Biparietal, 10 cm

**Figure 7.15** Arrangement of the meninges showing how cerebral veins traverse them. If much intracranial movement occurs, the arachnoid moves with the brain but the dura stays with the skull. Hence the vein can be torn at the arrowed sites.

(arteries paler than veins) course over it diving into each lobule as an end vessel.
• *Maternal surface.* Lobules of compressed villi (like seaweed out of water) separated from each other by sulci.

*Maternal side of the placental circulation*
Maternal blood is in vessels except in the placental bed where it is in contact with foreign tissues (syncytiotrophoblast of villi). Spiral arteries (about 200) lead blood from the uterine arteries to the placental bed pool. Maternal blood spurts under arterial blood pressure, loses way against a mass of villi and passes laterally, pushed by *vis a tergo* to the placental bed veins scattered over the floor of the placental bed.

Measurement of blood flow to the placental bed has been very difficult because it involved direct measurement in animals (unphysiological) or indirect methods with electromagnetic flow meters in humans (imprecise). Now indirect measurements with Doppler ultrasound allow more precise non-invasive flow studies in humans.

Maternal blood flow to the uterus is 100–150 ml/kg/min in late pregnancy, of which 80–85% goes to the placenta.

*Abnormal implantation*
• *Placenta accreta.* Villi penetrate decidua just into the myometrial layer; difficulty in separation.
• *Placenta increta.* Villi penetrate deeply into myometrium. Even more difficult to separate.
• *Placenta percreta.* Villi penetrate to subperitoneal myometrium. Impossible to separate.

The three diagnoses above cannot usually be differentiated clinically. They are pathological ones made at sectioning a uterus after removal.
• *Placenta praevia.* Implantation in the lower segment of the uterus.

## Umbilical cord

At term the umbilical cord is about 50 cm long, 2 cm in diameter. It contains two arteries and a vein which is derived from the left umbilical vein of the embryo. (The right one usually disappears.) For types of cord insertion, see Fig. 7.16.

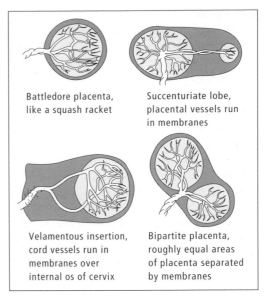

Battledore placenta, like a squash racket

Succenturiate lobe, placental vessels run in membranes

Velamentous insertion, cord vessels run in membranes over internal os of cervix

Bipartite placenta, roughly equal areas of placenta separated by membranes

**Figure 7.16** Types of umbilical cord insertion.

**Box 7.1 Diagnostic uses of checking amniotic fluid**

• Chromosome content of amniocytes and fetal skin cells in genetic diseases
• Rhesus effect measuring bilirubin breakdown products
• Metabolic upset of the fetus
• Infection of the amniotic cavity in premature rupture of membranes
• Respiratory maturity by measuring the lecithin–sphingomyelin ratio

Arteries spiral and give a cord-like appearance. Possibly their pattern wrapped around the vein allows their pulsations to help massage blood back along the umbilical vein. The vessels are packed and protected by a viscous fluid—Wharton's jelly.

There are no nerves in the cord or placenta. Hence ligation and cutting the umbilical cord does not hurt the fetus.

## Amniotic fluid

This surrounds the fetus.

- Produced:
  - in early pregnancy: from amnion over placenta and sac;
  - in late pregnancy: from fetal urine as well.
- Volume:
  - increase to 38 weeks; 500–1500 ml.
- Osmolality:
  - decreases in late pregnancy.

- Creatinine:
  - increases in late pregnancy.
- Acid–base:
  - normally accumulation of $CO_2$ and fixed acid causes a slight reduction in pH (about 7.15–7.20).

Amniotic fluid can be removed at amniocentesis and used to diagnose a number of factors (Box 7.1).

---

## Self-assessment

**7.1** Fill in the blanks in the following sentences from the list below.

In pregnancy the maternal cardiac output increases principally because of a greater (1) _____. Haemoglobin concentrations decrease because of an increased (2) _____ despite an increased (3) _____. The uterus grows by (4) _____ with a blood flow at term of (5) _____ ml/kg/min.

(a) 100–150
(b) red cell volume
(c) stroke volume
(d) 200–250
(e) hypertrophy
(f) plasma volume
(g) pulse rate
(h) red cell mass
(i) mitosis
(j) mean haemoglobin concentration

**7.2** Which of the following statements are true?
(a) Fetal haemoglobin shifts the oxygen dissociation curve to the right of that for haemoglobin A.
(b) At birth, changes in the neonatal circulation enable the entire circulating volume to enter the pulmonary tree.
(c) In fetal life oxygenated blood from the umbilical arteries flows directly to the left side of the heart.
(d) During fetal life the lungs are filled with amniotic fluid.
(e) Exposure to teratogens is more likely to cause congenital abnormalities in the first trimester of pregnancy.

**7.3** The functions of the placenta include which of the following?
(a) Transfer of oxygen from the mother to the fetus.
(b) Transfer of urea from the mother to the fetus.
(c) Prevention of premature labour.
(d) Transfer of nutrients from the fetus to the mother.
(e) Regulation of fetal metabolism of insulin and glucose.

**7.4** The smallest diameters of the fetal skull include which of the following?
(a) Mentovertical.
(b) Submentobregmatic.
(c) Suboccipitobregmatic.
(d) Biparietal.
(e) Occiptofrontal.

# Chapter 8

# Bleeding in pregnancy

## Miscarriage or abortion

An abortion is the expulsion of the products of conception before the 24th week of pregnancy. The word abortion is often considered by women to be a procured termination of pregnancy, legal or criminal. Hence, the softer term miscarriage is better used for the spontaneous event. A simple classification is helpful in understanding the various terms used (Fig. 8.1).

## Causes of spontaneous miscarriage

These are maternal, fetal and possibly paternal or genetic.

## Maternal causes

### General
- Age.
- Obesity.
- Acute febrile illness.
- Septicaemia with infection of the fetus.
- Severe hypertension or renal disease.
- Diabetes.
- Hypothyroidism.
- Trauma.
- A surgical operation.
- Emotional shock, perhaps more in folklore than actuality.

Drugs like ergot, quinine and lead may be taken to induce abortion. They are not very effective and the risk of poisoning is great.

### Local
- Uterine fibroids.
- Congenital uterine malformations.
- Incompetence of the internal os:
  - congenital;
  - acquired after difficult dilatation of the cervix.
- Hormone deficiency:
  - progesterone—the corpus luteum usually produces progesterone which helps embedding of the embryo;
- systemic lupus erythematosus;
  - anti-phospholipid syndrome.

## Fetal causes

- Genetic abnormalities.
- Congenital malformations.
- Faulty implantation.

### Congenital and genetic malformations
Examination of the chromosomes in material from spontaneous abortion shows gross abnormalities in over half—often the embryo has failed to develop or has been absorbed. In these cases, miscarriage usually takes place at about eight weeks. Ultrasound shows that the amniotic sac contains no

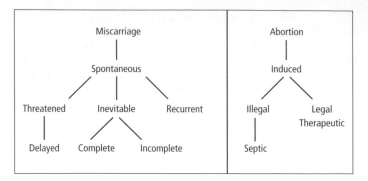

**Figure 8.1** A simple classification of the terms used.

embryo. In other cases, gross malformation of the fetus is shown.

### Faulty implantation
The embryo may become implanted in an unfavourable site in the uterus, for example in the isthmus, cervical canal or in the uterine cornu. Most of these cases end in spontaneous miscarriage; rarely the pregnancy continues.

## Incidence of spontaneous miscarriage

The frequency depends on the definition:
• in clinically diagnosed pregnancies 15–20% will miscarry in early pregnancy;
• non-development of the blastocyst within 14 days occurs in up to 50% of conceptions.

## Clinical features and management of spontaneous miscarriage

### Threatened miscarriage

*Symptoms*
• Scanty uterine bleeding preceded by symptoms of pregnancy.
• Pain is usually absent; there may be backache or slight uterine contractions.

*Examination*
• The breasts may be active.
• The uterus is enlarged corresponding with dates of amenorrhoea.

• The cervix is closed.
• There is no pelvic tenderness.

*Differential diagnosis*
• Delayed miscarriage when the uterus is smaller than expected. Check with ultrasound.
• Ectopic pregnancy when pain generally precedes bleeding.
• Dysfunctional uterine bleeding—where no signs of pregnancy.

Ultrasound can show a sac (five weeks), an embryo and the fetal heart beat (six weeks). Human chorionic gonadotrophin (hCG) can be measured in blood or urine.

*Treatment*
Treatment is usually rest until fresh bleeding has ceased.

After bleeding has ceased, the woman should avoid exertion and intercourse till after the 12th week of pregnancy. Progesterone therapy is ineffective, but still used.

### Inevitable miscarriage

*Symptoms*
Bleeding and pain are characteristic, bleeding is heavier than in threatened miscarriage. There may be crampy, low abdominal pains and an escape of amniotic fluid.

*Examination*
• Uterus enlarged.
• The internal os of the cervix is dilated. Prod-

ucts of conception may be felt in the cervical canal. Once this has occurred, miscarriage is inevitable.

*Treatment*
Before 12 weeks' gestation, evacuate the uterus under general anaesthesia in an operating theatre.

After 12 weeks, allow miscarriage to take place spontaneously, but be prepared to evacuate the uterus if it is incomplete. If bleeding is severe, Syntometrine should be given, 5 units/0.5 mg intramuscularly.

## Incomplete miscarriage

An incomplete miscarriage occurs when some of the products of conception are retained in the uterus. These are usually parts of the placenta or chorionic tissue attached to the uterine wall.

*Symptoms*
• Continued bleeding after a period of amenorrhoea.

*Differential diagnosis*
• Threatened miscarriage.
• Ectopic pregnancy.
• Dysfunctional uterine bleeding.
Ultrasound may help to clarify the diagnosis.

*Treatment*
• Conservative management.
• Evacuation of the uterus in the operating theatre.

## Complete miscarriage

If all the products of conception have been passed and the uterus is empty, the miscarriage is complete. There is little bleeding, the uterus is small with the cervix closed or merely patulous in a multiparous woman.

No treatment is required provided the differential diagnosis of ectopic pregnancy has been excluded (see p. 100).

## Delayed or missed miscarriage

The embryo dies in early development and is retained there and/or the sac continues to develop. The early embryo is commonly reabsorbed leaving an empty sac—a blighted ovum (a term with unpleasant connotations for the parents and is best avoided when talking to the patient and her partner).

*Symptoms*
• At first those of pregnancy, but these disappear.
• The breasts become soft.
• Dark brown vaginal discharge.
The cervix is closed and the uterus smaller than would be expected; hCG levels drop in 7–10 days.

*Differential diagnosis*
• Tubal mole.
• An incomplete miscarriage.
• A complete miscarriage.
Ultrasound will confirm the diagnosis.

*Treatment*
• Surgical evacuation. This should be offered if an embryo with an equivalent size of >8 weeks is present.
• Medical treatment. Evacuation of the uterus can be successful in 50% of cases by giving vaginal or oral prostaglandins every three hours until miscarriage takes place.
• Expectant management. This is usually safe and effective if the sac is empty or the embryo is <8 weeks in size. The sac usually reabsorbs with minimal bleeding but it may take several weeks and the patients should be offered regular follow-up until miscarriage is complete.

## Recurrent miscarriage

Three consecutive spontaneous miscarriages constitutes recurrent miscarriage. This may be primary where the woman has borne no viable child, or secondary. The most important associations are:
• Maternal:
  (a) antiphospholipid syndrome (APS) (40%);
  (b) polycystic ovaries (Chapter 3) (50%);

(c) incompetence of the cervix (5%);
- trauma of the cervix;
- previous difficult labour;
- repeated dilatation of the cervix;
- operations of the cervix.

(d) congenital malformation of the uterus (1%);

(e) genetic—most commonly a balanced translocation in one parent (3%).

### Management

This depends on the time in pregnancy when it occurs. She is wise to abstain from exertion, intercourse and travelling until after the 14th week. The pregnancy should be monitored by ultrasound to ensure that the fetus is present and developing normally. Late recurrent miscarriage after the 12th week is often due to incompetence of the cervix which may require suturing prophylactically (Fig. 8.2).

If the woman is found to have APS, then treatment with aspirin and heparin during pregnancy improves the take-home-baby rate from 10% to 40%.

### Investigations

**1** APS lupus anticoagulant and anticardiolipin antibodies are measured and repeated after 6 weeks. Two positive results are needed to confirm the diagnosis.

**2** PCOS, LH, FSH, testosterone (d 3–8), ultrasound scan.

**3** Cervical incompetence and congenital abnormalities—hysterosalpingography and transvaginal ultrasound scan may show an incompetent cervix or uterine anomaly.

In pregnancy, transvaginal ultrasound is usually helpful in showing the same deficiency and/or changes in the cervical length and dilation.

**4** Karyotype of both parents.

Between pregnancies hysterosalpingography may show an incompetent internal os. This may also reveal a congenital malformation of the uterus.

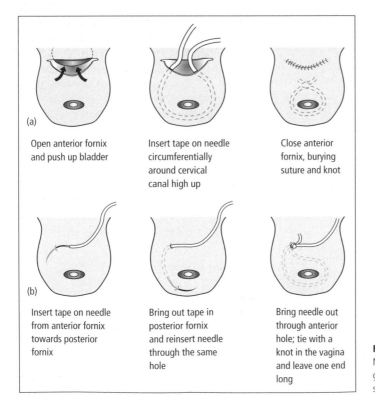

(a)
Open anterior fornix and push up bladder

Insert tape on needle circumferentially around cervical canal high up

Close anterior fornix, burying suture and knot

(b)
Insert tape on needle from anterior fornix towards posterior fornix

Bring out tape in posterior fornix and reinsert needle through the same hole

Bring needle out through anterior hole; tie with a knot in the vagina and leave one end long

**Figure 8.2** (a) The Shirodkar and (b) Macdonald sutures, performed under general anaesthetic. If they work, they should be removed at 38 weeks.

## Counselling after miscarriage

Counselling is often needed because a spontaneous miscarriage may lead to bereavement even though the event was too early in pregnancy for a viable baby to be born. The woman and her partner should receive an explanation of what happened and of the possible cause of the miscarriage if it is known. If there is a treatable cause, such as uterine fibroids, treatment of this should be discussed even though the operation itself may be best postponed for about three months.

The couple are often anxious to have another pregnancy. In most normal cases, where no serious cause is identified, there is no reason why they should not immediately, that is, as soon as the woman has had a normal period or two. Commonly given advice to wait 3–6 months has no logical basis.

Parents find it helpful to know the chances of a sucessful pregnancy next time (see Box 8.1).

## Criminal abortion

Under the Offences Against the Person Act 1861, any attempt to procure abortion by the woman herself or by another person is a felony, irrespective of whether she is in fact pregnant. The position of termination of pregnancy under the Abortion Act is considered in Chapter 5.

Abortion may be procured by:
- drugs;
- instruments passed into the uterus;
- foreign bodies—slippery elm bark introduced into the cervix;
- injections of soap or douching with soap or antiseptic solutions.

| Box 8.1 Chances of a live birth in a subsequent pregnancy | |
|---|---|
| No. of miscarriages | % |
| • One | 85 |
| • Two | 75 |
| • Three or more | 60 |
| Unless APS diagnosed | |
| • No treatment | 10 |
| • Aspirin and heparin | 40 |

Criminal abortion is dangerous:
- drugs may cause poisoning;
- infection can easily be introduced;
- risk of severe haemorrhage can occur;
- embolism with air or soap solution.

The doctor called to deal with a woman who has had a criminal abortion is bound to respect her confidence. He or she should not inform the police or any other person unless the woman dies or appears likely to do so, when a dying declaration should be obtained. Deaths must be reported to the coroner (see also p. 79).

## Septic abortion

Infection of the uterine cavity following an abortion leads to septic abortion. It can occur after spontaneous miscarriage, but most cases result from criminal interference with non-sterile instruments.

Spreading infection leads rapidly to salpingitis, pelvic peritonitis, pelvic cellulitis, septicaemia and pyaemia. Infection with *tetanus* will give the typical features of the disease and can be fatal. Infection with *Clostridium welchii* is not uncommon in criminal abortions; the picture is that of severe infection with shock and tachycardia. Such cases need prompt and efficient treatment preferably in an intensive care unit.

*Symptoms*
- A history of abortion, often criminal.
- Pelvic infection and septicaemia.
- Fever.
- Pelvic tenderness with foul discharge from the uterus and bleeding.
- Neutrophil leucocytosis is found on the blood count.
- The haemoglobin level may be reduced.

*Treatment*
- Admission to hospital.
- Swabs should be taken for cultures from the cervix and blood culture taken in seriously ill patients.
- Adequate doses of antibiotics should start at once; a combination of amoxycillin, clindamycin

and metronidazole may be used initially. A change of antibiotic may be needed when the cultures and sensitivities become available.

• Full intravenous supportive measures and steroids may be needed.

• If the products of conception are retained, the uterus should be evacuated. This should be done at once if there is severe bleeding, otherwise it is preferable to wait 24 hours to allow the antibiotics to take effect.

# Ectopic pregnancy

Ectopic pregnancy is one outside the uterine cavity, the commonest site being the fallopian tube. It may also occur, although rarely, in:

• uterine cornu;
• ovary;
• cervix;
• abdominal cavity;
• broad ligament.

For practical purposes, ectopic pregnancy will be considered as tubal pregnancy.

*Incidence*
Estimates of the incidence of tubal pregnancy vary. In the UK it is 0.5%. In other countries, especially in Africa, it may be as high as 1% because of the higher prevalence of chronic tubal disease.

*Causes*
The ovum is fertilized in the fallopian tube and reaches the uterus in about five days. Anything that delays the passage of the fertilized ovum to the uterus can result in tubal pregnancy, such as intrauterine device (IUD) and progesterone-only pill (POP) (see Box 8.2).

---

**Box 8.2 Risk factors for ectopic pregnancy**

Pelvic inflammatory disease (PID)
Previous pelvic surgery
Previous ectopic pregnancy
Intrauterine device (IUD)
Progesterone only pill (POP)
Depoprovera
Emergency contraception
Sterilization

---

*Salpingitis* is the commonest predisposing cause. This may not be so severe as to cause complete closing of the tube, but it may destroy tubal cilia, kinking or narrowing the tube. Chlamydia is now the commonest organism associated with tubal damage. The woman is often unaware that she has had a tubal infection. *Tuberculous salpingitis* is an important but, in the UK, rare cause, for it damages the tube but often leaves it patent.

*Congenital malformation* of the tube may lead to crypts and diverticula providing sites for ectopic implantation (very rare).

*Pathology*
The muscular walls of the tube do not allow the embryo to grow beyond a certain size. The trophoblast gradually invades and erodes the tubal wall which, unlike the endometrium, is not prepared for implantation. Blood vessels are damaged and eventually bleeding takes place.

A tubal pregnancy may terminate in a number of ways.

• *Absorption*—in a few cases it is possible that absorption of a very early tubal pregnancy occurs.

The embryo dies in the tube, with a small amount of bleeding, and is partly absorbed.

• *Tubal abortion*—part or all of the products of conception are expelled from the tube into the peritoneal cavity.

• *Tubal rupture*—this is the most dramatic and best known termination of a tubal pregnancy, though in fact less common than absorption or tubal abortion. There is acute intraperitoneal haemorrhage from erosion of an artery. The pregnancy is often implanted in the narrower isthmus of the tube.

• *Secondary abdominal pregnancy*—this is the rarest outcome of all. The embryo is expelled complete from the tube and acquires a secondary attachment in the peritoneal cavity. It can occasionally go on to a full term abdominal pregnancy. Many cases of children delivered from the peritoneal cavity by laparotomy have been reported, particularly in the West Indies.

*Clinical features*
The picture of ectopic pregnancy is:

• *Amenorrhoea*—this can be 4–8 weeks' duration, but may present before amenorrhoea is noticed.
• *Pain*—typically constant and often unilateral due to spasm of the tubal muscle. There may be referred shoulder pain via the phrenic nerve from blood in the abdominal cavity.
• *Vaginal bleeding*—when a pregnancy implants in the tube, the uterine endometrium is still converted into decidua. When the embryo dies, the decidua in the uterus separates. The bleeding is usually scanty, less than a normal period and dark brown in colour.
• *Faintness* or even *shock* with an acute rupture.

UNRUPTURED ECTOPIC PREGNANCY

This may present with:
• slight activity of the breasts;
• slight tenderness over one side of the uterus.

On bimanual examination, the uterus is slightly enlarged and the cervix is soft. There may be dark blood oozing from the external os. The pregnant tube is usually not palpable. There will be cervical excitation with tenderness on the side of the ectopic.

On bimanual examination, the tubal mass is rarely felt as a diffuse boggy swelling. If it is of any size, it displaces the uterus to the opposite side of the pelvis.

ACUTE RUPTURE OF A TUBAL ECTOPIC

This presents as an acute abdominal emergency with:
• collapse;
• severe abdominal pain;
• pallor, rapid pulse and hypotension;
• blood may track up under the diaphragm giving shoulder pain;
• the abdomen is slightly distended, tender and rigid;
• on vaginal examination, the uterus is soft and may be enlarged but is very tender;
• a tender tubal mass may not be palpated because of the extreme tenderness and guarding.

## Investigations

• *Ultrasound* is helpful. While it may not always show the embryo or its sac in the tube, findings may include:
  • an empty uterus with thickened decidua;
  • fluid (blood) in the pouch of Douglas;
  • a multi-echo mass in the region of the tube.
• *Progesterone levels* are commonly low because the pregnancy is failing.
• *Serum bhCG* is usually lower than expected for gestation and on serial measurements increases by less than 60% over 48 hours.
• *Laparoscopy* is the ultimate investigation to make the diagnosis with direct vision.

*Differential diagnosis*

The diagnosis is from any other acute abdominal catastrophe such as rupture of a viscus or acute peritonitis. The clinical picture is so typical that in most cases diagnosis presents no difficulty. Other diagnoses which may confuse are:
• inevitable miscarriage;
• bleeding with an ovarian cyst;
• pelvic appendicitis;
• acute salpingitis.

*Treatment*

The treatment of tubal pregnancy is removal of the pregnancy and sometimes the affected tube by laparoscopy or laparotomy. If the tube is patent and not seriously damaged, it may be possible to conserve it and thus leave the woman with a chance of conception later in life.

Laparoscopy techniques exist to:
• kill the embryo with a direct injection of methotrexate or mifepristone allowing absorption so requiring no surgery on the tube;
• incise the swollen tube over the ectopic pregnancy, aspirate the embryo, and achieve haemostasis (salpingostomy).

In a case of severe haemorrhage, the patient must be taken immediately to the operating theatre. Little time should be wasted in attempting resuscitation which can prove useless and may only increase bleeding. An intravenous drip should be set up and a blood transfusion given as soon as possible. It is sometimes possible later to collect the extravasated blood from the peritoneal cavity with a Cellsaver and return it to the circulation.

In most cases the affected tube should be removed; an exception may be made if the woman desires children and the other tube is already missing or seriously diseased. The disadvantage of conservation is the increased risk of recurrence of ectopic pregnancy.

Tubal pregnancy and normal intrauterine pregnancy may occur simultaneously in rare circumstances, most commonly after assisted conception.
• Medical treatment with methotrexate can be used if the hCG level is less than 5000 iu/l and the ectopic mass is less than 4 cm in diameter on ultrasound scan. There should be no symptoms or signs of rupture.

## Hydatidiform mole

Hydatidiform mole is a benign tumour of both parts of the chorion; the cytotrophoblast and the syncytiotrophoblast may be found in varying proportions. The villi undergo cystic or hydropic degeneration and a certain amount of bleeding almost always occurs.

Hydatidiform moles vary greatly in their rate of growth, in the amount of chorionic gonadotrophin produced and in the amount of invasion of the uterine wall.

Only rarely can a fetus be found, but hydatidiform degeneration may occur in the placenta. The birth of a living fetus with a hydatidiform mole has been described.

### Incidence
In the UK one in 2500 pregnancies, but much commoner in the Far East.

### Clinical features
The typical clinical features are amenorrhoea followed by continuous or intermittent vaginal bleeding. The other symptoms of pregnancy occur, often exaggerated; vomiting may be severe and early pre-eclampsia can develop. The uterus is often larger than the dates would suggest and feels very soft and boggy. Theca lutein cysts may develop in the ovaries.

Vesicles of the mole may be passed spontaneously and this is diagnostic of the condition.

### Investigations
Chorionic gonadotrophin excretion in urine is often greater than other pregnancies; while levels of 40000 to 60000 iu/l are common, concentrations of over 100000 iu/l are generally diagnostic of a mole. Ultrasonic examination is reliable in showing the absence of a fetus with the characteristic picture of snowflakes or soap bubbles (bright sunlight shining through the washing-up water).

### Treatment
The uterus must be emptied completely in all cases. If there seems to be spontaneous evacuation, the uterus must still be carefully aspirated and curetted, the specimen being sent for histology examination.

An intact mole may be dealt with by suction evacuation under cover of continuous oxytocin i.v. drip, curetting gently to remove all the mole. Intravenous Syntometrine must be given to minimize bleeding. Suction evacuation is safest and carries less risk of perforation than curettage.

Dangers include:
• haemorrhage which can be profuse;
• sepsis;
• perforation of the uterus;
• air embolism;
• incomplete evacuation of the uterus.

A second aspiration or curettage may be needed two weeks later to be sure that the mole has been completely removed.

### Follow-up
The woman should be followed-up by regular estimations of urinary hCG for at least a year and should avoid pregnancy for six months after hCG levels have returned to normal. Tests should be carried out monthly for the first six months and after that every two months. Persistence of hCG after one month may suggest incomplete evacuation of the uterus or malignant change. Persistence is an indicator for chemotherapeutic treatment with actinomycin D or methotrexate to prevent choriocarcinoma.

During the period of follow-up, the woman should not take the contraceptive pill but use barrier methods of contraception.

In the UK, follow-up is undertaken in specialist centres.

## Invasive mole

In some cases of hydatidiform mole, there may be great trophoblastic activity with penetration of the uterine wall. This can still be a simple invasive mole causing uterine enlargement and bleeding with a positive pregnancy test; these may require hysterectomy.

In severer cases trophoblast penetrates into the parametrium and leads to internal haemorrhage. The level of hCG is very high. These cases require urgent hysterectomy.

## Choriocarcinoma

This malignant tumour invades the uterine wall and metastasizes widely through the bloodstream. Rarely primary tumours are found in the ovary or testis as a form of teratoma.

It is fortunately an unusual tumour; about 40% follow hydatidiform mole, 40% follow abortion and 20% pregnancy at term. Conversely, a hydatidiform mole may go on to choriocarcinoma in

4–5% of women with a mole, compared with 0.0002% after normal pregnancy.

*Clinical features*
Uterine bleeding is the commonest symptom. Secondaries may appear rapidly and are most often found in the lungs, the uterus and the vagina, but they can involve the liver and the central nervous system. The levels of hCG are very high, often above 1000000 iu/l.

Choriocarcinoma is sensitive to cytotoxic drugs and is now curable in the majority of patients. Those with low-grade disease treated with methotrexate can retain their fertility and have further successful pregnancies. Assay of hCG in serum or urine is used as a tumour marker and reduction in its levels is a test of cure.

Chemotherapy is best given in units which specialize in its use and various combinations of drugs are given; cisplatin is the first line of attack and may be combined with methotrexate, vincristine, cyclophosphamide and actinomycin D.

With modern treatment, hysterectomy is now rarely indicated except with massive tumours causing severe bleeding or when the response to chemotherapy is poor.

**Self-assessment**

**8.1** A woman presents with her second miscarriage. Which of the following pieces of information should she be given in respect of miscarriage?
- (a) It is unlikely that she has done/taken anything to cause the miscarriage.
- (b) She has a 75% chance of miscarrying again.
- (c) She may try again for a pregnancy after one normal period.
- (d) She has a 25% chance of miscarrying again.
- (e) The majority of miscarriages are due to an abnormality in the baby.

**8.2** Which of the following are risk factors for ectopic pregnancy?
- (a) Combined oral contraceptive pill (COCP).
- (b) Progestogen only pill (POP).
- (c) Subserosal fibroids.
- (d) Chlamydia.
- (e) Corpus luteal cyst.

**8.3** Which of the following statements are true of a hydatidiform mole?
- (a) May be associated with early onset pre-eclampsia.
- (b) Is more common in the UK than in the Far East.
- (c) Should be treated with methotrexate.
- (d) Should be followed up for a minimum of one year in a specialist centre.
- (e) Is associated with a higher than average hCG concentration.

**8.4** Which of the following is true of choriocarcinoma?
- (a) There is early spread to bones.
- (b) Cisplatin is the chemotherapeutic agent of choice.
- (c) Hysterectomy is only indicated if there is severe bleeding.
- (d) After hydatidiform mole the risk of choriocarcinoma is 40%.
- (e) After hydatidiform mole the risk of choriocarcinoma is 4%.

# Chapter 9

# The antenatal period

The aims of antenatal care are to bring the mother and child to labour in the best possible condition. They are:

**1** A screening process applied to the entire pregnant population to detect subgroups at higher risk for complications of pregnancy.

**2** Suitable diagnostic procedures to determine who are really at risk.

**3** The management of high-risk pregnancies.

**4** The educational preparation of the couple for childbirth and the rearing of the infant.

## Diagnosis of pregnancy

### Symptoms

#### Amenorrhoea

The monthly shedding of the endometrium is prevented by higher progesterone levels from the persistence of the corpus luteum. Pregnancy is dated from the first day of the last normal menstrual period (LNMP) even though conception does not occur until about 14 days later. Any bleeding after the LNMP should be considered as abnormal.

#### Nausea and vomiting

Nausea occurs in 80% of nulliparous and 60% of multiparous women. For many pregnant women this is the first sign of pregnancy with the symptoms occurring even before the first period is missed.

The nausea and vomiting usually disappears by 16 weeks' gestation and lessens in severity after about 12 weeks. Although some women are sick first thing in the morning, it is not unusual to find that vomiting may occur at any time of the day. Commonly some biscuits or sweets help prevent nausea.

There is usually no accompanying metabolic upset, women do not feel ill all the time, and it does not affect their daily activities. They do not usually require hospitalization. Specific causes may include urinary tract infection or ingestion of iron tablets.

#### Breast symptoms

Breast enlargement accompanied by tingling of the skin and nipples. Montgomery's tubercles develop from between six and eight weeks' gestation and colostrum may be secreted from the nipples after about 12 weeks' gestation.

#### Urinary symptoms

From six weeks' gestation onwards, many women experience increased frequency of micturition. This is due to:

- Increased renal blood flow in the early stages.

- Pressure on the bladder from the growing uterus in later pregnancy.

## Signs

### Uterus

- An increased softness and enlargement of the uterus can be felt on bimanual vaginal examination from 6–8 weeks of gestation.

### Breasts

- Increased in size and feel warm.
- The areolae darken.
- Montgomery's tubercles develop.
- Tortuous skin veins dilate.

## Investigations

### Pregnancy test

Animal pregnancy tests and early crude immunological tests have now been replaced by accurate, sensitive tests involving monoclonal antibodies. Human chorionic gonadotrophin (hCG) is a glycoprotein hormone that contains two carbohydrate side chains: alpha ($\alpha$) and beta ($\beta$). The $\alpha$ subunit is identical to that of follicle stimulating hormone (FSH), luteinizing hormone (LH) and thyrotrophin (TSH). The $\beta$ subunit is immunologically specific. hCG is secreted by the trophoblast cells of the fertilized ovum and later by the definitive placenta.

Modern tests can detect hCG levels as low as 25 iu/l, before the time of the missed menses. Such tests can be performed in two minutes and are unaffected by urine contaminated by proteinuria, or bacterial contamination. Only a few drops of urine are required. The tests come in a variety of kits which can be bought in any chemist and are based on a colour change occurring if hCG binds to the monoclonal antibody embedded in the absorbent paper. Two main sorts are available: a double band of blue or a central spot of pink indicates a positive test while a single band of blue or absence of a pink spot indicates a negative pregnancy test.

### Ultrasound

Real-time ultrasound machines will detect an intrauterine gestation sac from five weeks of amenorrhoea, with fetal heart activity becoming visible at six weeks and a fetal pole visible at seven weeks.

Transvaginal probes enable a better resolution image than transabdominal ultrasound allowing the diagnosis of an intrauterine pregnancy to be made one week earlier (5–6 weeks).

## Antenatal visits

The current method of antenatal care was established 80 years ago but is now subject to change. In particular, the visits in mid-pregnancy (12–34 weeks) may be reduced.

Traditionally, the woman is seen monthly from the booking visit until 28 weeks, fortnightly until 36 weeks and then weekly until delivery. A reduction in the number of visits does not affect the outcome of pregnancy (Table 9.1) and is very popular with women.

The aim of the visits is to screen the low-risk population by means of history, examination and investigation; then antenatal care for high-risk

Table 9.1 The spacing of antenatal visits by traditional and by modern care

| Traditional (gestation in weeks) | Modern |
| --- | --- |
| 6–12 | 8–12 |
| 16 | |
| 20 | 20 |
| 24 | |
| | 26 |
| 28 | |
| 30 | |
| 32 | 32 |
| 34 | |
| 36 | 36 |
| 37 | |
| 38 | 38 |
| 39 | |
| 40 | 40 |
| 41 | 41 |

women may be carried out on a more frequent basis.

The following scheme applies to all women and is an attempt to identify risk factors.

## The first visit

Ideally the booking visit should be at 8–12 weeks' gestation. More frequently now the woman's history is being taken in her own home by a community midwife.

## History

**1** Establish the reliability of the LNMP (Box 9.1).
- Was the woman sure of the dates?
- Was the cycle regular?
- Was the woman on oral contraceptives within two months?
- Was there bleeding in early pregnancy?

Any of the above circumstances render prediction of expected date of delivery (EDD) from LNMP unreliable and later ultrasound examination is needed to determine dates.

**2** History of maternal disease, e.g. hypertension, diabetes mellitus.

**3** Family history, e.g. diabetes mellitus, tuberculosis, hypertension, multiple pregnancy or the birth of a congenitally abnormal baby, inherited disorders.

**4** Past obstetric history. This involves listing all the pregnancies in chronological order together with the following details (see Box 9.2):

(i) Deliveries after 24 weeks regardless of outcome.

(ii) Miscarriages and ectopic pregnancies:
- First trimester (less than 12 weeks) or second trimester.
- If second trimester, were they:
  (a) Relatively painless, associated with early rupture of the membranes suggesting cervical incompetence.
  (b) Associated with pain and bleeding suggestive of premature placental separation.
  (c) Associated with the delivery of a dead, macerated baby, an intrauterine death.

(iii) List all therapeutic abortions, their reason, gestation and method by which they were performed.

**5** Drug history. Note all drugs taken in the pregnancy so far.

**6** Allergies. Note allergies to medication, food or Elastoplast.

**7** Social history:
- Detail the woman's alcohol, tobacco and illicit drug intake giving appropriate advice.
- The woman's marital status, her occupation and that of her partner.
- The living conditions.
- Social support—family, friends.

## Examination

In the absence of a relevant history and with the routine use of ultrasound, there is little need to examine the pregnant woman's pelvis. Most doctors

---

**Box 9.1 Establishing the expected date of delivery (EDD) from the LNMP**

|  | *Example* |
|---|---|
| **1** Take date of 1st day of LNMP | 21 September 2003 |
| **2** Take away 3 months and add a year | 21 June 2003 |
| **3** Add 7 days | 28 June 2004 |
| **4** This is the EDD | |

*Do not use if*
- Dates uncertain
- Cycle not regular (i.e. outside range of 24–35 days)
- Been on oral contraception within 2 months

---

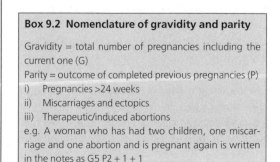

**Box 9.2 Nomenclature of gravidity and parity**

Gravidity = total number of pregnancies including the current one (G)
Parity = outcome of completed previous pregnancies (P)
i)   Pregnancies >24 weeks
ii)  Miscarriages and ectopics
iii) Therapeutic/induced abortions
e.g. A woman who has had two children, one miscarriage and one abortion and is pregnant again is written in the notes as G5 P2 + 1 + 1

and midwives, however, would still perform the following examinations:

1 Maternal blood pressure.

2 The respiratory system.

3 The breasts to check for:
- Lumps.
- Inverted nipples, which may require advice for breast feeding.

4 The spine for kyphosis or scoliosis.

5 The abdomen looking for scars, masses and, if the pregnancy is sufficiently advanced, the size of the uterus.

6 The legs looking for varicose veins.

7 Vaginal examination is not usually required at a booking visit but sometimes is done:
- To confirm the pregnancy.
- To check uterine size. } If ultrasound not available.
- To exclude uterine or ovarian masses.
- To take a smear if the patient has not had one within the last three years, although this is often left until the postpartum visit.

## Investigations

### Urine

1 Proteinuria—renal disease.

2 Glucose—diabetes.

3 White blood cells—response to infection.

4 Nitrite—bacteria.

### Blood

1 Haemoglobin.

2 Red cell indices, particularly the mean corpuscular volume (MCV). } Anaemia.

3 ABO and Rhesus (Rh) group (if negative need for Anti-D).

4 The presence of atypical antibodies.

5 Sickle cell screen particularly if the patient is Afro-Caribbean.

6 Haemoglobin electrophoresis, looking for thalassaemia if the patient is Asian or Mediterranean in origin.

7 Test for hepatitis antigens.

8 Test for rubella antibodies.

9 Human immunodeficiency virus (HIV) test. All women after appropriate counselling should be offered an HIV antibody test but the following patients are at high risk:
- Women from or with partners from sub-Saharan Africa.
- Drug abusers or partners of drug abusers.
- Women who have bisexual partners.
- Women with haemophiliac partners.
- Women who have had a blood transfusion overseas.

In places where HIV is more prevalent, universal testing is performed with an opt-out policy. In the UK this includes London and Edinburgh.

10 Screening test for syphilis (usually VDRL, Venereal Disease Research Laboratory test). If positive, more specific tests are required.

## General advice for healthy pregnancy

1 Establish a rapport between the woman and the antenatal clinic staff.

2 Show the woman where she can discover more about her pregnancy and delivery from:
- books available;
- parentcraft classes;
- relaxation classes;
- video and TV programmes.

3 Discuss the social welfare benefits available.

4 Make arrangements for the medical social worker to see the woman if there are any difficulties such as care of the other children or housing.

5 Advise a visit to the dentist reasonably soon, as dental care in pregnancy is free, and there is an increased prevalence of tooth decay and gingivitis in pregnancy.

6 Give dietary advice. This should be simple advice as most people in the UK have a more than adequate diet. The idea of eating for two should be discouraged and, in general, pregnant women need only an additional 500 kcal (2100 J) a day to ensure normal fetal growth.

Vegans may require specialized advice from the dietitian in order to ensure adequate nutrition throughout the pregnancy especially for certain amino acids. Similarly, some Asian women may need dietary advice or supplements of vitamin D as a consequence of living in the cloudy Northern Hemisphere.

**7** Advise the woman to stop smoking since it increases the risk of intrauterine growth retardation and delayed fetal maturation.

**8** Advise the woman to stop drinking alcohol or cut down on her intake.

**9** Advise the woman to avoid unpasteurized products, soft cheese and paté as these have been associated with intrauterine death secondary to listeriosis.

**10** Advise the woman to be careful when dealing with cats' litter by avoiding emptying the tray and using rubber gloves because of the risk of acquiring toxoplasmosis which may lead to mental retardation in the fetus.

**11** Consider providing iron supplementation. The routine of prophylactic iron supplements in pregnancy is controversial. Many obstetricians only provide iron if the woman has a haemoglobin of less than 10.5 g/dl or a MCV of less than 84 fl at the booking visit. Additional indications may be for multiple pregnancies or the previous pregnancy within 2 years.

Most women's haemoglobin level will fall by about 1 g/dl due to haemodilution that occurs in pregnancy.

If iron is given, it should be taken with meals as it is only absorbed in the ferrous state and this is best achieved in the presence of vitamin C.

In the non-pregnant state, about 10% of iron is absorbed and this is thought to double in pregnancy. When supplementation is given, you should aim to give at least 100 mg of elemental iron a day.

**12** Vitamin supplements. These are not usually required by women receiving an adequate diet. An exception is folic acid as it is often only barely sufficient in many diets. The requirements in pregnancy rise from 50 µg a day to 300 µg a day. Many women are therefore given prophylactic iron tablets that also contain folic acid (500 µg a day.) Folic acid supplements have been shown to reduce the incidence of neural tube defects (NTDs) when taken preconceptually and up to 14 weeks' gestation.

## Special visits

### To be performed at all visits

**1** Check the history of recent events and ensure that the baby is moving.

**2** Examine:
- Blood pressure.
- The growth of the uterus and its contents can be assessed by measuring the symphysiofundal height (SFH; Fig. 9.1). Normal growth is 1 cm per week ±2 cm, e.g. at 32 weeks the SFH should be 30–34 cm. Less than 30 cm may indicate growth retardation or oligohydramnios; greater than 34 cm may indicate a multiple pregnancy, polyhydramnios or macrosomia. Clinical assessment by palpation is rather a crude method with only 40% of small babies accurately detected and of these only 60% will still be small for dates at birth.

The SFH is measured by palpating the fundus, a tape measure is placed under the left index finger and laid over the abdomen to the top of the symphysis which should be felt for gently as it can be tender. The tape measure should be face down to prevent cheating (making the measurement fit the gestation). Beyond 26 weeks the following should be noted in the notes:
- lie (longitudinal, oblique, transverse) (Fig. 9.2);
- presentation (cephalic, breech, none) (Fig. 9.3);

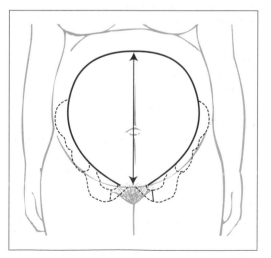

**Figure 9.1** The symphysiofundal height (SFH).

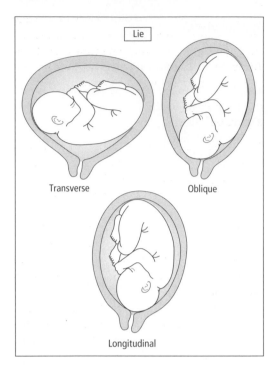

Figure 9.2 Diagrammatic representation of the possible lies of a baby.

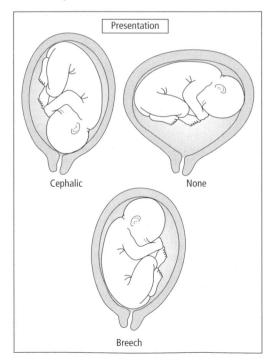

Figure 9.3 Diagram of the possible presentations of a baby.

• engagement (one-fifth palpable, see p. 160);
• liquor volume (normal, polyhydramnios, oligohydramnios);
• fetal heart auscultation with a hand-held Doppler (from 14 weeks) or pinard stethoscope (beyond 30 weeks).
• Test the urine for protein and glucose. This is also traditional and, in the absence of hypertension, it is less worthwhile testing for protein.

## Additionally at 26–28 weeks

• Check the haemoglobin.
• If the woman is Rh-negative also check for the presence of Rh antibodies. Give anti-D.
• Many now screen for gestational diabetes by doing random blood sugar at 28 weeks' gestation.
• Check the lie and presentation of the fetus.

## Additionally at 34 weeks

• Check haemoglobin level.
• If the patient is Rh-negative, check for the presence of antibodies. Give anti-D.
• If the presentation is cephalic, is the head engaged?

## Between 41 and 42 weeks

• Examine the cervix to assess the chances of success of induction if this is needed and do a membrane sweep if the cervical os is open; 70% of women will go into spontaneous labour within 48 hours.

## Advice to mothers

Apart from the dietary and social welfare information that should be available to the woman when she books, the following should be enquired about specifically.

### Intercourse

There is no restriction to intercourse during pregnancy unless the woman bleeds from the vagina or has placenta praevia. Mechanical problems may occur in late pregnancy so that alterations in the position of intercourse may become necessary, for example the woman may be more comfortable on top.

## Alcohol

Alcohol crosses the placenta readily and so can affect a fetus as much as an adult. Excessive drinking in pregnancy is associated with the fetal alcohol syndrome, characterized by a short nose with a low bridge, small eyes with a narrow palpebral fissure and mental retardation.

No ill-effects have been described with an alcohol intake below 4 units a week.

## Rest and exercise

Even in normal pregnancy, the extra weight carried by the woman may increase her sense of tiredness and lethargy. Sensible exercise such as walking and swimming or organized exercise to which the woman is accustomed (e.g. aerobics) should be allowed in pregnancy.

## Travel

The woman should only travel over distances which are comfortable to her.

Air travel is probably better than train for long distances, but airlines can refuse to carry women over 34 weeks' gestation for international flights and over 36 weeks' gestation for domestic travel. They are the final arbiters, not the travel agents.

## Clothes

Women should be advised to wear what looks good and feels comfortable.

Maternity brassieres are often not required until late pregnancy, but women should be advised to move into them as soon as they feel that their present brassiere is inadequate for support.

## Bathing

The woman should bathe as she wishes. Avoid vaginal douching in pregnancy.

## Bowels

Pregnancy tends to make women constipated because of the progestogenic effect of relaxing smooth muscles. This is best overcome by increasing fluid intake, fresh fruit and by the use of foods rich in fibre. Laxatives should not be used unless the constipation becomes symptomatic.

## Onset of labour

Many nulliparous women have no idea what to expect; up to 10% of women who present with pains are subsequently proved not to be in labour.

Advise that the onset of labour is usually accompanied by one of the following:

**1** Regular painful contractions coming from the small of the back and radiating to the lower abdomen. Nulliparous women are usually advised to come into hospital when such contractions are occurring once in every 5–10 min.
**2** A bloody or mucous show. This is not necessarily a sign of labour. If accompanied by uterine contractions women should be advised to contact their midwife or delivery unit.
**3** Rupture of the membranes accompanied by a gush of amniotic fluid. In this case, women should be advised to come into hospital because of the risk of cord prolapse.

It should be emphasized that it is much better for a woman to come into hospital if she thinks she is in labour. Even if she is not, many of the causes of uterine pain may be serious and should be evaluated in the maternity unit.

## Psychological preparation

Pregnancy and delivery are a worry to most women. Commonly there is a fear of:
• The unknown.
• Giving birth to an abnormal baby.
• Giving birth to a dead baby.
• The pain that accompanies labour.

Many women's fears can be alleviated by proper antenatal preparation and by encouraging them to ask questions at the antenatal clinic. Women and their partners should be encouraged to attend talks about childbirth and subsequent rearing of their children. The antenatal clinic is a busy place, but doctors and midwives should never appear to be rushed and should encourage women to express their fears or anxieties and to ask questions.

## Parentcraft classes

The aim of these classes is to help women and their partners to prepare for labour, delivery and the care of their newborn baby. Couples should be encouraged to attend together.

The following areas are covered:
1 Stages of labour.
2 Possible abnormalities of labour.
3 Methods of delivery.
4 Pain relief.
(a) Natural methods—teaching the woman exercises.
- In the first stage, slow breathing between contractions and quick shallow breathing during contractions.
- In the second stage, women are taught expulsive breathing that involves fixing the diaphragm and the upper abdomen.
(b) Inhalational gases ($N_2O$).
(c) Transepithelial nerve stimulation (TENS).
(d) Regional local anaesthesia: epidural.
(e) Acupuncture/hypnotherapy.
(f) Opiates—these are no longer recommended.
5 Place of birth.
- Hospital                      90%
- GP/midwifery unit        5%
- Home                          5%

Five percent choose in early pregnancy to deliver at home but only 2% actually deliver there. 40% of prigravida will be transferred mostly in labour because of failure to progress in the first or second stage of labour. This can be very distressing for all concerned. They must be counselled that regional anaesthesia, resuscitation of the newborn and treatment of a postpartum haemorrhage will be more difficult compared with delivery in hospital.

Women in their first pregnancy often have very high expectations of having a normal labour and delivery which can be unrealistic. They may write detailed birth plans (virtually never written by women in their second or third pregnancy) outlining their desired management of labour. It is important to try to make their expectations realistic otherwise the mother (and her partner) may experience profound disappointment, anger and a sense of failure which may affect both her ability to care for her newborn baby and increase her risk of postnatal depression.

## Assessment of fetal well-being

The obstetrician is responsible for the care of two patients in labour, one of them being the fetus. The hidden patient is guarded by the following barriers:
- *Anatomical.* These can be overcome to some extent by ultrasound imaging.
- *Physiological.* These need an understanding of the interaction between fetal and maternal physiology.
- *Psychological.* These need an explanation to the mother, her relatives, and often medical and midwifery staff to overcome the in-built resistance to investigating the unborn.

## Screening for neural tube defects (NTDs) and Down's syndrome

### Serum α fetoprotein

NTDs account for 50% of congenital abnormalities. Some hospitals offer a blood test at 15–17 weeks to measure maternal serum α fetoprotein, although the majority of these defects are now detected by high resolution real-time ultrasound routinely performed at 18–20 weeks' gestation.

### The triple test

Whilst a high α fetoprotein result may indicate an increased risk of the baby having a NTD, a low result is associated with an increased risk of Down's syndrome. This is not a highly specific or sensitive test and, combined with the measurement of hCG and oestriol, (expected to be raised and lowered respectively in the presence of Down's syndrome) makes a screening test aimed at detecting those babies at high risk of Down's syndrome. The results are expressed as medians of the mean and related to the age and weight of the mother. The test result is given as a risk and a test is considered positive if the risk is greater than 1:250. The test is gestation dependent so the woman must have a dating scan to confirm the gestation of the baby and she must be aware that the result only gives the risk of the baby having Down's syndrome and this is not a diagnosis. The test will detect seven out of 10 babies with Down's syndrome but may give a false positive result (i.e. a high risk with a normal baby) or a false negative result (i.e. a low risk with an abnormal baby). Women with a positive result are offered amniocentesis to get fetal cells and so make a definitive karyotypic diagnosis.

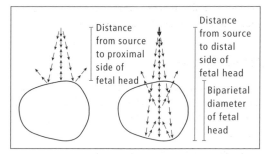

**Figure 9.4** From the combined source and receiver, the transducer, the ultrasound impulses go out in straight lines. Only those which strike reflective surfaces at right angles will return along the same path. Hence the highest and lowest points of the fetal skull may be determined. The distance between them can be measured to a sensitivity of 1 mm.

## Nuchal translucency

More recently, a test becoming increasingly used is the measurement of the nuchal (behind the neck) fat pad of the baby. The measurement is done by ultrasound scan at between 11 and 13 weeks. It gives a risk, similar to that of the triple test, but can pick up fetuses with other trisomies or congenital heart disease. Since it is done earlier the women whose fetuses are at high risk of abnormality may be offered chorionic villus sampling.

## Routine anomaly ultrasound scanning (18–20 weeks)

Most hospitals in the UK now offer a routine ultrasound examination at 18–20 weeks' gestation. The aim of this ultrasound examination is:
• To establish gestational age.
• To exclude major structural abnormalities of the fetus.
• To diagnose multiple pregnancy.

A small pulse of ultrasound is sent into the tissues and a recorder in the same transducer, then detects the echoes. The distance between tissue boundaries can be assessed by determining the differences in time taken for the echoes to return from each boundary (Fig. 9.4).

At the 18–20-week routine ultrasound visit, the following are assessed:

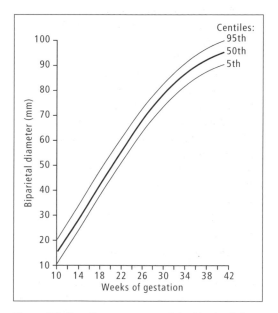

**Figure 9.5** Growth measurement of the biparietal diameter to determine the gestational age.

• The biparietal diameter (BPD; Fig. 9.5).
• The head circumference (HC).
• The abdominal circumference (AC).
• Femur length (FL).

These measurements are used to confirm the gestational age of the fetus. The EDD may be changed if the measurements are more than two weeks greater or smaller than the 50th centile at 18–20 weeks.

The later the scan is done the less accurate dating by ultrasound becomes and caution should be exercised before changing the EDD if the first scan is done after 22 weeks.

The ultrasound scan will detect the following:

• Multiple pregnancy.

• Placental site—particularly low-lying placenta (5% at 20 weeks but 0.5% at 34 weeks when the scan should be repeated).

• Fetal congenital abnormalities:

  • Anencephaly (absent top of the head and brain).

  • Spina bifida.

  • Double bubble of dilated stomach and duodenum in duodenal atresia (common in Down's syndrome).

  • Some cardiac abnormalities (Fallot's tetralogy, ventricular septal defect (VSD), atrial septal defect (ASD)).

  • Hydrocephaly.

  • Renal pelvic dilatation (outflow obstruction—urethral valves in boys).

• Sacral agenesis (insulin-dependent diabetics).

• Major limb defects (dwarfism).

• The ultrasound scan is the first time that parents see their baby and it is known to increase the bonding that they feel towards their baby.

## Third trimester assessment

### Maternal assessment of fetal movement

• The mother counts ten fetal movements entering them on a chart (Fig. 9.6). She is asked to start counting fetal movements from 9.00 a.m. and then to record the time by which she has felt ten movements. If this is later than 9.00 p.m. she is asked to report for further examination with a cardiotocograph (CTG).

Current evidence suggests that maternal appreciation of fetal movements is of value in high-risk pregnancies but does not seem to prevent unexplained stillbirths in pregnancies thought to be at low risk.

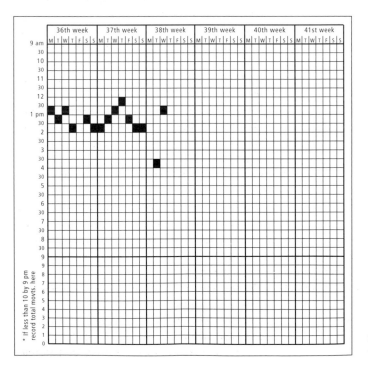

**Figure 9.6** The Cardiff count-to-ten fetal activity chart (see text).

## Biochemical tests

These tests have largely been replaced by biophysical methods of monitoring fetal health because of:
• A wide range of normal values obtained in pregnancy.
• The errors in laboratory measurement.
• The need, in most cases, for serial testing.
These tests used to include measurement of oestriol and human placental lactogen (HPL) but are rarely used in modern obstetric units.

## Biophysical methods

These may be considered as:
1 Short-term methods.
   • The biophysical profile.
   • The CTG.
   • Doppler studies of the fetal circulation.
2 Medium-term methods.
   • Measurements of fetal growth.
   • Doppler measurements of the uteroplacental circulation.

### Short-term methods

*The biophysical profile*
Ultrasound examination of the following features composes the biophysical profile:
• Fetal movements.
• Fetal breathing movements.
• Fetal tone.
• The amniotic fluid volume.
• The CTG.
Each element is scored 0, 1 or 2 over 40 minutes giving a maximum possible score of 10. A score of <6 is evidence of fetal compromise and delivery should be considered.

The biophysical profile is not used routinely in the UK, but is useful in high-risk pregnancies particularly after intrauterine growth retardation has been detected. Measurement of the amniotic fluid volume is one of the most sensitive measures of fetal well-being and a significant reduction is associated with a poor outcome for the baby.

*The CTG*
An antenatal record of the fetal heart rate is recorded with Doppler ultrasound. In addition, fetal movements and uterine activity are measured by an external pressure transducer. A mnemonic, DR C BRAVADO, has been developed to ensure a more standard evaluation of the CTG by doctors and midwives. The date (D) and reason/risk (R) for doing the CTG should be recorded on the CTG printout as well as the name, date of birth (DOB) and hospital number of the patient. The frequency and strength of contractions (C) should be recorded in the woman's notes or on the partogram (see p. 160).

The essential features of the CTG are:
1 *The baseline rate* (BR). Between 110 and 160 beats/minute (bpm), with a variability of 5–15 bpm. Rates outside these limits are extremely rare antenatally.
   • Baseline bradycardia usually suggests congenital heart disease.
   • Fetal tachycardias are seen in the presence of anything that causes a rise in the maternal pulse rate such as a maternal pyrexia. In the absence of a maternal cause, the fetal tachycardia should be taken as a sign of fetal distress.
2 *Acceleration* (A). In a 20-minute recording, the fetus normally produces an acceleration at least twice (Fig. 9.7). An acceleration is a rise in fetal heart rate of 15 bpm above the baseline that is sustained for more than 15 seconds.

A CTG that shows two or more accelerations in a 20-minute period is considered reactive. Non-reactive traces should not last more than 20 minutes in the third trimester.
3 *Variability* (VA) (Fig. 9.8). The fetal heart rate from 26 weeks is controlled by a balance between the sympathetic and parasympathetic nervous system resulting in a natural variability of 5–15 bpm.

Baseline heart rate variation of less than 5 bpm is rarely seen antenatally although it may follow drugs such as diazepam or night sedation.

In the absence of drugs it may indicate fetal distress.
4 *Decelerations* (D). Antenatal decelerations in the fetal heart rate that are not associated with contractions are of serious significance and should

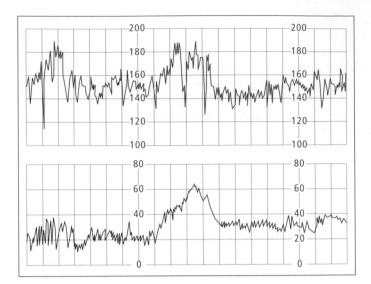

**Figure 9.7** Acceleration of fetal heart rate (above) with uterine contraction (below).

**Figure 9.8** Antenatal CTG showing loss of baseline variability.

indicate delivery taken in association with other factors.

**5** *Overall impression* (O). Reassuring or non-reassuring. This final conclusion leads the doctor or midwife to make decisions about the management of the pregnancy. Senior medical staff must be involved in the decision making if the CTG is non-reassuring as it may reflect fetal distress. It should be remembered that the CTG is only one of many parameters for assessing fetal well-being and even non-reassuring CTGs are sometimes associated with a perfectly healthy, well oxygenated, baby. Examples of non-reassuring CTG traces are shown in Chapter 12.

There is no universal agreement as to how frequently the CTG should be performed. As with many other things in obstetrics, it should be planned and interpreted in the light of the woman's circumstances, e.g. if there has been a small unexplained antepartum haemorrhage (APH) only a daily CTG is required, but a growth-retarded baby in a woman with severe hypertension may warrant two or even three CTGs per day.

At present, the predictive value of a normal CTG is in doubt.

*Doppler waveforms from the fetal circulation*

If sound is aimed at a moving target, the echoes that return from the target will have shifted in frequency—the Doppler shift. The blood cells moving in the umbilical artery can be readily detected by Doppler ultrasound and in normal pregnancies produce the waveform shown in Fig. 9.9a.

If resistance increases in the placenta, e.g. in pre-eclampsia, Doppler-shifted frequencies are not recordable in the last part of diastole (absence of end-diastolic frequencies). Figure 9.9b demonstrates this phenomenon.

In a few babies, there may be a reversal of frequencies in end-diastole (Fig. 9.9c) indicating that blood which should be flowing towards the placenta for exchange of $O_2$ and nutrients is flowing backwards towards the baby. This means that the baby may die soon and delivery should be expedited.

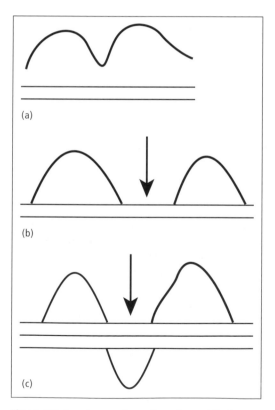

**Figure 9.9** Doppler waveforms from the umbilical artery reflecting resistance to flow (impedance) in the fetal vessels of the placenta. (a) Normal. (b) Loss of end-diastolic frequencies (arrowed)—increased resistance. (c) Reversed frequencies (arrowed)—much increased resistance.

### Medium-term methods

*Measurements of fetal growth*

Measurements of fetal growth are best achieved by measurements of the head circumference and the abdominal circumference. Real-time ultrasound can be used to determine fetal growth in one of three ways:

**1** To determine size when the fetus is thought clinically to be small.

**2** As a screening test for small babies. Some hospitals now offer a second ultrasound examination at 30–34 weeks' gestation to measure the fetal abdominal circumference. If this is not low, the baby only has a small chance (approximately 10%) of being small for gestational age (SGA) at birth.

**3** Serial measurements of fetal growth. Women at risk of having a SGA fetus should have serial ultrasound (fortnightly) to document the growth velocity of their babies.

*Doppler waveforms from the uteroplacental circulation*

Waveforms may be recorded from the maternal arcuate arteries, the first branches of the uterine arteries.

Failure of invasion results in a persistence of a high-resistance waveform (a notch) rather than the development of the usual low-resistance waveforms. Women with persistently high-resistance waveforms have a high probability of developing pre-eclampsia and an asymmetrical SGA fetus.

Antioxidants (vitamin C and E) have been shown to reduce the incidence of pre-eclamptic toxaemia/pregnancy-induced hypertension (PET/PIH) (see Chapter 10).

## Definition of terms

There is much confusion in the obstetric literature over the terms used to signify that the baby is small. These terms are:

• *Low birth weight (LBW)*. This term is used for a baby with a birth weight of <2500 g. This term is most useful on a worldwide basis where gestational age at delivery is often unknown. It is obvious that a baby who is <2500 g at birth may be preterm, or small, or both. Neonatal paediatricians have extended this classification to very low birth weight (VLBW) babies which indicates a birth weight of <1500 g and extremely low birth weight (ELBW) babies with a birth weight of under 1000 g.

• *Intrauterine growth restriction (IUGR)*. IUGR is the presence of a pathology that is slowing fetal growth, which if it could be removed would allow the resumption of normal fetal growth. There are no tests available antenatally or postnatally to determine whether a baby has truly suffered from IUGR although the ratio of the HC:AC on ultrasound scan (USS) may help.

• *Small for gestational age (SGA)*. This is a statistical definition used if the infant's birth weight is below a certain standard for the gestational age. There is no universally agreed standard and such lower limits as the tenth, the fifth and the third centile, alternatively two standard deviations from the mean have all been used. As the definition is statistical, one should expect for example that 10% of the normal population of babies have birth weights of less than the tenth centile. To interpret the birth weight, it is necessary to have charts derived from the local population being measured.

The term SGA is also applied antenatally when the growth or size of the fetus falls below statistically determined limits on population-derived charts.

## The SGA fetus

In broad terms, impairment of fetal growth can be:

• Symmetrical SGA (Fig. 9.10). In this case the measurements of the fetal head and abdominal circumference are equally small. The baby is a miniature baby. The vast majority of these babies represent the biological lower limits of normal. Causes of symmetrical SGA are shown in Table 9.2.

• Asymmetrical SGA (Fig. 9.11). This is a rarer form of impaired fetal growth, the causes of which are also shown in Table 9.2. The abdominal circumference slows its growth relative to the increase in head circumference. This is secondary to the fetus using the stores of brown fat normally laid down around the liver for nutrition of the baby in the first few days of life. In many cases, abnormal growth is associated with absence of end-diastolic flow in the umbilical circulation. Such babies are at risk of antenatal hypoxia which may result in stillbirth, neonatal death or major mental disability.

The differential growth patterns in these fetuses result from a redistribution of fetal blood flow. In response to underperfusion in the intervillous

**Figure 9.10** Symmetrical SGA measurements of (a) fetal head circumference (HC) and (b) fetal abdominal circumference (AC). HC: AC ratio = 1.0.

**Table 9.2** Causes of babies who are small for gestational age (SGA)

| Symmetrical SGA (60%) | Asymmetrical SGA (40%) |
|---|---|
| Race (white > black > Asian)<br>Sex (boy > girl)<br>Maternal size<br>Toxins<br>• alcohol<br>• cigarettes<br>• heroin<br>• methadone<br>Congenital infections<br>• cytomegalovirus<br>• parvovirus<br>• rubella<br>• syphilis<br>• toxoplasmosis<br>Malnutrition | Poor maternal response to<br>• pregnancy<br>• pre-eclampsia<br>• poor trophoblast invasion<br>Cigarettes<br>Drug abuse<br>Chromosomal and congenital abnormalities |

**Figure 9.11** Asymmetrical SGA measurements of (a) fetal head circumference and (b) fetal abdominal circumference.

space, there is an increase in resistance to blood flow within the fetal circulation. This means that blood returning from the placenta to the fetus takes the path of least resistance and is diverted to the fetal brain, coronary arteries and adrenals. Initially, this is to the benefit of the fetus but, if it continues for too long, then the fetal bowel, kidneys and liver become ischaemic resulting in the complications of asymmetrical SGA babies: necrotizing enterocolitis, renal failure and failure of coagulation due to insufficient production of coagulation factors by the liver.

## Management of SGA

### Symmetrical SGA

Most SGA fetuses represent the biological lower limits of the normal range and only require serial measurements of ultrasound growth performed on a fortnightly basis. If the baby demonstrates normal growth (see Fig. 9.10), no further action is necessary.

The only problem posed for the obstetrician is to recognize those few babies that are congenitally abnormal or infected. The following actions are recommended:
• Check maternal blood for infections that are known to cross the placenta (syphilis, toxoplasmosis, rubella, parvovirus and cytomegalovirus).
• Search the fetus carefully with ultrasound looking for structural markers that may suggest a chromosome abnormality. If these are present the baby should be karyotyped, usually by means of a fetal blood sample obtained from the umbilical cord (cordocentesis). This is of value even in the third trimester as it is well known that fetuses with trisomies are prone to fetal distress in labour. If the trisomy is lethal then, after discussion with the parents, a Caesarean section may not be advised should such distress develop.

### Asymmetrical SGA (IUGR)

Management should be:
• Fortnightly ultrasound measurements of head circumference and abdominal circumference to determine growth rate.

The amniotic fluid volume should be measured by determining the height of the largest column of fluid or the addition of a column from the four quadrants of the uterus giving an amniotic fluid index. The former is normally between 2 and 8 cm. Less than 2 cm suggests increasing fetal compromise.
• Doppler waveforms from the umbilical circulation. If these are normal they should be repeated on a weekly basis. Delivery is not indicated in the presence of normal umbilical artery waveforms. Absent end-diastolic flow should indicate delivery in a fetus that is considered to be viable, >24 weeks, >500 g.
• In the absence of Doppler waveforms, immediate fetal well-being should be monitored by daily CTGs and maternal counting of fetal movement. Delivery is indicated for cessation of fetal growth over a 4-week period, for abnormalities of the CTG, significant reduction in fetal movements.

### Self-assessment

**9.1** Mrs Walker is 36-weeks pregnant in her first pregnancy. Please examine her and give your conclusions to the examiner. (Mannequins are available to practise on, although ideally you should perform the examination on a woman in the antenatal clinic, having asked her permission to do so first. Remember that you should always have a female chaperone with you whenever you examine a woman.) As you examine the woman run through the examination and present to a clinician or fellow student who will score against the checklist in Answers to self-assessment questions, p. 312.

**9.2** Which of the following investigations are performed at the first antenatal visit in the UK?
(a) Toxoplasmosis.
(b) Rubella.
(c) Cytomegalovirus (CMV).
(d) Syphilis.
(e) Hepatitis A.

**9.3** Which of the following are used as indicators of fetal well-being beyond 24 weeks of pregnancy?
(a) Liquor volume.
(b) Fetal lie.
(c) Fetal movements.
(d) Uterine artery dopplers.
(e) Umbilical artery dopplers.

**Self-assessment** *Continued*

**9.4** A woman presents at 12 weeks of pregnancy. She has had two livebirths at term, delivered a live baby at 21 weeks who died within a few minutes of birth, one pregnancy loss at 8 weeks and an intrauterine death at 25 weeks. Which one of the following correctly expresses her gravidity and parity?

(a) Gravida 6 Para 4 + 1.

(b) Gravida 6 Para 3 + 2.

(c) Gravida 5 Para 3 + 2.

(d) Gravida 5 Para 4 + 1.

(e) Gravida 6 Para 5 + 0.

# Chapter 10

# Diseases of pregnancy

## Hyperemesis gravidarum

*Incidence*
Less than 1 : 1000 pregnancies in UK; a rare condition in the endogenous population.

*Aetiology*
• Hormonal—rapid increase in hCG and progesterone; hypothyroidism.
• Reflex—a chemosensitive trigger zone which stimulates the vomiting centre.
• Ketosis—after excess vomiting, build up of ketones exacerbates the vomiting and a vicious circle develops.
• Hydatidiform mole—very high hCG levels.

*Progress*
Can lead to:
• Dehydration.
• Hypovolaemia.
• Electrolyte depletion.
• Vitamin deficiency, particularly thiamine.
• Death from liver failure or the end processes of the above.

*Presentation*
• Cannot retain food or fluid.
• Weight loss because of loss of body fluid and burning up of fat.
• Haemoconcentration and unstable acid–base balance.
• Ketosis.

*Management*
1 Exclude other diseases:
• Urinary infection.
• Hiatus hernia and gall bladder disease.
• Obstructive gut lesions.
• Central nervous system (CNS)-expanding lesions.
2 Exclude obstetric cause:
• Multiple pregnancy.
• Hydatidiform mole.
• Acute yellow atrophy of the liver.
3 Restore fluid and electrolyte balance intravenously (i.v.).
4 Specific anti-vomiting drugs, e.g. cyclizine or Maxolon.
5 Thiamine to prevent Wernicke's encephalopathy.
6 Steroid therapy—being assessed.
7 Psychological treatment—most respond to suggestion. If not, formal psychotherapy is needed.
8 Therapeutic abortion—very rarely required.

## Hypertensive disorders of pregnancy

Hypertension has these risks:
• In the *mother*.
• Cerebrovascular accident.
• Renal failure.
• Heart failure.
• Coagulation failure.

- Liver failure.
- Adrenal failure.
- Eclampsia: a generalized convulsive disorder like epilepsy but which is peculiar to pregnancy.
- In the *fetus*:
  - Asymmetrical intrauterine growth restriction.
  - Placental abruption.
  - Iatrogenic preterm delivery.

### Definitions

The currently internationally agreed definition of hypertensive disease in pregnancy is:

- Pregnancy-induced hypertension (PIH): hypertension occurring for the first time after 20 weeks' gestation.

Hypertension in pregnancy is defined as one of the following:

- Blood pressure of 140/90 mmHg on two occasions more than 4 hours apart.
- A rise of more than 30 mmHg in systolic blood pressure over the booking blood pressure.
- A rise of more than 15 mmHg in diastolic blood pressure over the booking figure.

PIH may be classified as:

- *Mild*: a blood pressure up to 140/100 mmHg without proteinuria.
- *Moderate*: a blood pressure up to 160/110 mmHg without proteinuria. In the absence of proteinuria PIH is rarely dangerous to mother or fetus.
- *Severe*: a blood pressure of more than 160/110 mmHg; and the presence of proteinuria (pre-eclampsia/pre-eclamptic toxaemia (PET)).

Proteinuria in pregnancy is defined as the following:

- More than 300 mg on a 24-hour collection of urine.
- Oedema associated with hypertension and proteinuria is a sign of worsening pre-eclampsia. Oedema alone is of little significance.

### Prevalence

This varies with the population but in the UK 10–15% of primigravid women will develop some form of hypertension. Of these, about 6% may be considered as suffering from PIH and 2% will develop pre-eclampsia.

PIH is almost entirely a disease of primigravidae. Pre-eclampsia only occurs in multigravid women under the following conditions:

- Those who have had it severely in the first pregnancy.
- Those who have changed their partner between pregnancies.
- Pregnancies complicated by hydatidiform mole.
- Multiple pregnancies.
- Gestational diabetes.
- Those with antiphospholipid syndrome.

### Aetiology

The precise mechanism is unknown; the following are recognized:

- Women who develop pre-eclampsia have a failure of the second wave of trophoblastic invasion.
- This failure probably leads to a local alteration of the prostacyclin:thromboxane ratio. Both these prostaglandins are produced by trophoblast and exert opposite effects. In PIH, the balance of the ratio appears to favour thromboxane. This leads to local vasoconstriction and platelet agglutination on already undilated vessels.
- The combination of the above two factors is associated with failure of the initial fall in peripheral resistance and hence blood pressure in midpregnancy is maintained—it normally shows a marked fall. Subsequent narrowing or clotting of the abnormal blood vessels leads to a further increase in peripheral resistance and hence hypertension.
- The narrowing of the blood vessels also leads to decreased perfusion of the intervillous space and hence the development of an asymmetrical small for gestational age (SGA) fetus.

Antioxidants (vitamin C and E) in pregnancy have been shown to reduce the prevalence of pre-eclampsia in women who are at high risk—previous early onset of PET, women with antiphospholipid syndrome.

### Clinical course

PIH usually presents in primigravidae in the late third trimester. It usually requires either no treatment or anti-hypertensive therapy alone while awaiting the onset of labour. Occasionally this progresses to the development of pre-eclampsia. A few women present with the symptoms and signs of pre-eclampsia and occasionally this can occur in the late second or early third trimester. The presence of symptoms, rising blood pressure or increasing proteinuria heralds the onset of fulminating pre-eclampsia and requires prompt treatment and delivery to prevent the development of eclampsia and renal/cerebral damage (Table 10.1).

## Mild disease

Women with mild PIH may be discharged from hospital and assessed as out-patients if:
• The blood pressure remains below 140/100 mmHg.
• They do not develop proteinuria.
• The fetus does not demonstrate asymmetrical SGA.

The woman's blood pressure should be monitored at least twice a week and fetal growth should be monitored fortnightly by ultrasound. If the condition does not deteriorate, it is difficult to justify induction of labour although few obstetricians

would be prepared to let these women go past 40 weeks' gestation.

## Moderate disease

All primigravidae who have a sustained blood pressure of 140/90 mmHg or more should be monitored in a day assessment unit or in hospital as the subsequent course of their disease cannot be predicted. In the absence of rapidly progressive disease, the following management features are relevant.

*Maternal*
**1** *Measurement of blood pressure.* There is no evidence that treating maternal blood pressure with anti-hypertensive drugs alters the course of the pre-eclamptic disease process or improves the prognosis of the fetus, but treatment is indicated to protect the maternal circulation. Sustained blood pressures of more than 160/100 mmHg would therefore indicate treatment, unless delivery was imminent. The current choice of therapy is oral

**Table 10.1** Pregnancy-induced hypertension.

|  | Mild | Moderate | Severe (pre-eclampsia) |
|---|---|---|---|
| *Symptoms* | None | Mild headache | Frontal headache |
|  |  | Oedema | Oedema ++ |
|  |  |  | Visual disturbance |
| *Signs* |  |  |  |
| BP | <140/100 | <160/110 | >160/110 |
| Proteinuria | None | None | ++ or +++ |
| Reflexes | Normal | Normal | Hyper-reflexia/clonus |
| Fundi | Normal | Normal | Occasional papilloedema |
| Renal | Normal | Normal | Decreasing urinary output |
| *Bloods* |  |  |  |
| FBC | Normal | Normal | Rising or falling Hb |
|  |  |  | Decreasing platelets |
| Urate | Normal | Slightly raised | Increasing |
| LFTs | Normal | Normal | Increasing |
| Clotting | Normal | Normal | Prolonged |
| *Fetus* | Normal | Normal/SGA | Asymmetric SGA |
| *Treatment* | None | Anti-hypertensives | Anti-hypertensives |
|  |  |  | Anti-epileptics/MgSO$_4$ |
|  |  | ? Delivery | Delivery |

FBC, full blood count; LFTs, liver function tests; SGA, small for gestational age.

methyldopa, nifedipine or labetalol but magnesium sulphate is now being used more.

**2** *Assessment of maternal renal function.* All patients should have:

- Urinary protein (daily).
- Plasma urea and electrolyte estimation (weekly).
- Plasma urate levels (weekly).
- Total urinary protein excretion (once).
- Liver function tests (twice weekly).
- Full blood count and clotting screen.

A rising urate (>0.35), urinary 24-hour protein excretion >300 mg/24 h or haemoglobin level indicates haemoconcentration. These are signs of fulminating pre-eclampsia and delivery should be considered. Rising liver enzymes (aspartate aminotransferase, AST; alanine aminotransferase, ALT), a falling haemoglobin and/or platelets are signs of the development of HELLP syndrome (Haemolysis, Elevated Liver Enzymes, Low Platelets) and are an indication for immediate delivery as these women are at high risk of developing eclampsia and liver failure.

FETAL WELL-BEING

- Real-time ultrasound assessment of fetal size. If this indicates asymmetrical SGA then carry out:

 (a) daily or twice daily cardiotocographs (CTGs) (minimum 1 hour each time);

 (b) a weekly examination of the umbilical circulation by Doppler ultrasound.

 (c) Doppler waveforms from utero-placental circulation.

In moderate disease, delivery is indicated for:

- Progression to pre-eclampsia.
- Declining maternal renal function.
- Fetal distress, which usually means an abnormal CTG or absence of end-diastolic flow in the Doppler measurement of the umbilical circulation.
- Placental abruption.

In the absence of the above features, most obstetricians would consider inducing the pregnancy after 38 weeks' gestation, if the cervix is favourable and neonatal facilities are adequate.

## Severe or fulminating pre-eclampsia

*Symptoms*
- *Frontal and often occipital headache* due to cerebral oedema. The headache is dragging or throbbing in nature and is worse when the woman is supine. It occurs classically first thing in the morning and resolves to some extent during the day if the patient is mobile.
- *Visual disturbances* due to oedema of the optic nerve or the retina consisting of black holes in the visual field or double vision.
- *Epigastric pain.* This is due to stretching of the liver capsule.

*Signs*
- *Hyper-reflexia and clonus.* This is due to the cerebral oedema and gives the clinical picture of an upper motor neurone lesion.

Hyper-reflexia, in obstetric terms, is defined as the ability to obtain the reflex away from the tendon that usually causes it, e.g. the knee jerk reflex occurs by tapping the anterior surface of the tibia rather than the infrapatellar tendon.

Clonus in obstetric terms is only considered serious if it is sustained for more than four beats.
- *A rapid rise in blood pressure.*
- *Rapid increase in proteinuria.*
- *Decreasing urine output.*

*Treatment*
This disease process starts to reverse as soon as the placenta is delivered and hence the solution to fulminating pre-eclampsia is to end the pregnancy. Before this happens, the maternal condition must be prevented from worsening:
- Control the maternal blood pressure. At present this is done by the use of i.v. hydralazine or labetalol.
- Prevent maternal fits with magnesium sulphate or i.v. diazepam.

Having controlled the blood pressure and reduced the risk of fitting, the baby should be delivered preferably vaginally but indications for Caesarean section are:
- An unfavourable cervix.
- An abnormal fetal position such as a breech presentation.

- Fetal distress.
- Abruption of the placenta.
- A failed induction.
- Difficulty in controlling the maternal blood pressure.

*Prognosis*

MATERNAL

In the absence of eclampsia, maternal mortality should be low, but it must be remembered that pre-eclampsia is one of the leading factors of maternal death, even in developed countries (7.5/10$^6$ maternities, 1997–99). Maternal morbidity may occur from subsequently badly managed fluid balance. If the woman can be helped over the first 48 hours after delivery without serious injury, then the disease rapidly gets better. This is usually indicated by a diuresis. Usually no permanent long-term renal or vascular damage follows pre-eclampsia.

FETAL

The perinatal mortality rate (PNMR) increases with the severity of the disease, but may be summarized as follows:
- Mild: no change in PNMR.
- Moderate: slightly increased depending upon gestation at birth.
- Severe: double PNMR.
- Severe pre-eclampsia superimposed on PIH: treble PNMR.

The morbidity to the baby is difficult to quantify as it depends upon the gestation at delivery and the fetal size (Chapter 23).

## Eclampsia

Eclampsia is characterized by epileptiform fits associated with hypertension of a moderate to severe degree. In the UK it is rare with a prevalence of about 1:3000 deliveries. Worldwide it is usually preceded by pre-eclampsia, but the quality of antenatal care in the UK now is such that three-quarters of cases of eclampsia occur without pre-existing recorded evidence of hypertension.

*Prevalence*

In the UK the disease is rare because of:

1 Better antenatal care which has led to earlier recognition of pre-eclampsia.
2 More aggressive treatment of pre-eclampsia which has lessened the incidence of subsequent eclampsia.
- The rate of eclampsia may be taken as a guide to antenatal care—to its availability, usage and quality.
- Less than 1% of women in the UK with moderate or severe PIH will go on to develop eclampsia.

*Aetiology*
- Cerebral oedema.
- Cerebral vasoconstriction.
- Cerebral hypoxia.
These lead to cerebral ischaemia and hence fits.

*Clinical course*

At present in the UK about 25% of women with eclampsia will have a fit before labour; most of the rest are likely to have a fit in the postpartum period. The character of the fit is very similar to an epileptic fit with a typical fit consisting of:
- Twitching: 30 seconds.
- Tonic phase: 30 seconds.
- Clonic phase: 2 minutes.
- Coma: 10–30 minutes.
Such fits may repeat frequently.

*Treatment*

AIMS
- Keep the woman alive during the fit.
- Prevent more fits.
- Deliver the baby.

PREVENTION
- Magnesium sulphate reduces the incidence and severity of fits.

DURING THE FIT
- Turn the woman on her side.
- Maintain the airway.
- Stop the fit by giving i.v. diazepam and magnesium sulphate.

• Prevent further fits. This is usually done by giving a continuous infusion of magnesium sulphate or diazepam.
• If the woman is not in hospital, arrange an emergency transfer giving adequate anticonvulsants to cover the journey.
• Lower the blood pressure by use of i.v. hydralazine, labetalol or magnesium sulphate.
• Deliver the baby. As with fulminating PIH, such women are best if the baby is delivered vaginally, as this speeds the recovery process. The indications for Caesarean section are those listed in the section on pre-eclampsia.

*Prognosis*

MATERNAL MORTALITY

In the UK death from eclampsia is rare with the woman more likely to die from the hypertensive effects on the cerebral circulation from a cerebrovascular accident.

FETAL MORTALITY

During an eclamptic fit: 300/1000. Overall: 150/1000 intrauterine deaths from hypoxia or neonatal death from prematurity.

## Rhesus (Rh) incompatibility (Box 10.1)

### Rh genes

The Rh genes are carried on a pair of chromosomes. There are six Rh antigens (*C, D, E, c, d, e*) of which *D* and *d* are the most important, for upon these depend whether a person is designated Rh-positive or Rh-negative.

The individual making these gametes may be heterozygous if some of the gametes contain *c, d, e* and others *C, D, E*, or the person may be homozygous if all gametes carry *c, d, e*.

There is no problem if the woman is Rh-positive, even if her partner is a Rh-negative man; if homozygous, all her children will be Rh-positive;

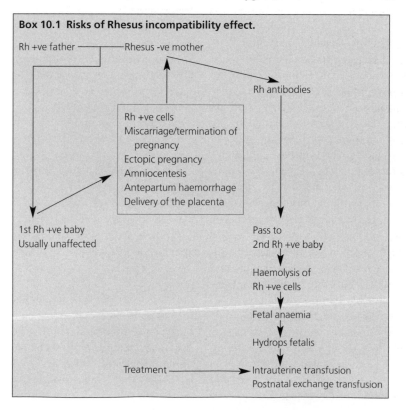

Box 10.1 Risks of Rhesus incompatibility effect.

Rh +ve father —— Rhesus -ve mother

Rh antibodies

Rh +ve cells
Miscarriage/termination of pregnancy
Ectopic pregnancy
Amniocentesis
Antepartum haemorrhage
Delivery of the placenta

1st Rh +ve baby
Usually unaffected

Pass to
2nd Rh +ve baby

Haemolysis of
Rh +ve cells

Fetal anaemia

Hydrops fetalis

Treatment —— Intrauterine transfusion
Postnatal exchange transfusion

if heterozygous, she may have a Rh-negative child but that is no problem.

Should she be Rh-negative and her partner homozygous Rh-positive (35% of the male population), she will always have a Rh-positive child and there may be problems.

He may be heterozygous Rh-positive (65% of the male population) producing equal numbers of Rh-positive and Rh-negative gametes having equal chances of giving his Rh-negative partner a Rh-positive or a Rh-negative child.

## Immunization

A Rh-positive mother cannot be immunized against the Rh factor and so there are no problems for her and her baby.

The Rh-negative woman can be affected if she is inoculated with Rh-positive blood. The Rh *gp* antigens evoke an antibody response against the Rh *gp* (most marked against the *D* antigen—anti-*D*).

In Rh-negative women the inoculation of Rh-positive cells can occur from:
• The passage of red cells from a Rh-positive baby.
• An incomplete cross-matched transfusion.

The former is more likely in a major fetomaternal bleed which may occur in the following situations: antepartum haemorrhage (APH), spontaneous miscarriage, ectopic pregnancy, therapeutic abortion, amniocentesis, external cephalic version (ECV), but most commonly during the third stage of labour when the placenta separates from the uterine wall.

In most Rh-incompatible pregnancies no antibody is formed until after the first fetomaternal bleed most commonly in the third stage of labour and, consequently, the baby of the first pregnancy is unaffected.

In subsequent pregnancies, if the fetus is Rh-positive, small fetomaternal bleeds may evoke a major secondary antibody response. Large amounts of antibody (immunoglobulin G (IgG)) cross the placenta and can cause increasingly severe Rh disease in successive pregnancies if the fetus is Rh-positive. The antibody weakens the envelopes of the fetal red cells, which are then broken down in the spleen. Depending on the speed and degree of cell breakdown, this can produce:

1 Fetal anaemia.
2 Hyperbilirubinaemia. *In utero* the excess bilirubin is removed across the placenta to the maternal circulation but following delivery the bilirubin accumulates and so the infant becomes jaundiced.
3 Oedema.

*Clinical picture*
This can vary.
• The fetus may die *in utero* if the anaemia is severe enough.
• The infant may be born grossly anaemic and oedematous with hepato-splenomegaly—hydrops fetalis. There is a rapid rise in bilirubin following birth. Jaundice develops rapidly within the first 24 hours of life.
• The infant can be anaemic and continues to break down red blood cells after delivery as the maternal Rh antibodies are still circulating in his blood, and so can become more anaemic and jaundiced during the postnatal period.

*Management*

PREVENTION
• Either give 500 iu anti-*D* immunoglobulin to all Rh-negative women at 26 and 34 weeks;
• Or be selective and give 500 iu anti-*D* immunoglobulin if she has a:
  • Therapeutic abortion.
  • Spontaneous abortion/ectopic pregnancy.
  • Amniocentesis.
  • Any bleeding in pregnancy/threatened miscarriage.
  • ECV.
  • After delivery at any gestation.

The former is now the recommended programme for prevention of Rh disease.

VARIABLE DOSES
• After delivery of a baby to a Rh-negative mother, the baby's blood group should be checked and a Kleihauer test performed on the maternal blood. Acid is added to the maternal blood; fetal cells are resistant to destruction in acid so the amount of fetal blood that has entered the maternal circulation can be calculated. If the baby's blood group is

positive the dose of anti-*D* is adjusted to ensure that all the Rh-positive fetal cells are destroyed without sensitizing the mother. This prevents the development of Rh disease in the next baby.

DETECT AT-RISK FETUS
- Maternal Rh screening, anti-*D* antibody titres.
- Ultrasound scan to detect hydrops fetalis — oedema of the skin, pleural effusion, ascites, hepato-splenomegaly, cardiac enlargement.
- Amniocentesis or cordocentesis is performed under ultrasound guidance. 10 ml of amniotic fluid (AF) or 5 ml fetal blood is removed. The content of bilirubin is measured by spectrometry (AF) or directly in the serum and the haemoglobin can be measured in the blood. If the bilirubin is raised in the amniotic fluid the need for a transfusion is calculated from a Lilley's at-risk graph.

*History*
1 Check history of:
   - Previous transfusion.
   - Jaundiced babies.
   - Exchange transfusions.
   - Hydrops.
   - Stillbirth or neonatal death.
2 Check all Rh-negative pregnant women for anti-*D* and, if above 20 iu/l, perform an indirect Coombs' test.
Check:
- On booking.
- If negative at booking, at 26 and 34 weeks.
- If positive at booking, at 20, 24, 28, 32 and 36 weeks or more frequently if rapidly rising.
If antibody titre rises above 1 : 8 by 20 weeks, do an amniocentesis.

To reduce risks carry out amnio/cordocentesis under ultrasound guidance. Remove 10 ml AF or 5 ml of fetal blood. Check for haemoglobin and bilirubin.
3 Check cord blood immediately after birth for:
   - ABO group and Rh group.
   - Haemoglobin.
   - Direct Coombs' test.
   - Bilirubin.

*Treatment*
- Intrauterine transfusion.
- Elect time of delivery.
- Exchange transfusion after delivery.
- Phototherapy after delivery.
- Top-up transfusion.

INTRAUTERINE TRANSFUSION
In very severe Rh disease the fetus can die *in utero* from anaemia and hydrops before he can be delivered. An intrauterine transfusion can prolong the life *in utero* of an infant to a gestation where the risks of prematurity are estimated as being less than those of the Rh disease. This can be done by an:
1 Intraperitoneal transfusion guided by ultrasound.
2 Umbilical vein transfusion guided by ultrasound.

Rh-negative blood is either transfused under ultrasound control into the fetal peritoneal cavity, or into an umbilical vein. Repeat as necessary, according to amniotic optical density, or fetal haematocrit. The intravenous route is becoming increasingly the preferred method.

CHOOSE TIME OF INDUCTION AND BEST METHOD OF DELIVERY
Balance the risks of prematurity (too soon) with that of worsening Rh disease (too late). Consider the risks of vaginal delivery and be prepared for a lower segment Caesarean section (LSCS). The paediatric team should be in close liaison and a senior paediatrician present at the delivery with fresh Rh-negative blood available.

RESUSCITATION AND EXCHANGE TRANSFUSION
Good resuscitation is essential. In an anaemic and premature infant, lung disease is common. It can be due to:
- Surfactant deficiency at very early delivery.
- Pulmonary oedema from anaemia and hypoproteinaemia.
- Hypoplastic lungs secondary to pleural effusions.
   In severe Rh haemolytic disease of the newborn, an umbilical artery catheter should be inserted as soon as possible to assess and control $Pao_2$ and pH.
- Central venous pressure should be measured.
- Drain pleural effusions and ascites at resuscitation.

INDICATIONS FOR EXCHANGE TRANSFUSION

**1** *Early:* Decision mainly based on cord haemoglobin (in addition consider history of previously affected babies).

- Cord haemoglobin <12 g/dl.
- Strongly positive Coombs' test.
- Cord bilirubin >85 μmol/l.

**2** *Late:* Usually done for hyperbilirubinaemia. The aims of exchange transfusion are:

- Treat anaemia.
- Washes out IgG antibodies.
- Decreases degree of haemolysis.
- Removes bilirubin.
- Prevents kernicterus.

CONTINUOUS PHOTOTHERAPY

For jaundice from birth, until bilirubin falling.

TOP-UP TRANSFUSION

A late anaemia can develop. If haemoglobin falls below 7 g/dl, give top-up transfusion. Prophylactic oral folate will be required.

# Genital tract bleeding in late pregnancy

Antepartum haemorrhage is defined as bleeding from the genital tract after the 24th week of pregnancy and before the onset of labour.

*Incidence*
5% of all pregnancies.

*Causes*

MATERNAL

- Placenta praevia: 30%.
- Abruptio placentae: 35%.
- Local cause in the vagina and cervix: 5%.
- Blood dyscrasias: <1%.
- Cause never found: 30%.

FETAL
Vasa praevia: <1%.

# Placenta praevia

A placenta which encroaches on the lower segment of the uterus. The lower segment can be defined as that part of the uterine wall which:

- Does not contract in labour but is stretched in response to contractions.
- Used to be the isthmus before pregnancy.
- Underlies the loose fold of peritoneum that reflects from the bladder.
- Is covered by a full bladder anteriorly.
- Is within 8 cm of the internal cervical os at term.

*Classification*
Box 10.2 shows the classical, contemporary and ultrasound classifications. Figure 10.1 shows the grades of severity of a placenta praevia.

*Aetiology*
Placenta praevia follows the low implantation of the embryo. Associated factors are:

**1** Multiparity.

**2** Multiple pregnancy.

**3** Embryos are more likely to implant on a lower segment scar from previous caesarean section. This increases the risk of placenta accreta/increta/percreta (see p. 93).

*Presentation*
- Nowadays most low-lying placentae or placenta praevia are diagnosed by ultrasound.

---

**Box 10.2 The classification grades of placenta praevia.**

I The placenta reaches the lower segment but not the internal os

II The placenta reaches the internal os but does not cover it

III The placenta covers the internal os before dilatation but not when dilated

IV The placenta completely covers the internal os of the cervix even when dilated

| Classical | Contemporary | Ultrasound |
|---|---|---|
| Grade I | Marginal ⎫ | Minor |
| Grade II | Lateral  ⎭ | |
| Grade III ⎫ | Central | Major |
| Grade IV ⎭ | | |

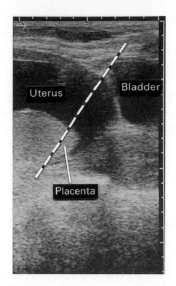

**Figure 10.2** Ultrasound scan showing posterior placenta praevia (Grade I) at 32 weeks' gestation. Dotted line is the junction of the upper and lower segments of the uterus.

**Figure 10.1** Grades of severity of a placenta praevia (see Box 10.2).

• Recurrent painless bright red vaginal bleeding.
• A persistent malpresentation or high head in late pregnancy.

An ultrasound scan will show the position of the placenta clearly within the uterus (Fig. 10.2). If the placenta lies in the anterior part of the uterus and reaches into the area covered by the bladder, it is known as a low-lying placenta (before 24 weeks) and placenta praevia after 24 weeks.

*Management*

ASYMPTOMATIC LOW-LYING PLACENTA
• About 5% of pregnant women will have a low-lying placenta when scanned at 16–20 weeks' gestation.
• The incidence of placenta praevia at delivery is about 0.5%, therefore in 9 out of 10 women the placenta will rise away from the cervix as the uterus grows.

• All women with a low-lying placenta diagnosed in early pregnancy should be rescanned at 34 weeks' gestation.
• There is no need to restrict work activities or sexual intercourse in women with a low-lying placenta on ultrasound unless they bleed.
• If the placenta praevia is still present at 34 weeks' gestation and is Grade I or II, the woman should be rescanned on a fortnightly basis but need not be admitted to hospital unless bleeding occurs.
• Clinically, a high presenting part or abnormal lie at 37 weeks implies that the placenta is covering the cervix and a Caesarean section should be performed electively.

PLACENTA PRAEVIA WITH BLEEDING
• Admit to hospital.
• Insert a broad-bore i.v. cannula and start an infusion of normal saline—if the woman is shocked start with a colloid infusion, e.g. Haemaccel.
• Take blood for cross-matching and haemoglobin estimation.
• If the woman is anaemic, she is no longer bleeding and the baby is <37 weeks then she should be transfused aiming for a haemoglobin of >10.5 g/dl.

This can be repeated as necessary until the baby reaches maturity when delivery should be by Caesarean section.

- *Avoid all digital vaginal examinations.* A gentle bivalve speculum examination should be performed to determine if blood is coming through the cervical os, especially if a placenta praevia has been suspected but not diagnosed definitely.
- Perform ultrasound as soon as possible because this is more precise.
- Cross-matched blood should be kept permanently available.
- Placental position and fetal growth should be monitored by fortnightly ultrasound scans.
- At 36–37 weeks' presentation, a final ultrasound should be performed and acted upon:

    (a) Grades III and IV placenta praevia should have a Caesarean section between 37 and 38 weeks' gestation by an experienced obstetrician particularly if the placenta is on the anterior wall of the uterus.

    (b) If the presenting part is below the lower edge of the placenta in Grade I, then it is safe to wait until labour and these women can be expected to deliver vaginally.

*Prognosis*

MATERNAL

Death from placenta praevia in the developed world is now extremely rare. If women are in hospital Caesarean section should be undertaken to prevent death from excessive bleeding. The major cause of death in women with placenta praevia now is postpartum haemorrhage (PPH). PPH is common because the lower segment does not contract and retract as in the upper segment, and therefore maternal vessels of the placental bed may continue to bleed after delivery. This may lead to an emergency hysterectomy if the bleeding cannot be stopped.

FETAL

Bleeding from placenta praevia is maternal in origin. The risk to the fetus is therefore mostly dependent upon the gestation at which it becomes necessary to deliver the baby.

# Placental abruption

This is bleeding from the placental bed of a normally sited placenta. It may occur as an antepartum or an intrapartum event.

*Classification*

MAJOR

This is clinically obvious and may result in the death of the fetus. It is also life-threatening to the mother and usually involves separation of more than one-third of the placenta.

MINOR

Premature separation of small areas of the placenta may result in placental infarcts. Several small abruptions may precede a large abruption. Much of the bleeding that occurs from an abruption is not discharged through the vagina and is known as concealed haemorrhage. Bleeding which is clinically obvious is revealed haemorrhage. Most times it is obviously mixed.

*Aetiology*

The causes of abruption are not known but the following factors are associated:

- Proteinuric hypertension.
- Multiparity. Fourth pregnancies carry a four times risk over first pregnancies.
- Trauma. ECV and seat belt injuries (rarely).
- Overstretched uterus (polyhydramnios, multiple pregnancy) at the time that the membranes rupture.
- Previous placental abruption. This increases the risk by two to three times.
- Raised maternal serum $\alpha$ fetoprotein in the absence of fetal malformation (6% risk).

*Presentation*

MAJOR

Women present with abdominal pain and varying degrees of shock. The blood loss that is visible (revealed haemorrhage) is often less than the degree of shock.

On examination:

**1** The uterus is woody hard; due to a tonic contraction.
**2** The fetal parts cannot be felt.
**3** The fetus may be dead.

MINOR

Minor abruptions are often not diagnosed until after delivery. They may present with:
• Mild abdominal pain associated with threatened preterm labour.
• Unexplained APH.
• Tenderness over one area of the uterus only.

*Complications*
Severe abruption may result in:
• Shock from blood loss due to a large retroplacental clot, often concealed.
• A disseminated intravascular coagulopathy (DIC).
• Oliguria or anuria due to hypovolaemia.

Minor degrees of placental abruption may result in impaired fetal growth and/or hypoxic ischaemic encephalopathy (HIE)—cerebral palsy.

*Management*
Major placental abruption is a life-threatening condition for both the mother and the baby.
If the fetus is still alive:
• Insert two large-bore i.v. cannulae and infusion of normal saline/colloid.
• Send 20 ml blood for cross-match of 4 units, haemoglobin and coagulation studies.
• Perform an immediate Caesarean section if necessary to save the baby's life (high risk of post-partum haemorrhage).
• Ensure adequate fluid replacement following the Caesarean section.
• Leave an indwelling urinary catheter in to monitor urinary output.
• Consider insertion of a central line to monitor maternal intravascular volume more closely.

If the fetus is dead, then the woman should be allowed to deliver vaginally. This usually happens rapidly (within 4–6 hours) as the abruption stimulates labour. If not in labour, rupture of membranes usually leads to a swift delivery. The relevant points of the management of labour are:

• Epidural analgesia is contraindicated because of the risk of coagulopathy, but a patient-controlled opiate infusion can be used.
• If a coagulopathy has developed (prolonged APTT, PTT, increased fibrin degradation products, low platelets) or the woman starts to bleed, she should be managed in the following manner in conjunction with a consultant haematologist.
  (a) Give 4 units of fresh frozen plasma.
  (b) Ask the blood bank to get 6 units of platelets ready.

The consumptive coagulopathy begins to improve immediately after the uterus has been evacuated of its contents. Marked abnormalities of the coagulation tests usually resolve within 4–6 hours of delivery of the placenta.

## Local causes of bleeding in late pregnancy

Urinary or anal bleeding may be reported as vaginal bleeding in error. They need exclusion and their own treatments.

## Cervicitis and vaginitis

• Occasional excessive infection (especially with *Candida*).
• Treat cause.

## Cervical polyp

• Scanty bleeding. Can be seen with speculum.
• Leave alone in pregnancy and treat later if necessary.

## Cervical ectropion

• Spotting of blood only. Can be seen with speculum.
• Leave alone in pregnancy and treat later if necessary.

## Varicosities of vagina

• Moderate bleeding in mid-trimester.
• Treat with pressure if close to vulva.

• Only ligate surgically in pregnancy if absolutely necessary; it is difficult.

## Cancer of cervix

• Rare but important.
• Irregular bleeding and discharge. Confirm diagnosis by biopsy.
• If before 24 weeks, hysterotomy and immediate Wertheim hysterectomy followed by radiation.
• If after 24 weeks, may await 32 weeks then Caesarean Wertheim hysterectomy followed by radiation.

## Blood dyscrasias

These are extremely rare. Bleeding may be seen in the following conditions.
• Idiopathic thrombocytopenia.
• Von Willebrand's disease.
• Leukaemia.
• Hodgkin's disease.
• Antiphospholipid syndrome.

*Management*
These conditions are usually known before pregnancy and are best managed in conjunction with a relevant specialist.

## Fetal bleeding

This occurs from rupture of vasa praevia when there is a velamentous insertion of cord vessels and these cross the cervical os.

*Diagnosis*
This condition usually presents with scanty bleeding at the time of membrane rupture. It may be associated with alterations in the fetal heart rate producing a sinusoidal pattern (see p. 169).

*Confirmation*
If there is time, the blood lost can be checked for fetal haem by its resistance to alkalinization (Kleihauer test). Alternatively the condition may be suspected when an ultrasound examination reveals the presence of a succenturate lobe on the opposite side of the internal os to the placenta.

*Treatment*
Deliver the fetus as soon as possible and prepare to transfuse.

## Polyhydramnios

Definition: an excess of amniotic fluid detected clinically. The range of normal volumes of fluid present is wide and varies with the duration of pregnancy. *Average* values for amniotic fluid are:
12 weeks: 50 ml;
24 weeks: 500 ml;
36 weeks: 1000 ml;
The normal range at term in a singleton pregnancy is large — 500–1500 ml.

*Diagnosis*
This is either clinical or by simple ultrasound. Other methods of measuring amniotic fluid *in situ* are too complex for routine use and often unreliable.

*History*
• Tenseness of abdomen.
• Unable to lie comfortably in any position.
• Dyspnoea, indigestion, piles and varicose veins.
• Decreased sensation of fetal movements.

*Examination*
• Increased symphysio-fundal height.
• Very tense, cystic uterus bigger than maturity (like a balloon filled with water).
• Difficult to feel any fetal parts.

*Investigations*
*Ultrasound.* The deepest column >8 cm or the amniotic fluid index is greater than the 95th centile.

*Differential diagnosis*
• Twins: laxer feel to uterus and too many fetal parts felt.
• Ovarian cyst: uterus displaced to one side in later pregnancy.
• Full bladder.
    All are resolved by ultrasound examination.

*Associations*

MATERNAL
• Diabetes.

FETAL
• Congenital abnormality; anencephaly; meningomyelocoele; upper alimentary atresia e.g. tracheoesophageal fistula.
• Twins (particularly monozygotic).

*Clinical course*

ACUTE
• Painful with tense uterus and oedematous abdominal wall.
• Primiparous.
• Pre-eclampsia.
• Often early (22–32 weeks' gestation).

CHRONIC
• Slower onset.
• Uncomfortable rather than painful.
• Last weeks of pregnancy.

*Management*

ACUTE
1 Bed rest.
2 Ultrasound to rule out twins or abnormality.
3 Release fluid from uterus.
  • If *fetus normal*: through abdominal wall with narrow-bore needle. Drain fluid off slowly until the woman is comfortable (500–1000 ml over 4–8 hours).
  • If *fetus abnormal* and viable—consider induction. If not viable—paracentesis.

CHRONIC
1 Bed rest.
2 Ultrasound to rule out twins and fetal abnormality.
3 Glucose tolerance test.
4 Sedation if very painful.
5 Treat underlying maternal condition.
6 If fetus normal, induce labour when indicated by fetal state *not* because of the polyhydramnios.
7 Watch for uterine dysfunction and postpartum haemorrhage (PPH) after labour.

# Oligohydramnios

A lack of amniotic fluid, a much rarer condition.

*Diagnosis*
• Uterus is small for dates (early).
• Uterus feels full of fetus (later).
• Ultrasound shows reduced amniotic fluid index (<2 cm columns).

*Fetal associations*
• Adhesions from fetal skin to amnion.
• Renal agenesis.
• Asymmetrical SGA.

*Clinical course*
• Labour often preterm.
• High fetal death rate.
• High rate of fetal abnormalities (e.g. dislocated hips and talipes).

# Obstetric cholestasis

Obstetric cholestasis only occurs in pregnancy and usually presents in the third trimester. It is more common in multiple pregnancies.

*Presentation*
• Itching, often generalized but commonly worst on palms and soles of feet.
• Absence of rash.
• Insomnia.
• Right upper quadrant pain.
• Malaise.
• Intolerance of fatty foods.

*Investigation*
Liver function test (LFT).
• Raised transaminase concentrations (ALT and AST).
• Raised bile salts.

*Risks*

MATERNAL
• Increased risk of PPH.

FETAL
- Increased risk of fetal distress.
- Increased risk of stillbirth over 38 weeks (18/1000 births).
- Double the incidence of premature labour.
- Increased risk of intracerebral haemorrhage.

*Treatment*
- Prophylactic Vitamin K until delivery because of reduced absorption leading to increased risk of PPH.
- Antihistamines, calamine, aqueous cream (for itching).
- Ursodeoxycholic acid—effective in reducing itching and usually returns liver function tests to normal or near normal. However it does not alter the outcome of pregnancy, but the symptoms become tolerable allowing the baby to mature to term in the majority of cases (37 weeks).

*Monitoring*

MATERNAL
- Weekly LFTs and clotting screen.

FETAL
- Alternate day CTG.
- Weekly liquor volume and umbilical artery Doppler.
- Fortnightly growth ultrasound scan.

*Delivery*
All women should be delivered at 37–38 weeks to try and prevent intrauterine death. Vaginal delivery is indicated in the majority of cases and it is rare for induction to fail even in primigravidas. As there is an increased risk of fetal distress the fetal heart rate should be monitored continuously electronically (CTG). Syntometrine / Syntocinon must be given with the birth of the anterior shoulder to reduce the risk of postpartum haemorrhage (PPH).

*Recurrence*
There is a high likelihood (>60%) of recurrence in subsequent pregnancies.

---

**Self-assessment**

**10.1** Which of the following statements are true?
(a) Pre-eclamptic toxaemia is defined as a rise in the diastolic blood pressure after 20 weeks of pregnancy by more than 15 mm/Hg from the booking blood pressure without proteinuria.
(b) Women with pre-eclampsia are at increased risk of developing gestational diabetes.
(c) Pre-eclamptic toxaemia is defined as a rise in the diastolic blood pressure after 20 weeks of pregnancy by more than 15 mm/Hg from the booking blood pressure with proteinuria.
(d) The most dangerous risk of pre-eclampsia for the mother is cerebral oedema leading to fitting.
(e) The most dangerous risk of pre-eclampsia for the mother is developing HELLP syndrome.
**10.2** A woman of 38 presents at 36 weeks in her first pregnancy with a headache. The symphysiofundal height is 35 cm, cephalic presentation with the head 4/5 palpable per abdomen. Her blood pressure is 174/112, pulse 82 beats per minute, temperature 36.7°C. The CTG is reassuring. Her reflexes are brisk bilaterally with 4 beats of clonus in each ankle. Which of the following is the most appropriate treatment?
(a) Magnesium sulphate infusion followed by delivery of the baby.
(b) Magnesium sulphate infusion with hydrallazine followed by delivery of the baby.
(c) Immediate delivery of the baby.
(d) Phenytoin infusion with hydrallazine followed by delivery of the baby.
(e) Diazepam with hydrallazine followed by delivery of the baby.
**10.3** Anti-*D* should be given to all women who are Rh negative in which of the following scenarios?
(a) Threatened miscarriage.
(b) Following the birth of a baby whose blood group is A negative.

**Self-assessment** *Continued*

(c) Following the birth of a baby whose blood group is A positive.

(d) Ectopic pregnancy.

(e) Medical termination of pregnancy.

**10.4** A woman of 28 presents at 34 weeks of pregnancy with constant abdominal pain and a small amount of bleeding. Her symphysiofundal height is 37 cm, her uterus is tender and firm. The CTG shows unprovoked decelerations. Her pulse is 108 beats per minute and her blood pressure 100/60 mm Hg. What is the most likely diagnosis?

(a) Placenta praevia.

(b) Cervical cancer.

(c) Von-Willebrand's disease.

(d) Placental abruption.

(e) Cervical polyp.

**10.5** Polyhydramnios is associated with which of the following?

(a) Gestational diabetes.

(b) Fetal renal agenesis.

(c) Pre-eclamptic toxaemia.

(d) Obstetric cholestasis.

(e) Tracheoesophageal fistula.

# Chapter 11

# Diseases in pregnancy

The majority of women who become pregnant are healthy and remain so throughout their pregnancy. A few women present with pre-existing medical disorders that may affect the pregnancy. Some disorders may arise during the pregnancy. Doctors should be aware of the effect that pregnancy may have on these disorders and their treatment.

## Urinary tract infection in pregnancy

During pregnancy the ureters are dilated and kinked because of:
• Increased progesterone levels which relax the smooth muscle.
• Mild obstruction of the lower ureters in late pregnancy.
  This encourages:
• Stasis of urine.
• Reflux of infected urine to the kidney evoking pyelonephritis.

## Asymptomatic bacteriuria

The presence of more than $10^5$ bacteria/ml of urine in the absence of symptoms.

*Incidence*
About 3% of pregnant women—increases with parity and age.

*Significance*
Asymptomatic bacteriuria is associated with a risk of:

• Acute pyelonephritis in pregnancy (30%).
• Structural abnormalities in the urinary tract (3–5%).

*Screening*
In early pregnancy, all women should have urine tested for either:
• The presence of white cells and nitrites, or;
• cultured for bacteria.

*Treatment*
The most common organisms grown are:
• *Escherichia coli*.
• *Proteus mirabilis*.
  These are usually sensitive to amoxycillin, trimethoprim or nitrofurantoin. A 5-day course of an antibiotic to which the organism is sensitive should be prescribed. This will result in a cure in more than 85% of women, but the urine should be recultured one week after treatment.
  A renal ultrasound and an intravenous (i.v.) urogram should be performed 3 months after delivery to exclude a structural urinary tract abnormality.

## Symptomatic infections

*Incidence*
1–2%; commoner in primigravidae.

*Symptoms*
- Dysuria (due to urethritis).
- Increased frequency (due to trigonitis).
- Backache, loin pains, night sweats and rigors (due to pyelonephritis).
- Headache, vomiting and muscle aches (due to pyrexia).

*Examination*
- The woman is usually pyrexial if the infection has involved the kidneys. In many cases this may be at levels of up to 40.5°C.
- If the woman has pyelonephritis she will be tender in the renal angles.

*Investigation*
A mid-stream specimen of urine (MSU) should be sent for:
- Dipstick for nitrites and leucocytes.
- Microscopy for white cells.
- Culture to determine the organism responsible.
- Sensitivity of organisms to antibiotics.

*Management*
All women who have renal angle tenderness or a pyrexia must be admitted to hospital because of the threat of preterm labour.
Management consists of:
1 Bed rest.
2 Ample fluid intake, at least 3 litres a day; if nauseated, give i.v.
3 Start a broad-spectrum i.v. antibiotic such as amoxycillin; may need changing when an organism's antibiotic sensitivities are known.
4 If the woman has pyelonephritis, do a renal ultrasound when she has recovered from the infection.
5 Keep her in hospital until the renal angle tenderness has disappeared.
6 The antibiotics can be given orally once temperature is normal. A complete 5-day course at least should be given. The urine should be recultured 5 days after the last dose of antibiotic has been given.

## Chronic renal disease

*Renal changes in normal pregnancy*
- Renal blood flow increases.
- Glomerular filtration rate (GFR) increases.
- Plasma concentrations of urea and creatinine fall in normal pregnancy.
- There is an increase in total body water that exceeds the increase in total body sodium, resulting in a decrease in plasma osmolality.
- There is a 25% fall in serum uric acid concentrations during the first two trimesters but this returns to pre-pregnant levels by the third trimester. Watch if using urate to monitor pre-eclampsia.

*Prognosis*
The outcome of the pregnancy is worse if:
1 The woman was hypertensive before pregnancy.
2 The woman had proteinuria before pregnancy started.
3 There is active progression of renal disease or it is associated with other medical conditions.
   Pregnancy probably has no long-term adverse effects on renal disease.

*Fetal prognosis*
- Normotensive women with chronic renal disease have 2–3 times greater risk of developing pre-eclampsia. In the absence of pre-eclamptic toxaemia (PET) perinatal mortality is not increased. If PET develops, the risk of fetal death is directly related to the gestation at delivery.
- Women with more severe renal disease have a high incidence of both PET and impaired fetal growth. Among women with pre-existing hypertension and proteinuria, the perinatal mortality rates approach 30%. Cause of death is from preterm delivery and complications associated with small for gestational age (SGA).

## Acute renal failure in pregnancy

This may be:
1 Tubular necrosis: this is largely recoverable.
2 Cortical necrosis: this is usually irrecoverable and these patients go on to need long-term dialysis or transplantation.

*Presentation*

**1** Oliguria: <500 ml/day (20 ml/hour), the minimum volume to remove catabolites.
**2** Anuria: the absence of urine.

*Aetiology in obstetrics*

**1** *Hypovolaemia.*
  • Severe pre-eclampsia.
  • Placental abruption.
  • Postpartum haemorrhage (PPH).
  • Hyperemesis gravidarum.
  • Miscarriage.
**2** *Gram-negative shock.* This may result from:
  • Pyelonephritis.
  • Chorioamnionitis.
  • Puerperal infections.
  • Septic miscarriage.
The usual organism is *E. coli*, but it may be *Clostridium*.
**3** *Nephrotoxins.* In modern obstetric practice these are rare. Illegal abortions may result in infection followed by haemolysis and renal failure.
**4** *Acute renal failure* associated with acute fatty liver of pregnancy. Rare; usually fatal.
**5** *Vomiting* in late pregnancy associated with jaundice. The disease occurs in many systems and renal failure, pancreatitis and colitis may occur.

*Management*

Three consecutive phases:

**1** *Oliguria*: lasts from a few days to a few weeks. Complete anuria is rare in acute tubular necrosis and usually suggests acute cortical necrosis or obstruction.
**2** *Polyuria*: markedly increased urine production that may last up to 2 weeks. The urine is dilute and metabolic waste products are poorly eliminated. Plasma urea and creatinine may continue to rise for several days following the increase in urinary output. Profound fluid and electrolyte losses can occur in this phase.
**3** *Recovery*: urinary volumes decrease towards normal and renal function improves.
  General management:
• Determine the cause.
• Insert a urinary catheter and maintain accurate fluid balance charts.

• Insert a central venous pressure line and measure the pressure.
  In pregnancy, central venous pressure should range from +4 to +10 cmH$_2$O. If this is low it suggests the cause of the renal failure is due to hypovolaemia and therefore the volume should be restored with up to 2 litres of normal saline followed by a plasma expander. Response of over 30 ml of urine in 1 hour should be seen within 1 hour of the fluid load.
• Send baseline investigations, including urea and electrolytes, liver function tests, serum amylase, plasma proteins, coagulation studies, and if required, perform an arterial blood sample for acid–base balance.
• If the patient is not hypovolaemic or does not respond to the fluid load, then the alternatives are as follows:
  (a) Conservative management. Give i.v. the volume of patient fluid output plus 500 ml/day. Monitor electrolytes and start dialysis if or when the patient is uraemic or hypercatabolic.
  (b) Intensive management using vasodilators and inotropes (renal dose dopamine). This requires the insertion of a pulmonary artery catheter and the monitoring of cardiac output. Vasodilators and inotropes are given and the patient is fluid-loaded.
• Involve intensive care physicians and the renal physician at an early stage.

## Anaemia

Anaemia can follow:
**1** Lack of production of blood: haemopoietic.
**2** Increased breakdown of blood: haemolytic.
**3** Blood loss: haemorrhagic.
  In pregnancy, most anaemia is haemopoietic when it may be due to lack of:
**1** Iron: iron deficiency anaemia.
**2** Folic acid: megaloblastic anaemia.
**3** Protein: iron deficiency anaemia.
  Normal levels of haematological indices are shown in Box 11.1.

## Box 11.1 Normal haematological values in pregnancy

| Blood | Range |
|---|---|
| Total blood volume (ml) | 4000–6000 |
| Red cell volume (ml) | 1500–1800 |
| Red cell count ($10^{12}$/l) | 4–5 |
| White cell count ($10^9$/l) | 8–18 |
| Haemoglobin (g/dl) | 10.5–13.5 |
| Mean corpuscular volume (fl) | 80–95 |
| Mean corpuscular haemoglobin ($\mu$g) | 32–36 |
| Serum iron ($\mu$mol/l) | 11–25 |
| Serum ferritin ($\mu$g/l) | 10–200 |
| Serum folate ($\mu$g/l) | 6–9 |
| Total iron-binding capacity ($\mu$mol/l) | 40–70 |
| Platelets ($10^9$/l) | 150–300 |

**Table 11.1** Indices of iron deficiency and megaloblastic anaemia.

| | Iron deficiency | Megaloblastic |
|---|---|---|
| *Blood film* | | |
| Red cells | | |
|   Size | N or ↓ | ↑ |
|   Hypochromia | ↓ | N |
|   Anaesocytosis | + | + |
|   Poikilocytosis | + | + |
| White cells | N | Leucopenia |
| | | Hypersegmented |
| | | |
| *Haematological values* | | |
|   Hb | ↓ | ↓ |
|   MCV | ↓ | N or ↑ |
|   MCHb | ↓ | N |
|   MGHbC | ↓ | ↑ |
|   Serum iron | ↓ | N |
|   Serum ferritin | ↓ | N |
|   Serum folate | N | ↓ |
| | | |
| *Marrow* | ↓ Iron stores | ↑ Megaloblasts |

# Iron deficiency anaemia (Table 11.1)

## Aetiology

### POOR INTAKE

- Diet deficient in iron-containing foods.

### POOR ABSORPTION

- Vomiting in pregnancy affects absorption.
- Increased pH of gastric juice.

- Ferric ions in gut instead of ferrous.
- Lack of vitamin C.

### INCREASED UTILIZATION

Demands of pregnancy. Total body iron measures about 3500 mg. Includes:

- Fetus and uterus: 500 mg.
- Increased maternal blood volume: 500 mg.

More if:

- Multiple pregnancies.
- Grand multiparity.
- Pregnancies close together.
- Vegetarian (particularly vegans).

### DIAGNOSIS

- Rarely made clinically unless woman is severely affected.
- May show pallor of conjunctivae.
- May have tiredness and oedema.
- Hb estimates must be done on all pregnant women at booking, and twice later in pregnancy, at 26 and 34 weeks.
- If level below 10 g/dl, diagnose anaemia, look for cause and treat.

## Treatment

### PREVENTATIVE

Regular iron-bearing foods in diet (Box 11.2). If needed, iron tablet supplements. Daily requirements are 100 mg elemental iron with 300 $\mu$g folic acid.

- See she gets them—give them to her at the clinics.
- See she takes them—ask at each visit.
- See they are effective—check Hb levels.

## Box 11.2 The iron-rich foods

*Animal*
Red meat—iron in haemoglobin and myoglobin
White meat
Fish } —iron in the myoglobin

*Plant*
Lentils
Dark-green leaf vegetables } moderate amount of iron only (rich in folates)
Beans of all sorts

CURATIVE

Depends on:

1 Degree of anaemia.

2 Duration of pregnancy.

3 Cause of iron deficiency:
   • Mild anaemia: Hb below 10 g/dl.
   • Severe anaemia: Hb below 8 g/dl.

   *Mild:*

1 Check that the woman is being given, and is taking, oral iron.

2 If so, increase oral iron; add vitamin C to aid absorption or try another preparation.

3 If she cannot swallow tablets, use liquid preparation.

4 If change of oral therapy does not improve, use intramuscular (i.m.) or i.v. preparation. Give total dose i.v. as a transfusion in 1000 ml of saline. Alternatively, iron dextran 250 mg is associated with a rise of Hb of about 1 g/dl. Give on alternate days, i.m. for six doses, with small test dose first to check anaphylaxis.

   *Severe and early:*

1 Admit to hospital and check that anaemia is solely iron deficient:
   • Blood film.
   • Serum iron.
   • Total iron-binding capacity.
   • Serum ferritin.
   • Serum folate.
   • Sickle/thalassaemia status.

2 Treat with oral, i.m. or i.v. therapy as required.

3 Check protein and vitamin intake adequate.

4 Check that improvement is maintained for rest of pregnancy.

   *Severe and late:*

1 If after 36 weeks, too late to rely on haemopoiesis to provide red cells in time to cover labour. Therefore transfuse slowly with packed red cell blood.

2 If Hb below 4 g/dl consider exchange transfusion.

3 Build up iron stores for puerperium by i.m. therapy.

## Folic acid deficiency anaemia

*Aetiology*

Folic acid required for building DNA in all tissues.

Hence demands are maximal when fetal tissue being made.

1 Poor intake:
   • Diet deficient in folates.
   • Vomiting in pregnancy.

2 Increased utilization:
   • Demands of pregnancy.
   • Rapid growth of fetal, placental and uterine tissues.
   • Worse if:
     (a) Multiple pregnancy.
     (b) Grand multiparity.
     (c) Fetal haemolysis (in Rh effect).
     (d) Infection.

Commoner in underdeveloped countries and combined with other forms of malnutrition.

*Diagnosis*

Sometimes made clinically.
• May be tired, breathless, oedematous.
• May have other signs of malnutrition.

*Haematology*

See Megaloblastic column, Table 11.1.

*Treatment*

PREVENTATIVE

Folic acid supplements in last 20 weeks of pregnancy (300 µg/day).

Theoretical risk of masking pernicious anaemia (PA) and its uncommon accompanying subacute combined degeneration (SCD) of the spinal cord. In practice, PA is very rare in those under 35 years and SCD almost unknown in the pregnancy age group.

CURATIVE

• Mild or moderate anaemia—folic acid 5–10 mg/day orally only.
• Severe anaemia—folic acid 5–10 mg/day i.m.:
   (a) oral iron          } both should be
   (b) blood transfusion  } given with care.

## Haemolytic anaemias

These can all be diagnosed before pregnancy at pre-pregnancy consultation.

## Haemoglobinopathies

### Sickle cell disease

*Aetiology*
- Abnormal Hb: typical original geography.
  (a) HbS (commonest): Middle East, Africa, USA, Caribbean and southern Europe.
  (b) HbC: Ghana.
  (c) HbE: South-East Asia.
  (d) HbD: Punjab.

*Diagnosis*
- Crises or infarcts:
  (a) Chest pain.
  (b) Sudden head or abdominal pain.
  (c) Joint pains.
- Bone marrow exhaustion.
  A crisis could be triggered by:
- Infection.
- Hypoxia.
- Dehydration.
- Trauma.

*Haematology*
- Low Hb.
- Sickling and target cells on blood film.
- Electrophoresis shows abnormal Hb patterns.

*Treatment*
- Detect early.
- Hydrate with intravenous fluids.
- Oxygen.
- Folic acid prophylactically 1–2 mg/day.
- Transfusion of red blood cells.
- Diuretic.
- Antibiotics.
  If crisis:
- Hydrate.
- Check Hb every 4 hours.
- Heparinize.
- Antibiotics.
- Consider exchange transfusion.
- If blood pressure rises rapidly, deliver.
- Splenectomy for some.

## Thalassaemia

*Aetiology*
Defective genes alter Hb side chains. May be $\alpha$ or $\beta$ which can either be:
- Homozygous—thalassaemia major: usually fatal before pregnancy age group. Sickle cell anaemia.
- Heterozygous—thalassaemia minor: commonest thalassaemia. $\beta$-Thalassaemia minor is the more serious especially if combined with any other abnormal Hb such as S or C.

*Diagnosis*
- Classically women from the Mediterranean countries but now widespread in the Middle and Far East. The woman usually knows about this and will mention it in the history.
- Globin chain synthesis studies.
- Occasionally a mild anaemia (MCV$\downarrow$ MCH$\downarrow$ MCHC=).
- Splenomegaly.
- Jaundice.
- Pain from bone infarcts (later in life—ulcers of legs).

*Haematology*
- Increased red blood cell fragility.
- Hb level low.
- Serum iron raised.

*Treatment*
1 No use giving iron alone (iron stores high) but folate helpful.
2 Cover haemolytic crisis with transfusions carefully.
3 Prevent stress if possible (e.g. hypoxia).
4 Treat infections early.
5 Beware coexistent:
  - Malaria.
  - Glucose-6-phosphate dehydrogenase deficiency.
  - Other abnormal Hb.
6 Deliver between crises.

## Haemorrhagic anaemia

Rare in temperate climates:

- Recurrent chronic gastrointestinal bleeding (peptic ulcer, piles).

Commoner in tropics:

- Recurrent chronic bleeding (e.g. tapeworms, hookworms).

*Treatment*
- Treat cause.
- Correct anaemia—as above.

# Heart disease

Frequency and severity of heart disease in pregnancy are diminishing in this country because:
- Most heart disease in this age group is rheumatic in origin.
- Rheumatic fever is much rarer in childhood with better housing and nutrition.
- Rheumatic fever is more effectively treated in childhood by chemotherapy.

*Aetiology*
- Rheumatic 80%: mitral valve affected 85%, aortic valve 10%, both 5%.
- Congenital 15%: septal defects and reversed shunts.
- All the rest 5%: ischaemic, thyrotoxic.

*Pathophysiology*
Pregnancy is a hyperkinetic state and is an extra load on the heart. If the heart is damaged, avoid other loads.
- Anaemia—blood is inefficient at oxygen transport.
- Pre-eclampsia—harder work if hypertension or oedema present.
- Arrhythmia—fibrillation is inefficient at delivering blood.
- Flare-up of rheumatic fever—not common but watch for and treat.
- Acute bacterial endocarditis risk increased because of irregular endothelium over heart valves; hence cover labour, surgery and dentistry with antibiotics.

*Cardiac complications in pregnancy*
1 With mitral stenosis:

- Pulmonary oedema.
- Right-sided congestive failure.

2 With aortic stenosis:
- Left-sided congestive failure. Rare to start *de novo*, in pregnancy.

3 Eisenmenger's syndrome.
- If right-to-left shunt—pulmonary hypertension.

4 Fallot's tetralogy.
- If right-to-left shunt, risk of cardiac failure.

5 Coarctation of aorta.
- Risk of rupture in late pregnancy or labour. Often repaired before; if well healed, no increased dangers.

6 Artificial valves—thrombosis.

*Management*

IN PREGNANCY
1 Diagnose early.
- History.
- Examination.

2 Assess severity early: ideally cardiologist and obstetrician to see woman together at same antenatal clinic.

Investigations:
- Electrocardiogram (ECG).
- Chest X-ray.
- Echocardiography.
- Maybe:
  (a) Catheter studies (pressure and blood gases).
  (b) 24-hour ECG.

Factors:
  (a) Age.
  (b) Severity of lesion.
  (c) Functional decompensation.

3 Book for hospital delivery and be prepared for bed rest in hospital.

4 Extra rest at home.

5 Continue anticoagulation if patient already on it. Consider subcutaneous heparin rather than oral anticoagulants unless plastic valve prosthesis. For these continue on warfarin.

6 Senior cardiologist, anaesthetist and obstetrician make labour plan and write it on hospital records. See that senior staff of each discipline are available to cover labour.

IN LABOUR

**1** Reduce extra work—good analgesia; probably epidural unless anticoagulated.
**2** Nurse head up: tilt bed or extra pillows.
**3** Antibiotics especially if a congenital heart lesion.
**4** Short second stage; maybe forceps or vacuum extraction.
**5** Give Syntometrine only if high risk of postpartum haemorrhage (PPH); otherwise not.
**6** Manage pulmonary oedema if it occurs.
- Tilt head up 35°.
- $O_2$.
- Aminophylline 0.5 g, i.v.
- Morphine 15 mg.
- Digitalis if arrhythmia or tachycardia.
- Diuretics—frusemide.

IN PUERPERIUM

**1** Rest:
- Keep in hospital longer.
- Check home conditions adequate—few stairs if possible.
**2** Physiotherapy to legs and gentle exercises.
**3** Breast feeding allowed unless cardiac condition deteriorated in pregnancy. It can be hard work, for only one person can do it and it means getting up at night.

*Prognosis*

MATERNAL

**1** Mortality: increased risk of death—9% of all maternal deaths in UK are associated with heart disease.
**2** Morbidity: increased risk of deterioration of heart condition. Used to be inevitable. This is not so if proper care is taken.

FETAL

Little increased risk if mother kept healthy. Watch for fetal risks from anticoagulation if relevant.

# Respiratory diseases

## Asthma

IN PREGNANCY

Often emotional factors are involved so asthma may worsen if pregnancy is resented. Continue all treatments started before pregnancy. Be careful of new therapies, e.g. budesonide teratogenic to some species; not known to be so in humans. Therefore use well-established drugs.
- Bronchial antispasmodics.
- Antibiotics.
- Steroids—inhaled or systemic.

Most asthmatics do not deteriorate in pregnancy but may in puerperium. No obvious correlation with hormone changes.

IN LABOUR

**1** Deliver so that mother's respiratory effort is minimal.
**2** May require extra antispasmodics in labour.
**3** If on steroids, hydrocortisone required to cover labour.
**4** Baby may be small for dates if asthma control was poor.

## Pulmonary tuberculosis

*Incidence*
Less than 1:1000 in UK; rare in endogenous population, higher in immigrants.

*Presentation*
- History of disease.
- Pick up on routine chest X-ray.

*Management*
**1** Notify any new cases to District Community Physician.
**2** Continue any antituberculous drugs already started in combination:
- Streptomycin.*
- INAH (isonicotinic hydrazide).

*Beware potential teratogenic effect in first trimester.

- Ethambutol.
- Rifampicin.*

**3** Bed rest.
**4** Surgery if needed in mid-pregnancy, avoiding first 14 and last 10 weeks.
**5** Follow up the family.

*Labour*
Delivery by most expeditious route (baby may be large).

*Mother*
**1** Allow breast feeding if no positive sputum bacteriology within 1 year and no chest X-ray signs of recent activity.
**2** Continue all drug treatments.
**3** Suppress lactation if baby has to be separated.
**4** Rest in hospital longer.
**5** Check community back-up services to give least effort to mother.
**6** Arrange for follow-up at chest clinic in case of tuberculosis flare-up.

*Baby*
**1** If mother has had bacteria in sputum within 1 year, separate baby from mother at birth. The mother must be warned during pregnancy that this will happen. If properly explained, she will realize it is a wise move.
**2** Give baby isoniazid-resistant BCG 0.05 mg at 7 days (unless premature). Await positive Mantoux before allowing baby back to mother (about 6 weeks).

## Endocrine diseases

### Thyroid disease

Pregnancy is a hyperdynamic state. Increased oestrogen levels cause enlargement of thyroid gland and an increased output of thyroid hormone. Since this is mostly in the form of protein-bound thyroxine, such patients are not hyperthyroid, for the active fraction is not increased.

*Beware potential teratogenic effect in first trimester.

### Hyperthyroidism

- Difficult to diagnose for the first time in pregnancy.
- If established beforehand, continue treatment, usually carbimazole, but keep dose as low as possible.
- Consider thyroidectomy if disease is increasingly difficult to control.

Operation is safe if mother properly prepared. Avoid radioactive-iodine testing because of fetal thyroid pick-up and retention. Maternal thyroid-stimulating IgG passes across placenta and may stimulate fetal thyroid, sometimes enough to cause neonatal thyrotoxicosis. This is unusual but can be predicted by testing maternal blood levels of IgG in late pregnancy.

### Hypothyroidism

- Rarely get pregnant if not on therapy.
- If treated, continue treatment, and be prepared to increase dosage.

## Pituitary disease

### Prolactinoma

- Women on long-term bromocriptine become pregnant.
- Oestrogen stimulation of pregnancy may cause enlargement of tumour; pressure on optic chiasma threatens vision.
- Check with computerized tomography (CT) scan. Prolactin levels raised but variable.
- A few tumours need treatment if they enlarge:
  (a) first bromocriptine;
  (b) then surgery.

### Hypopituitarism

- Mostly starts in puerperium after pituitary vein thrombosis following PPH.
- Study each pituitary-controlled function separately and treat those deficient.
- If mother treated, baby does well.

## Diabetes

Diabetes is a metabolic disease which results from an underproduction of insulin by the pancreas. This results in disturbances of carbohydrate, fat and protein metabolism and leads to a sustained rise in blood glucose.

During pregnancy, diabetes may be one of the following types:

**1** Pre-existing diabetes which is usually insulin-dependent.

**2** Gestational diabetes or an impaired glucose tolerance test discovered for the first time in pregnancy.

### Glucose homeostasis in pregnancy

- In normal pregnancy, fasting glucose blood levels are maintained at 4–5 mmol/l.
- To maintain the glucose level, however, there is a doubling in the secretion of insulin in the second and third trimesters of pregnancy. Pregnancy represents a relatively insulin-resistant state.
- The insulin resistance is due to the placental secretion of oestrogen, progestogen and human placental lactogen together with a change in peripheral insulin receptors.
- Glucose crosses the placenta by facilitated diffusion resulting in a fetal glucose level of approximately 1 mmol/l less than its mother.
- The facilitated diffusion system is saturated at maternal levels of 11–12 mmol/l. Therefore the fetus is probably never subject to levels of greater than 11 mmol/l.

## Established diabetes mellitus

Occurs in 1–2% of the pregnant population.

*Effects of pregnancy on the diabetes*
- Insulin requirements increase during pregnancy and rapidly fall to pre-pregnancy levels after delivery.
- Pregnancy aggravates proliferative diabetic retinopathy. Ideally any retinopathy should be treated before pregnancy.
- Women with diabetic nephropathy are more likely to develop pre-eclampsia and to have poorer renal function during pregnancy, but there are few adverse long-term effects on renal function.
- There is a high incidence of asymmetrical SGA and preterm delivery.
- Diabetic neuropathy and vascular disease are rare in pregnancy.

*Effects of poorly controlled diabetes on the pregnancy*
- Diabetes is associated with an increased risk of first trimester miscarriages.
- Second trimester miscarriages, due to fetal death.
- Congenital abnormalities. By ×3, 50% neural tube defects, 30% cardiac abnormalities. Diabetics tend to show a predominance of multiple malformations and caudal regression appears exclusively in diabetics.
- Pregnancy-induced hypertension.
- Preterm delivery.
- Polyhydramnios.
- Macrosomic infants which may result in difficulties at delivery particularly shoulder dystocia.
- Sudden intrauterine death in the last 4 weeks of pregnancy. This appears to be confined to babies who are macrosomic.
- Perinatal mortality ×2–3. This can be reduced to background levels with good diabetic control.

*Effects of diabetes on the infant*
- Macrosomia: birth weight for gestational age exceeds the 90th centile.
- An increased risk of birth trauma, because of shoulder dystocia.
- An increased risk of asphyxia during delivery.
- An increased risk of respiratory distress syndrome (RDS) compared with babies of similar gestation.
- Hypoglycaemia. The fetal pancreas secretes high levels of insulin during pregnancy to cope with the passage of glucose from the mother. After delivery, the glucose source is removed, but the pancreas continues to secrete extra insulin resulting in hypoglycaemia.
- Hypercalcaemia.
- Hypothermia. Infants with diabetic mothers have large surface areas and so lose heat rapidly. Although they have more fat than the normal baby,

this is yellow fat and is not the thermogenic brown fat.

• Hyperbilirubinaemia. Infants with diabetic mothers are plethoric due to polycythaemia and the excess red blood cells break down after delivery causing jaundice.

*Management*

There is increasing evidence that good control of diabetes around the time of conception, and the first weeks after, reduces the incidence of congenital abnormalities and of miscarriage. Good control throughout pregnancy reduces many of the complications but has little effect on macrosomia (approximately 30%).

*Pre-pregnancy care*

• All insulin-dependent diabetics of reproductive age should take adequate contraceptive precautions until ready for pregnancy.

• Stress the need for pre-pregnancy counselling and planning:

(a) If they are on oral hypoglycaemic agent they should be changed to insulin.

(b) Twice-daily insulin regimens are the minimum acceptable for pregnancy. The best control of diabetes is achieved by giving a long-acting insulin at night and then by using a short-acting insulin to cover each meal throughout the day.

• Women should be taught to monitor their own blood sugar by BM Stix or Dextrostix. The monitoring should preferably be done by using an electronic glucose meter.

• Blood sugar should be monitored first thing in the morning, 1 hour before each meal and 1 hour after the biggest meal of the day.

• The aim is to maintain the blood sugar between 4 and 9 mmol/l.

• $HbA_1$ level should be checked after 6 weeks on the above regimen and should be less than 8%.

*Pregnancy management*

This should ideally be in a joint clinic in which women are seen by a diabetic physician with an interest in obstetrics and an obstetrician with an interest in diabetes.

• The aim is to maintain normoglycaemia as described above, throughout the pregnancy. This may lead to an increase in the number of hypoglycaemic attacks but these are not harmful to the fetus.

• The fetal death rate with hyperglycaemic coma is as high as 25%.

• The woman should be seen fortnightly throughout her pregnancy.

• Management of pregnant diabetics can normally be achieved at home especially if a specialist diabetic nurse is available to give advice over the telephone or to visit the patient's home.

• At each antenatal visit the following should be checked:

(a) The woman's diabetic record of home monitoring should be reviewed.

(b) The blood pressure.

(c) Symptoms suggestive of infection, particularly in the urinary tract.

(d) Fetal growth by clinical means and by reviewing the ultrasound results.

• The insulin requirements will increase markedly during pregnancy. In the first trimester they are usually static but then increase rapidly until 34 weeks, when they may then stabilize. Women should be taught to change their own insulin dosage.

*Ultrasound investigations*

**1** At 7 weeks' gestation to confirm fetal life and the number of fetuses.

**2** At 16–20 weeks' gestation a detailed scan for structural abnormalities.

**3** At 22–24 weeks' gestation to look specifically for cardiac abnormalities.

**4** Insulin-dependent diabetes alone is not an indication to perform karyotyping.

**5** Monthly fetal growth and amniotic fluid volume monitored. Figure 11.1 demonstrates the pattern of growth that is observed in babies who are destined to be macrosomic.

*Delivery*

• Aim to allow spontaneous labour but induce soon after expected delivery date (EDD).

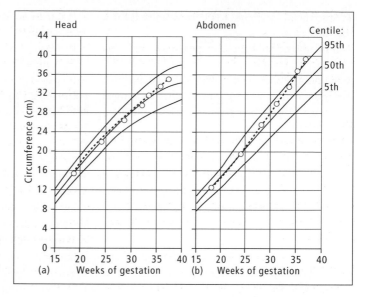

**Figure 11.1** Ultrasound growth charts showing a case of fetal macrosomia. (a) Head circumference. (b) Abdominal circumference.

• Caesarean section should only be carried out on obstetric grounds.
• Control of diabetes during labour is achieved by i.v. insulin infusion together with i.v. glucose. The woman's blood glucose is checked every hour by means of BM Stix, and should be 4–10 mmol/l.
• She should be encouraged to have an epidural as pain and fear release catecholamines which are gluconeogenic.
• Labour should be accelerated with Syntocinon if readings are more than 2 hours to the right of the partogram (see Chapter 13).
• A senior obstetrician should be present at the delivery because of the risk of shoulder dystocia.
• The incidence of Caesarean section in insulin-dependent diabetics is 2–3 times higher than the normal population because of:
  (a) Failed induction.
  (b) Fetal distress in early labour.
  (c) Disproportion (macrosomia).
  (d) An abnormal lie.

*Immediate care of the baby*
A paediatrician should be present at the delivery of all babies of insulin-dependent diabetic mothers. The following features are important:
• Resuscitate the baby if required.
• Dry the baby and keep it warm.

• Perform a BM Stix estimation of glucose from a heel prick at: 30 minutes, 1 hour, 4 hours, 8 hours, 12 hours and 24 hours.
• To prevent hypoglycaemia feed the baby early with glucose solution.
• Treat low values of blood glucose (less than 1 mmol/l) with an i.v. infusion of glucose. Some babies are resistant and may need to be given i.m. glucagon.
• Carefully examine the baby for congenital abnormalities.
• Measure the serum bilirubin on the 2nd day as this is when the hyperbilirubinaemia usually starts.

## Gestational diabetes

This is defined as the onset of diabetes or the appearance of abnormal glucose tolerance for the first time during pregnancy. A small proportion of these women will remain diabetic after delivery.

Gestational diabetes is not associated with congenital abnormalities. Main effects are:
• Development of polyhydramnios.
• Increase in the incidence of preterm labour.
• Production of macrosomia.
  It can be screened for in the following ways:

**1** Glucose tolerance test (GTT) on women at high risk (Box 11.3).
**2** Oral glucose load and a single blood sugar estimation 2 hours later.
**3** Random blood sugar at 28 weeks' gestation 2 hours after the last meal. Women who have high blood sugars are then given a glucose tolerance test.

THE GLUCOSE TOLERANCE TEST

This is a 50-g oral load of glucose in a flavoured drink. Fasting values of >5.8 mmol/l or 2-hour values of >7.8 mmol/l require further testing.

*Treatment*

There is no consensus view on treatment except that oral hypoglycaemics are contraindicated. The following outline is suggested:
• Home monitoring by means of an electronic glucose monitor.
• Fasting and 1 hour blood sugar after each meal on at least 2 days a week.
• No treatment required if the fasting blood sugar level is <5.5 mmol/l and the postprandial figures are <9 mmol/l.
• If higher levels are involved, the woman should start a simple carbohydrate-restricted diet. In addition to checking her blood sugars twice a week, also test her urine for ketones.
• If the simple diet does not achieve the required blood sugar levels, a twice daily regimen of medium- and short-acting insulin.

• If ketosis occurs the diet should be relaxed and start insulin.
• Ultrasound scan for fetal growth and amniotic fluid volume at least monthly.
• If no evidence of excessive fetal growth, spontaneous labour can be awaited up to 42 weeks' gestation. Women with ultrasound signs of macrosomia should be induced at term although some obstetricians perform a Caesarean section at 38–39 weeks' gestation.
• Control of blood sugar in labour is important. Those on insulin antenatally should have the same i.v. glucose and insulin regimen as insulin-dependent diabetics.
• With the delivery of the placenta, the insulin requirements soon disappear.
• There is evidence that women who have gestational diabetes have about a 40% chance of becoming diabetic in the long term, the risk doubling if the woman is obese. In the latter case, once breast feeding is ceased, the woman is given strict dietary advice and advised to lose weight.
• Gestational diabetes usually recurs in future pregnancies but this is not inevitable.

# Epilepsy

All anticonvulsant medications carry a small risk of teratogenicity. However, the risk of epileptic fits to the pregnancy outweighs the risk of teratogenicity, although some women may need a change in their medication in the first trimester to sodium valproate or phenytoin.

*Management*
• To reduce the teratogen risk, women should be advised to take the higher dose of folic acid (5 mg) preconceptually and throughout pregnancy.
• All women should be offered a fetal cardiology scan to detect congenital heart disease which, together with neural tube defects are the commonest congenital abnormality associated with antiepileptic medication.
• Vitamin K from 36 weeks to reduce the risk of postpartum haemorrhage.

---

**Box 11.3 High-risk features for abnormal glucose tolerance in pregnancy**

Maternal weight >90th centile (BMI >30 kg/m$^2$)
Previous big baby (>4.5 kg)
A first degree relative with diabetes
Glycosuria
   Once at <20 weeks
   Twice at >20 weeks
Previous unexplained stillbirth or neonatal death
Polyhydramnios
Fetal macrosomia on ultrasound

---

• Four to six weekly measurement of drug concentrations. The physiological increase in plasma volume commonly reduces the circulating drug concentration to below the therapeutic range. This increases the risk of epileptic fits which can be harmful to the mother and fatal to the fetus. If the level is below the therapeutic concentration then the dose is increased and the levels rechecked 2 weeks later.

> **Box 11.4 Reasons why appendicitis is a serious concern in pregnancy**
>
> **1** Underdiagnosed for it is not considered
> **2** Undertreated due to fear of abdominal operations in pregnancy
> **3** Appendix pushed out of right iliac fossa and becomes a general abdominal organ
> **4** Omentum does not wall off inflamed organ
> **5** Cortisol levels high, therefore poor inflammatory response.

## Abdominal pain in pregnancy

Diagnosis depends mostly on history and examination with very few investigations helping.

### Early pregnancy

#### Pelvic causes

**1** Miscarriage.
  • Spontaneous: crampy pain with contractions.
  • Induced: pain with sepsis.
**2** Ectopic pregnancy.
  • Pain from: stretch, leak of blood from ostium of tube, or rupture.
**3** Fibroids.
  • Pain from red degeneration—most common in mid-trimester.
**4** Ovarian cysts.
  • Pain from: rupture, twisting, or bleeding into cyst.
**5** Ligament stretch.
  • Pain from tension or haematoma.
**6** Impaction of the uterus.

#### Extrapelvic causes

**1** Vomiting in pregnancy.
  • Pain from abdominal wall muscle overstretch.
**2** Urinary infection.
  • Pain from bladder irritation and back pressure on kidney.
**3** Appendicitis (Box 11.4).
  • Pain from: peritoneal irritation, peritonitis, or rupture.

### Late pregnancy

#### Pelvic causes

**1** Labour (intermittent).
  • Pain from myometrial contractions.
**2** Hydramnios (constant).
  • Pain from stretch.
**3** Abruptio placentae (constant).
  • Pain from myometrial damage and stretch.
**4** Ruptured uterus (constant).
  • Pain from haemorrhage into peritoneal cavity.
**5** Ovarian cyst accident—rupture, haemorrhage, torsion.

#### Extrapelvic causes

**1** Rectus haematoma.
  • Pain from tissue stretch and irritation of tissues by blood.
**2** Fulminating pre-eclampsia (epigastric pain).
  • Pain from stretch of peritoneum over swollen liver.
**3** Cholecystitis.
  • Pain from gall bladder distension and inflammation.
**4** Peptic ulcer.
  • Pain from associated gastritis and acid irritation of submucosal tissues.
**5** Appendicitis—see p. 243.
**6** Pyelonephritis.
  • Pain from inflammation of pelvis or kidney.
**7** Ureteric stone.
  • Pain from renal colic due to obstruction.

**Management of abdominal pain**
• Make diagnosis accurately from history and ex-amination and act soon.
• Use ultrasound with vaginal probe if considered helpful.
• Be prepared to use a laparoscope in early pregnancy.
• Do not consider laparotomy to be dangerous in pregnancy.
• A pregnancy in a woman with an intra-abdominal inflammatory disease will not be harmed by prop-er surgical treatment. The fetus is more likely to be damaged if the proper operation is delayed.

# Infections in pregnancy

Any infection producing a pyrexia may cause mis-carriage or preterm labour.

Three groups of infections are particularly im-portant in pregnancy:
1 Genital tract infections.
2 Infections that cross the placenta.
3 Urinary tract infections.

## Genital tract infections

### Syphilis

All pregnant women are still screened for syphilis because, while the disease is rare, appropriate treat-ment can prevent congenital syphilis. Treponemas readily cross the placenta.

*Serological tests*
These fall into two groups:
1 *Non-specific tests.*
  • The Wassermann reaction (WR).
  • The Venereal Disease Research Laboratory (VDRL) slide test.
  • The rapid plasma reagin (RPR) card test.
False-positive tests may be seen with: chronic inflammatory diseases, yaws, narcotic abuse and pregnancy.
2 *Specific tests.*
  • The *Treponema pallidum* haemagglutination test (TPHA).

• The fluorescent *Treponema* antibody test (FTA).

These two tests are specific for *T. pallidum* and become positive some 2 weeks after the initial infection. They remain positive for ever once the patient has had the disease and do not produce biologically false-positive tests.

*Effects on the fetus*
1 Untreated early syphilis may result in neonatal death or stillbirth in 50%.
2 Congenital syphilis results in lasting neurologi-cal and skeletal damage.

*Management*
• *T. pallidum* is extremely sensitive to penicillin. Adequate treatment in early pregnancy protects the fetus. Even if the infection is only discovered in late pregnancy, treatment should still be given.
• Penicillin 1.2 mega-units i.m. for 10 days.
• Pregnant women who are allergic to penicillin should be given erythromycin 500 mg orally every 6 hours for 15 days.
• The woman should be followed by the genito-urinary physicians who should contact her sexual partners.

### Herpes genitalis

Herpes simplex virus (HSV) is a large DNA virus entering through a mucocutaneous surface, then migrating along nerves.

*Symptoms*
• The first attack of herpes genitalis is usually acutely painful.
• Vesicles break down to form shallow ulcers on the cervix, labia, perineum or the perianal areas.
• There is inguinal lymphadenopathy.
• Recurrent attacks are less severe; many give warning symptoms of a tingling sensation.

*Diagnosis*
• The lesions are usually clinically obvious.
• Ulcers should be scraped and the scrapings sent for viral identification.

*Effect on the newborn*
• Herpes neonatorum may kill up to 50% of those who get encephalitis but it is rare. A third of those remaining will have some residual neurological damage.
• The infection is acquired during the process of delivery or by ascending infection if the membranes have been ruptured for more than 4 hours.

*Treatment*
• Active infection in late pregnancy or early labour: consider Caesarean section to avoid herpes neonatorum.
• Acyclovir may be used in pregnancy.
• Acyclovir is used widely for the infant with herpes infection.

## Vaginal streptococcal infections

β-Haemolytic streptococcal (βHS) infections may cause:
1 Preterm rupture of the membranes and preterm labour.
2 Severe postpartum sepsis, particularly following Caesarean section.
3 Overwhelming neonatal sepsis that may lead to death.
  • About 20% of women will carry group B streptococci in the vagina. About 2% of these women will give birth to an infected infant and about 30% of these could die from overwhelming sepsis.
  • Screening all pregnant women for the infection is not practical.
  • All women presenting with preterm rupture of the membranes should have a sample of the amniotic fluid sent to identify the organism. If present, the baby should be delivered immediately with penicillin cover.
  • A woman who is known to be a carrier for βHS should be given prophylactic i.v. penicillin V during labour.

## Listeriosis

Between 1% and 5% of pregnant women will carry *Listeria monocytogenes* in the rectum. The organism may in addition be acquired in pregnancy from eating unpasteurized cheese and from cooked meats. It may produce the following symptoms:
• Maternal diarrhoea accompanied by a pyrexia.
• Premature labour.
  Listeriosis septicaemia of the preterm infant acquired at birth may be rapidly fatal and may occur in the presence of few symptoms in the mother.

*Treatment*
Ampicillin i.v.

## Infections that cross the placenta

The placenta acts as an efficient barrier against some infections in the mother. The following, however, are not uncommonly found in pregnant women and often cause serious consequences to the fetus:
• Syphilis (see p. 152).
• Rubella.
• Cytomegalovirus.
• Toxoplasmosis.
• Human immunodeficiency virus (HIV).
• Parvovirus.

### Rubella

The widespread policy of vaccinating schoolgirls and more recently all children means that German measles (rubella) is becoming rarer. All pregnant women are tested for the levels of rubella antibodies at the antenatal clinic; if they are seronegative, they are offered vaccination in the puerperium.
  Rubella rapidly crosses the placenta and may cause:
• Mental retardation and microcephaly.
• Cataract.
• Congenital heart disease.
• Deafness.
• Hepatosplenomegaly with thrombocytopenia if the mother is infected in the last half of the pregnancy.
  Women suspected of having acquired rubella in early pregnancy should have a rubella-specific IgM test. If positive, then the options available are:

**1** Termination of pregnancy. This applies particularly if the primary infection was less than 10 weeks' gestation as more than half of the babies will be affected.

**2** A chorionic villus sample. Electron microscopy and modern immune methods may be able to determine if the virus has crossed the placenta. This test can be performed at 11–14 weeks' gestation.

**3** A fetal blood sample at 18–20 weeks' gestation (cordocentesis) to determine if the fetus is IgM-positive for rubella. If negative, the patient can be reassured. If positive, it confirms that the fetus has been infected but does not guarantee that it is affected. Most would ask for a termination of pregnancy on these grounds.

## Cytomegalovirus (CMV)

CMV infection is now the most common perinatal infection in both the UK and USA. The most serious manifestations associated with primary maternal infection include:
- Stillbirth.
- Hepatosplenomegaly and jaundice.
- Thrombocytopenia.
- Microcephaly.
- Chorioretinitis.
  CMV may be acquired:
- In childhood from other children's saliva, tears, urine or stool.
- As an adult by sexual contact or blood transfusions.
- In the perinatal period by direct transmission across the placenta.

By the time pregnancy occurs, about 75% of women will be immune to CMV. Of women who acquire CMV in pregnancy, some 5% have a seriously damaged infant. Unlike rubella, there is no vaccination against the disease.

If the disease is suspected, it can be confirmed by looking for the IgM specific to CMV. Transplacental passage is not inevitable and the organism may be sought in the fetus by means of chorionic villus sample (early) or fetal blood sample (late) (see rubella).

## Toxoplasmosis

*Toxoplasma gondii* comes from parasites in cats' intestines. Human infection occurs as a result of eating poorly cooked meats that contain tissue cysts or which have been exposed to infected cat faeces. Infection readily crosses the placenta. In the mother, it may be asymptomatic, or produce a glandular fever-like illness. Transplacental infection may cause:
- Microcephaly or hydrocephaly.
- Cerebral calcification leading to epilepsy and cerebral damage.
- Chorioretinitis.

The disease is diagnosed in the mother by finding an IgM specifically against toxoplasmosis. The mother can be treated by spiromycin to prevent further transplacental passage of the organism. Fetal infection may be diagnosed by fetal blood sampling and the search for specific IgM.

There is treatment available for the fetus through the mother but many women are offered a termination if their fetuses are infected.

## Human immunodeficiency virus (HIV)

Pregnancy may allow mild immunosuppression of the T cell type leading to a theoretical fear of exacerbation of HIV illness in pregnancy. This has not been borne out in clinical practice.

The fetus can be infected antenatally by the passage of HIV across the placenta. About 15% of babies born to mothers who are HIV-positive will remain HIV-positive at 6 months of age. It is estimated that 50% of these fetuses infected *in utero* will be dead from AIDS by 2 years.
- Women in high-risk groups (see p. 108) should be offered HIV testing after appropriate counselling.
- HIV can be isolated from cervical secretions and therefore the baby may be infected at birth. Delivery should be by elective Caesarean section to reduce transmission. Stillbirth is more common beyond term.

HIV may be passed in breastmilk and so women in the UK with HIV should be advised not to breastfeed.
- There is little evidence that asymptomatic HIV infection has any significant effect on pregnancy

complications or the long-term outcome of women who are HIV-positive.

• Women who are HIV-positive need special care in the antenatal clinic, at delivery and in the puerperium, especially as they often have major psychosocial problems.

• Treat an HIV-positive woman in pregnancy and pre-Caesarean section with zidovudine (Retrovir) because it passes to the fetus and greatly reduces the risks of HIV infection in the newborn.

• The risk of health workers acquiring infection is small but delivery presents problems to the staff because the woman's blood and body products may contain live virus. In consequence, extra barrier precautions are taken.

• Knowledge of the HIV status of newborn babies of high-risk women is essential in planning their vaccination policy against other infections. Vaccination with live attenuated vaccines should be avoided.

## Hepatitis B

Hepatitis B virus is transmitted by contaminated blood products and by sexual intercourse. Transplacental rates of transmission are low amongst Europeans (<5%) but higher amongst Asians (40–90%). Rates of transmission are greater in women who are hepatitis B surface antigen positive.

The baby may be born apparently normal but develop hepatitis problems later. Rates may be reduced by both passive immunization with hepatitis B IgG and active immunization with hepatitis B vaccine.

## Uterine conditions in pregnancy

### Retroversion

Retroversion is the normal position of the uterus in 20% of women. If pregnancy occurs in a retroverted uterus:

• It usually comes upright as it enlarges.

• If tethered in the pouch of Douglas by old adhesions, it may enlarge by anterior sacculation.

• If the uterus is tethered it may grow and impact below the promontory of the sacrum. Growth can continue for a short time but soon there is:

  • Backache from pressure on the sacral peritoneum.

  • Retention of urine from stretching of urethra by displacement of bladder into abdomen.

  Unless this is relieved, the pregnancy will miscarry.

*Management*
1 Indwelling catheter and continuous drainage.
2 Uterus often slides up into the abdomen. Once up, it will not go back so no pessary is required.
3 Manual manipulation *per vaginum* under general anaesthesia below 16 weeks.

## Pelvic tumours

### Fibroids

Seen more commonly in the pregnancy age group among Afro-Caribbean women.

*Diagnosis*
Firm bosselated swellings detected usually in early pregnancy. Later they soften and are difficult to locate. Ultrasound can usually detect fibroids (see p. 231).

*Complications*
1 Miscarriage (usually submucosal fibroids).
2 Pressure:
  • On pelvic wall veins (oedema of legs), thrombosis.
  • On bladder (increased frequency).
3 Red degeneration:
  • Venous blood supply may be cut off and fibroid becomes stuffed with blood. Local pain and tenderness. May lead to premature labour.
  • If diagnosed correctly, analgesia and bed rest allow resolution.
  • If in doubt, do laparotomy to check. If red degeneration seen, leave alone. Myomectomy during pregnancy is contraindicated.

**4** Malpresentation:
  • Oblique or transverse lie may persist because of position of fibroids.
**5** Obstruction to labour:
  • Very rarely happens, because lower uterine fibroids usually ride up into the abdomen when lower segment is formed and stretched.
  • If cervical fibroids obstruct, Caesarean section must be performed, but do not do myomectomy at the same time because of risk of heavy bleeding.
**6** Dysfunction:
  • Masses of fibrous tissue distort the smooth transmission of contractile impulses through the uterus.

## Ovarian cysts

In pregnancy:
• Corpus luteal cysts: 70%.
• Benign mucous or serous cystadenoma: 20%.
• Dermoid cyst: 5%.
• Malignant tumour: 1%.

*Diagnosis*
Mobile mass alongside or displacing uterus in early pregnancy. Ultrasound can usually help diagnosis.

*Complications*
**1** Rupture of cyst.
**2** Torsion of cyst.
**3** Bleeding into cyst.
**4** Obstruction in labour (rare).

*Management*
If any cyst over 10cm diameter is detected, it should be removed. Try to do this in the middle trimester of pregnancy. Excise because:
• It may be malignant.
• It may undergo any of the above complications in labour or the puerperium.

---

**Self-assessment**

**11.1** Which of the following statements are true?
  (a) Women with gestational diabetes commonly present with ketoacidosis.
  (b) Women with a first degree relative suffering from Type 1 diabetes are at increased risk of developing gestational diabetes.
  (c) Women with pre-existing Type 1 diabetes are at increased risk of developing pre-eclamptic toxaemia.
  (d) Gestational diabetes is most commonly controlled by diet alone.
  (e) Gestational diabetes usually requires insulin therapy.
**11.2** Gestational diabetes is associated with an increased risk for the fetus of:
  (a) Unexplained stillbirth beyond 40 weeks of pregnancy.
  (b) Hypoglycaemia following birth.
  (c) There is an increased risk of shoulder dystocia.
  (d) Congenital abnormality.
  (e) Neonatal jaundice.
**11.3** Common causes of anaemia in pregnancy include:
  (a) Vitamin B6 deficiency.
  (b) Vitamin K deficiency.
  (c) Folate deficiency.
  (d) Vitamin B12 deficiency.
  (e) Iron deficiency.
**11.4** Which of the following statements are true?
  (a) Women with β-haemolytic streptococcus are at increased risk of going into premature labour.
  (b) Babies born to women with β-haemolytic streptococcus are at increased risk of hypoglycaemia.
  (c) β-haemolytic streptococcus is a vaginal commensal in up to 20% of women.
  (d) Women with β-haemolytic streptococcus should be treated with penicillin during labour.
  (e) Women with β-haemolytic streptococcus should be treated with penicillin antenatally to prevent infection in the neonate.

# CHAPTER 12

# Normal labour

Labour is the expulsion of the fetus and placenta from the uterus and is traditionally divided into three stages, unequal in length (Fig. 12.1).

## Stages

**1** *The first stage, dilatation*—from the onset of labour until the cervix is fully dilated. More recently it has been divided into two phases:
- The *latent phase* of effacement of the cervix: to 3 cm dilation.
- The *active phase* of active cervical dilatation: from 3 cm to full dilation.

**2** *The second stage, expulsive*—from full cervical dilatation to birth of the baby.

**3** *The third stage, placental*—from birth of the baby to the delivery of the placenta.

## Changes in pelvic organs during labour

**1** The cervix becomes effaced and dilates fully.

**2** The uterus and vagina become one elongated tube.

**3** The pelvic floor muscles are stretched backwards.

**4** The bladder becomes an abdominal organ and the urethra is lengthened.

**5** The bowel is compressed.

## Uterine action

The fetus is propelled down the birth canal by the action of the myometrium. Normal uterine activity is fundally dominant, so waves of contraction pass down from each cornu to the lower uterine segment.

During labour, contractions increase in frequency and strength. Contractions are painful and this may be due to:
- Hypoxia because of the duration of the contraction.
- Compression of the nerve endings in the myometrium.
- Cervical stretch and dilatation.

The patterns of propagation of the uterine activity start at each cornu and travel caudally. Labour starts with contractions about one in every 20 minutes increasing to one in every 2–3 minutes. The upper uterine segment contracts and retracts so that the lower segment and later, the cervix, is pulled over the baby's head rather like putting on a tight polo-neck sweater.

Figure 12.2 illustrates the intrauterine pressures that are achieved during normal labour.

## Mechanism of labour

In humans, the cause of labour is unknown. The following facts are accepted:

**Figure 12.1** Average length of stages of labour in a nullipara.

**Figure 12.2** Intrauterine pressure patterns.

- Oestrogens increase uterine muscle activity whilst progesterone suppresses it.
- In late pregnancy the fetal adrenal glands produce much more dehydroepiandrosterone sulphate (DHEAS) which is converted by the placenta into oestrogen. This encourages uterine contractions.
- The decidua releases prostaglandins (PGs), mainly $PGE_2$ and $PGF_{2\alpha}$. Such PGs cause minor uterine contractions which result in further hypoxia of the decidua and so further PG production.
- The final common pathway for a contraction is an increase in the cytosol-free calcium which causes a joining together of actin and myosin. This is common to all involuntary muscle contractions.
- Oxytocin, released from the posterior pituitary, cannot be detected in the blood in early normal labour. The release of oxytocin is dependent upon a monosynaptic reflex, initiated when the presenting part presses on the pelvic floor.

## The uterus in the first stage

**1** Uterine muscle fibres contract and retract, so they do not return to their original length after contraction but remain shorter.

**2** There is a heaping up and thickening of the upper uterine segment while the lower uterine segment becomes thinner and stretched.

**3** The cervix is pulled up and the canal is effaced so its length diminishes.

**4** The cervix is pulled up and open and so the os is dilated.

These changes often start with the painless Braxton Hicks' contractions of late pregnancy so that by the beginning of labour the cervix is often already partially effaced and a little dilated particularly in multiparous women.

## The uterus in the second stage

**1** A diminution in the transverse diameters because of:
- Pulling up of the lower segment.
- Straightening out of the fetus.

**2** The fetal head is forced into the upper vagina which now forms a continuous tube with the uterus and a fully effaced cervix.

**3** As well as uterine contractions, expulsive efforts are made by the mother using:
- The abdominal wall muscles.
- The fixed diaphragm, thus raising intra-abdominal pressure.

**4** Voluntary efforts are not essential; paraplegic women and those with epidural analgesia have normal deliveries. Pushing is instinctive, and very satisfying to the woman who then assists at her own delivery.

## The uterus in the third stage

**1** The uterine muscles contract so constricting the blood vessels passing between the fibres, and thus preventing excessive bleeding (Fig. 12.3).

**2** The placenta separates at the delivery of the fetus when the uterus contracts sharply in size. Haemostasis is mostly mechanical immediately after delivery, with muscle fibres kinking blood vessels. During pregnancy and most of the labour the placental bed and the placenta are roughly the same size. With the fetus removed, the area of the placental bed is reduced to about half that of the placenta (Fig. 12.4). The placenta is therefore sheared off and is finally expelled from the uterus by contractions passing down into the lower segment.

The signs of descent of the placenta in the uterus are:
- The uterus becomes hard.
- The umbilical cord lengthens.
- There is a show of blood.

**Figure 12.3** Uterine blood vessels become constricted when the surrounding muscle fibres contract.

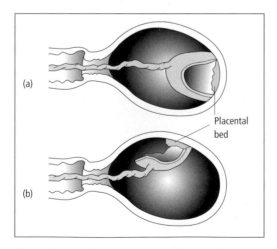

**Figure 12.4** (a) The commoner mechanism of placental separation in which the whole organ separates from its bed and balloons inside out into the uterine cavity. (b) Less commonly, the placenta separates at one side of the disc and is peeled off as the uterine muscle contracts and makes the placental bed much smaller in area.

# Management of normal labour

## Diagnosis of labour

The onset of labour is defined as regular painful uterine contractions that cause cervical change. By definition it is often a retrospective diagnosis.

## Admission

**1** 97% of women in the UK deliver in the hospital or midwifery/general practice-run maternity unit.
**2** Women should be advised to come into hospital when:
- Uterine contractions are occurring every 5–10 minutes.
- Their membranes rupture and amniotic fluid is released.
**3** Assuming the woman had full antenatal care, on admission and her records are available:
- A short history of labour is taken.
- A brief examination is performed including the following:
  (a) check the blood pressure;
  (b) determine the lie and presentation of the fetus;
  (c) determine the degree of engagement of the presenting part;
  (d) perform a vaginal examination to assess the degree of effacement and dilatation of the cervix.
- The woman is offered a warm bath.

## First stage of labour

Progress in labour is monitored by descent of the fetal head together with dilatation of the cervix. As little or nothing is known about the rate of cervical dilatation prior to admission to the labour ward, the partogram is started on admission.

The partogram (Fig. 12.5), used by most maternity units, is an easy, graphical method of assessing the progress of labour and helps facilitate handover between midwives. It contains the following information:

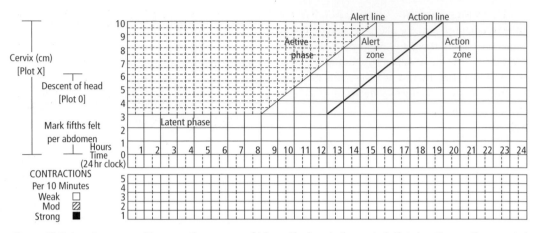

**Figure 12.5** A partogram used to assess the progress of labour. The lines in the cervical dilated section are the expected patterns of cervical dilatation in labour showing a slow latent phase and faster active phase. If dilatation crosses the action line then the patient should be reviewed and/or an ARM and syntocinon infusion started to accelerate labour.

**Figure 12.6** The expected normal progress and descent of fetal head through pelvis. Engagement, the maximum head diameter passing through the inlet of the pelvis.

**1** High-risk factors—obstetric, paediatric or anaesthetic.

**2** A record of the fetal heart rate. Higher risk women have continuous electronic fetal heart rate monitoring (EFM) by the cardiotocograph. Low-risk women usually have the fetal heart rate measured with a Pinard's stethoscope every 15 minutes, immediately following contractions. These records are plotted on the partogram.

**3** The cervicogram: graphical record of the rate of cervical dilatation.

**4** Descent of fetal head.

**5** Frequency, duration and strength of uterine contractions are recorded.

**6** If membranes are ruptured, the amniotic fluid colour.

**7** The volume of maternal urine that is produced, tested for ketones and protein.

**8** A record of the drugs given, in particular analgesics.

**9** Maternal blood pressure, pulse and temperature.

After the first examination the following should be plotted:

**1** The amount of the fetal head that can be palpated per abdomen in terms of fifths of the head descent. Figure 12.6 illustrates the system of fifths.

**2** The cervical dilatation (1 cm/hour beyond 3 cm).

**3** A line of expected cervical dilatation should then also be plotted. The WHO have produced an international partogram with two parallel straight lines plotted at 1 cm/hour. The first line represents the expected progress of a normal labour. If cervical dilatation falls below the first line and reaches/crosses the action line then an artificial rupture of the membranes (ARM) should be performed. If progress after 2 hours is not parallel to the action line then syntocinon should be started to make the contractions stronger and more frequent. Labour should then follow the action line, if it does not then a Caesarean section is indicated.

The level of descent of the presenting part should be checked and plotted every hour, whilst vaginal examinations may be performed every 3–4 hours. As long as the rate of cervical dilatation stays on or to the left of the nomogram, labour progress is considered to be normal.

## Care of the patient

• The woman should not be left alone during labour. Ideally there should be a midwife present with her throughout. In addition, many women choose to have their partner, companion or relative present.
• Analgesia should be given sufficient for the woman's need (p. 162).
• She should be encouraged to pass urine frequently. If the woman cannot void and the bladder becomes palpable in abdomen, she should be catheterized.
• Light snacks, soup or cool fluids are offered.

## Second stage of labour

**1** During the expulsive stage, the woman is encouraged to push with uterine contractions. If she is sitting propped up, this is done, by taking a deep breath and holding it, putting her chin on her chest, and pulling on the backs of her knees. Women usually achieve two or three expulsive pushes during each uterine contraction.
**2** Monitoring progress in the second stage of labour is by vaginal assessment of the lowest part of the presenting pole related to the ischeal spines. This applies until the presenting part becomes visible.
**3** Inhalation analgesia should be offered if the woman needs it. With organized pushing, many women do not require pain relief.
**4** Episiotomies are no longer performed routinely but are indicated for the following reasons:
• Fetal distress.
• Most operative vaginal deliveries.
• The presence of a rigid perineum which, in the opinion of the midwife, is delaying delivery.
• If an experienced midwife believes that there is going to be a major perineal tear.

Minor tears (1° and some 2°) often do not need suturing and heal well.
**5** If an episiotomy is to be performed, local anaesthetic (lignocaine 1% plain) is injected into the subcutaneous tissues of the vagina and perineum as the head distends the perineum. Just prior to crowning, a right mediolateral episiotomy is usually performed. With slow extension of the head the episiotomy does not extend.
**6** When the head is delivered, it is allowed to rotate (restitute) and then lateral traction is applied in the direction of the mother's anus which allows the birth of the fetal anterior shoulder.
**7** Now give 0.5 mg of Syntometrine intramuscularly (i.m.) to aid delivery of the placenta.
**8** The baby's head is raised towards the mother's abdomen so the posterior shoulder passes over the perineum and the rest of the baby usually then slips out.
**9** The baby's mouth and nasal passages are usually sucked free of mucus with a mechanical mucus extractor. The mouth should be cleared before the nose as aspirating the nose often causes the baby to inhale.
**10** The umbilical cord is clamped twice, and divided between the clamps. In developed countries, hospital units now use disposable plastic umbilical clamps, although Spencer Wells forceps suffice.
**11** The baby usually starts breathing within 1 minute of delivery. The baby may be given to the mother immediately if she so wishes but should be wrapped in a prewarmed blanket first.

## Third stage of labour

**1** Syntometrine has been given with the delivery of the anterior shoulder. Signs of placental separation are now no longer awaited before applying controlled cord traction.
**2** The operator's left hand is placed above the symphysis pubis and guards the front wall of the uterus to prevent uterine inversion.
**3** The umbilical cord is grasped in the operator's right hand and steady traction is applied until the placenta is delivered down into the vagina and into a kidney dish.
**4** The membranes usually follow the placenta and

can be removed by gentle rotation of the placenta helping them to peel off the uterus.

**5** The placenta and membranes are checked for completeness.

**6** Blood loss should be estimated; it is usually between 100 and 300 ml.

**7** Any tear or episiotomy should be carefully repaired under local anaesthetic with absorbable sutures such as Vicryl/Dexon (Fig. 12.7). Massaging the perineum with almond oil, prior to delivery, has been shown to reduce the risk of tearing.

## Pain relief in labour

• Labour is usually painful. Relief of pain is better given before the woman feels the pain of the contractions.

• Careful timing of analgesia is as important as correct dosage.

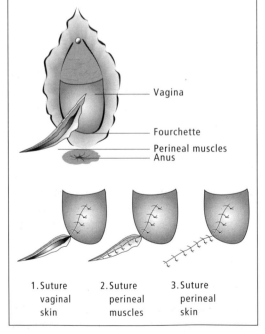

**Figure 12.7** Repair of an episiotomy.

## Drug analgesia

### Nitrous oxide

This is self-administered, pre-mixed with $O_2$ (50% of each), in Entonox machines. Inhalation should start as each contraction is felt and before the woman feels pain (Fig. 12.8) for it takes some seconds to work.

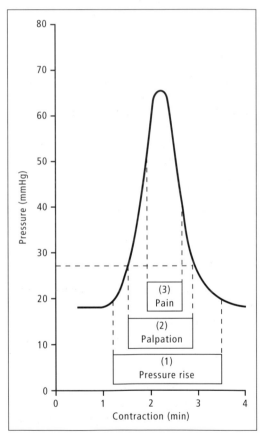

**Figure 12.8** Pressure recording of contraction in late labour: (1) tocograph pressure readings show contraction for 2.5 minutes; (2) clinical abdominal palpation diagnosis shows it for 1.5 minute; (3) pain is felt by the woman for 45 seconds.

## Pethidine

Pethidine has been used for many years as an analgesic in labour. Many units have now withdrawn it because of evidence that it is a poor analgesic and can have a prolonged depressant effect on neonatal respiratory effort.

• Synthetic analgesic and antispasmodic.
• Dose: 50–150 mg i.m.;
        50–100 mg i.v. (slowly, for it can cause nausea).
• Use in first stage. Try to avoid giving within 2 hours of expected delivery if possible because of depression of neonatal respiration.
• Can cause drop of maternal blood pressure.
• Causes nausea in 20%. Give anti-emetic.

## Morphine

• An alkaloid of opium. Stronger analgesic with no antispasmodic action. Used for the pains of occipitoposterior positions and long labours.
• Dose: 10 mg i.m.
• Morphine depresses the neonatal respiratory centre, and should be avoided for 2 hours before delivery if possible.
• May cause maternal vomiting (about 15%) so give anti-emetic (e.g. Phenergan 25 mg or Fentazin 5 mg).

## Diamorphine (heroin)

• Very powerful opiate. Good for anxious mother or long labour.
• Dose: 5–10 mg i.m.
• Depresses neonatal respiratory centre if given within 3–4 hours.
• Still used in Scotland and north of England.
*Note*: Barbiturates, tranquillizers and sedatives given in labour are *not* analgesics. They often potentiate analgesics and help progress by their own properties.

## Non-drug analgesia

Increasing numbers of women are turning to non-pharmacological methods of pain relief. Pain is such a subjective symptom that anything which helps a woman and does not put her or her fetus at increased risk should be explored. Maybe these methods cause the release of endorphins and so postpone the need for more formal analgesia; this reduces the total dose, giving the woman a greater sense of self-participation.

## Water

Immersion in warm water so that the woman becomes weightless reduces the sensation of pain and many women find passing the first stage of labour in a birth pool or large bath very helpful and soothing. Some women choose to stay in the water for second stage and delivery. In this situation the baby is monitored using a special Doppler/sonicaid which are waterproof. When the baby is born it is vital that the water is at 37°C and the baby is brought to the surface quickly so that it does not take its first breath underwater. The main risks for the infant are of drowning and infection and, although both of these are rare, they can be fatal.

## Relaxation

The woman should take training in pregnancy. The method works best if there is a sympathetic attendant to guide in labour (e.g. partner). It is safe for mother and fetus.

## Hypnosis

If both woman and attendant are trained, this can give good pain relief. It is expensive on attendant's time and only works for susceptible women. If it works, it is very safe for the fetus.

## Acupuncture

Some women opt for acupuncture in labour. The effects are very variable from one person to another and the need for several needles in various points of the body limits mobilization which many women find unacceptable.

## Transcutaneous nerve stimulation (TENS)

Small pulses of electrical vibration to the muscles of the back, from a portable battery-driven pack, provide distraction therapy. Some find it helpful in the early stages of labour. Even though it might not work for full labour, it could postpone the need for a stronger, more depressant, analgesia and so its use should be encouraged if women want to try it. However, labour ward staff must know how to work the machines and be sympathetic to their use.

## Anaesthesia

Depression of the central or peripheral nervous system to prevent transmission and reception of painful impulses.

### General

Total anaesthesia induced by injection (e.g. pentothal) and followed by inhalation (e.g. nitrous oxide or cyclopropane) results in an unconscious patient completely under the anaesthetist's control.

In labour one of the risks is regurgitation of acid stomach contents and their inhalation into the lungs producing aspiration pneumonia (Mendelson's syndrome). To avoid this:
- Have as empty a stomach as possible.
- If really necessary, ensure stomach is empty—pass a tube.
- Reduce acidity of stomach contents—give sodium citrate (30 ml) or $H_2$ blocker, e.g. ranitidine.
- Once induced, pass cuffed endotracheal tube.
- Tilt head up for intubation and 'use cricoid pressure.
- Only skilled senior anaesthetists deal with women in labour.

General anaesthesia is useful for operations such as an emergency Caesarean section when speed is essential.

## Regional

Nerve roots are blocked at their outflow.

### Spinal block
- Heavy nupivercaine into subarachnoid space.
- Give at L3–4, put woman in head-up position.
- Blocks $T_{11}$–$S_1$.
- Used once only usually for operative delivery (e.g. Caesarean section).
- Good anaesthetic used increasingly in UK.

### Epidural block
- Bupivacaine 1% or Marcain 0.25–0.5% through a cannula inserted into peridural fat. Affects nerve roots $T_{11}$–$S_4$.
- Pain relief rapid, lasting 2–3 hours.
- Repeated doses can be given; therefore used for pain relief in labour.
- Requires expert anaesthetist (Fig. 12.9).
- Loss of sensation from the uterus means the woman needs help in the second stage to recognize uterine contractions.
- Using a constant infusion of bupivacaine with fentanyl reduces the density of the block and allows some mobilization for the woman (walking epidural).

**Figure 12.9** An epidural block. The outer cannula is removed and the flexible plastic catheter remains in peridural space.

*Complications*

• A serious complication of the epidural block is puncture of the dura and so unwittingly performing a spinal anaesthetic with a big needle. This could lead to nerve blockage and stopping respiration if the anaesthetic agent flows up into the thoracic region. Such a complication is watched for carefully by an experienced anaesthetist; it occurs in 1 : 500 cases.

• A rarer complication is infection which might enter through the skin to the peridural area.

**Caudal block**

• Localized epidural through sacral hiatus.
• Gives good anaesthesia for operative deliveries but only 80% effective.

## Local

### Pudendal

• Block pudendal nerve with Xylocaine 0.5 or 1% as its two or three branches circumnavigate the ischial spine; given either through vagina or through perineal skin. Numbs the area on the right only as shown in Fig. 12.10, and therefore needs a field block as well.

• Used for outlet manipulations in the second stage of labour, e.g. easy forceps delivery.

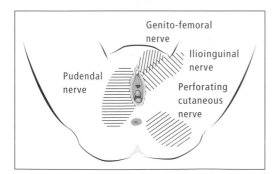

**Figure 12.10** The sensory nerve supply of the skin of the perineum. While the pudendal nerve principally supplies this area, other nerves are involved and need consideration in anaesthetizing the perineum locally.

### Field block

A local infiltration of the nerve endings in the vulva and labia:
• Prior to episiotomy or its repair.
• As an adjunct to pudendal block.

Proper analgesia and anaesthesia in labour work best when the woman and her partner have been instructed antenatally and have had a chance to learn about the methods available. She should talk to other women who have benefited by analgesia. All this is then applied by sympathetic attendants who look to the needs of the individual woman and tailor the therapy to her needs, preferably preventing pain being felt rather than trying to remove it after it has arrived.

## The fetus during labour

During labour the fetus descends down the birth canal and is then delivered. The process is conventionally broken down into the series of mechanisms detailed below, but these merge with each other and are inseparable.

*Flexion*
Uterine activity is fundally dominant; the line of force is down the fetal spine and causes flexion of the fetal head. The head then engages when the presenting diameter passes through the pelvic brim. In the majority of cases this is in the right occipitotransverse position.

*Descent*
Further uterine activity causes the fetal head to descend through the pelvic brim to the mid-cavity.

*Internal rotation*
Due to the angle of inclination between the lumbar spine and the pelvis (about 135°), the fetal head engages in the pelvis with one parietal eminence lower than the other (asynclitism). The leading parietal eminence is pushed into the pelvic floor with uterine contractions. When the uterus relaxes, the reaction from the pelvic floor muscles causes the fetal head to rotate until the head is no longer asynclitic. The head rotates from the

right occipitotransverse position at engagement to become direct occipitoanterior (Fig. 12.11).

### Further flexion

Further descent through the pelvis causes the chin to be forced tightly up against the fetal chest. The fetal occiput comes to lie behind the maternal symphysis pubis and the chin comes down to the lower part of the birth canal.

### Extension

Further descent pushes the fetal head forward and gradual extension of the fetal head occurs distending the perineum. With more extension, the widest diameter passes through the vulval introitus (crowning) and the head is born by extension at the fetal neck.

### Restitution and internal rotation

As the head is born, the shoulders enter the maximum diameter (the transverse diameter) of the maternal pelvic inlet. As they descend through the canal, one shoulder leads because of the angle of inclination. This causes the shoulders to rotate (just as the head did in internal rotation) and, as they do so, the head (outside the body now) rotates 90°. The shoulders now lie in the anteroposterior diameter behind the maternal symphysis pubis, the head rotates to its usual alignment with the shoulders.

### Delivery of the body

By assisted lateral flexion of the fetal head, the anterior shoulder is made to slip under the pubis and is born. The posterior shoulder and the rest of the body follows usually very easily.

During each uterine contraction, the maternal blood supply to the intervillous space is severely reduced and may be cut off. This reduces the fetal $O_2$ supply and allows less time for exchange of waste products from the fetus to the mother. Most normal fetuses can stand intermittent hypoxic ischaemia but preterm babies and those who are SGA may run into danger at this time. In consequence, the fetus often needs to be carefully monitored during labour.

## Monitoring the fetus during labour

There has been much recent controversy about the value of EFM in labour. There is probably little value in continuous EFM in low-risk pregnancies. Such women may have a short (20 minutes) cardiotocograph recording on admission to the labour ward. If the CTG is normal thereafter the fetal heart is listened to every 15 minutes with a Pinard stethoscope/sonicaid.

There is a high risk of hypoxia in the following circumstances so continuous EFM is required:
• Preterm infants (less than 37 weeks' completed gestation).

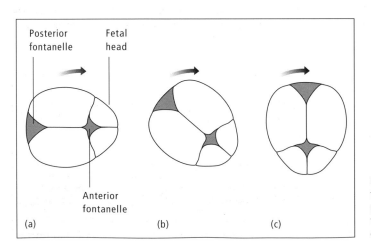

Posterior fontanelle

Fetal head

Anterior fontanelle

(a)  (b)  (c)

**Figure 12.11** Internal rotation of the fetus. (a) Inlet: right occipitotransverse position. (b) Mid-cavity: right occipitoanterior position. (c) Outlet: direct occipitoanterior position.

- Fetuses that are or are suspected to be SGA.
- Multiple pregnancies.
- Breech presentations.
- Women with epidural analgesia.
- Women with Syntocinon augmentation of labour.
- Women who have been induced.
- Women who are hypertensive.
- Women with major medical disorders, including diabetes.
- Women who develop meconium staining of the amniotic fluid during labour.
- Women who undergo a trial of uterine scar.
- If a fetal heart abnormality is recorded with the Pinard stethoscope/sonicaid.

## Continuous electronic fetal heart rate monitoring

In all modern labour wards, this is performed with either:

**1** An external fetal heart rate monitor with Doppler ultrasound echoing off movements of the fetal cardiac walls or the cardiac valves.

**2** An electrode attached to the fetal scalp (Fig. 12.12) showing the fetal heart rate derived from the fetal ECG.

Either of these provides the fetal heart rate and this is recorded on a continuous trace. In normal labour, this should be between 110 and 160 beats/minute (see p. 115). EFM is used as a screening test to detect those babies who are developing metabolic acidosis. The diagnostic test is to perform a fetal scalp sample and measure the scalp pH.

Changes in the fetal heart rate may be classified into three groups.

*Speed of heart rate*

**1** A *fetal tachycardia*. Figure 12.13 demonstrates a fetal tachycardia of about 170 beats/minute. The causes of this might be:

- A maternal tachycardia due to pyrexia, pain, fear or dehydration.
- Fetal hypoxia.

(a)                                        (b)

**Figure 12.12** Fetal scalp electrodes for (a) clipping onto or (b) screwing into the skin of the fetal presenting part thus providing electrical continuity.

**Figure 12.13** A CTG demonstrating an uncomplicated, moderate, baseline tachycardia. The baseline is 170 beats/minute. The reduced variability is a feature of the tachycardia. This trace was due to a maternal pyrexia in labour consequent upon a urinary tract infection.

**Figure 12.14** A CTG demonstrating a moderate baseline bradycardia. The baseline is 100 beats/minute. No cause for this was found.

**Figure 12.15** A CTG demonstrating loss of baseline variability.

Management is to exclude or correct a maternal cause and, if the tachycardia persists, a fetal blood sample should be performed.

**2** A *baseline bradycardia*. Baseline bradycardias are uncommon and provided they are in the 110–120 beats/minute range and there is baseline variability they are not of serious significance (Fig. 12.14). Bradycardias of <110 beats/minute in labour are often due to congenital heart block.

*Baseline variability*

Terminology in this area is difficult because of the way in which the machinery records the heart rate. Most external Doppler machines group average beats and so the term beat-to-beat variation should be reserved for fetal heart rate traces that are obtained by fetal scalp electrodes where true beat-to-beat measurements are made.

The variation in fetal heart rate from one beat to the next (baseline variability) is due to the balance between the parasympathetic and the sympathetic nervous system. In normal labour this varies by 5–15 beats either side of the baseline.

The major variations of baseline variability are:

**1** *Loss of baseline variability*. This is illustrated in Fig. 12.15 and may be caused by:
- Administration of drugs to the mother including pethidine, diazepam and many anti-hypertensive agents, especially β-blockers.
- Fetal sleep especially in early labour.
- Fetal hypoxia. In the absence of maternal drugs, loss of baseline variability should lead to a fetal blood sample.

**2** *Increased baseline variability* (sinusoidal rhythm). This is illustrated in Fig. 12.16 and usually is of serious significance. The causes of it are as follows:
- Fetal asphyxia.
- Fetal anaemia, e.g. due to Rh incompatibility.

*Intermittent variations*

**1** *Accelerations* (see Fig. 9.7, p. 116) are intermittent periods in which the fetal heart rate is raised

**Figure 12.16** A CTG demonstrating minor sinusoidal rhythm. The baseline is 110 beats/minute.

**Figure 12.17** Type I or early deceleration.

quite markedly above the baseline. They are a sign of fetal health.

**2** *Decelerations.* Decelerations are intermittent changes in the baseline and fall into four categories:

• Early decelerations.

These are illustrated in Fig. 12.17 and are due to vagal stimulation following head compression as the fetus descends the birth canal. They usually have no significance and do not require a fetal blood sample unless the fetus is preterm.

• Late decelerations.

These are illustrated in Fig. 12.18. They differ from early decelerations in that they are U-shaped, start more than 30 seconds after the contraction has started and continue after the contraction has finished. They are thought to be metabolic in nature and always warrant a fetal blood sample.

• Variable decelerations.

These are also of two types:

(a) *Isolated variable decelerations* (Fig. 12.19). These are commonly seen in labour following the use of a bed pan or after an epidural top-up. They may also result from umbilical cord compression and will usually disappear if the woman is turned on her side. Provided the fetal heart rate trace returns to normal the baby is not asphyxiated and fetal blood sampling is not required.

(b) *Recurrent variable decelerations* (Fig. 12.20). The important features to note are that the decelerations vary both in shape and in their relationship to the uterine contraction. The most common cause of these is cord compression. Either the cord is compressed between the presenting part and the pelvic side walls or the cord is around the fetal neck or a limb. Usually they do not indicate a fetal blood sample but, if

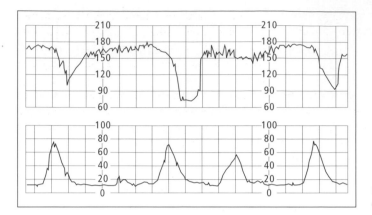

**Figure 12.18** Type II or late deceleration.

**Figure 12.19** Oxytocin-induced profound deceleration.

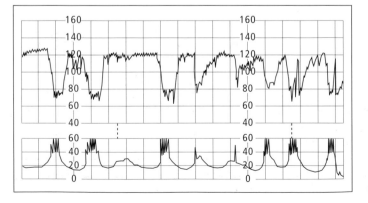

**Figure 12.20** Variable decelerations.

associated with meconium or a change in the baseline heart rate, one should be performed.

## Passage of meconium

Stimulation of the vagus *in utero* causes the fetal gut to contract and the anal sphincter to relax so that meconium (fetal stool) is passed into the amniotic fluid. Meconium is made up of swallowed cells in late pregnancy and alimentary tract cells, all of which are stained with bile.

With a normal fetal heart rate trace, the fetus is unlikely to be hypoxic, but if the fetal heart rate trace is abnormal when meconium is passed, then a fetal blood sample (FBS) should be performed.

## Fetal blood sample

Fetal blood sampling is a diagnostic test for fetal acidosis. A bead of blood is taken from the fetal scalp and the pH and base deficit can be measured.

During a uterine contraction:
• Maternal blood flow to the intervillous space is vastly reduced or may even cease.
• Passage of $O_2$ from the mother to the fetus is reduced and thus the fetus may become hypoxic.
• The fetus withstands these periods of hypoxia by employing anaerobic metabolism. To do this, the fetus must mobilize glycogen from liver and muscle stores to produce glucose as an energy source.
• Anaerobic metabolism results in the production of large amounts of lactic acid and an increase in the arterial $CO_2$. In normal circumstances, the rise in arterial $CO_2$ is buffered, mostly by fetal bicarbonate.
• Between contractions the lactic acid and the buffered $CO_2$ are passed back to the mother who excretes them.
• If glycogen stores are poor (the preterm or those with SGA), other sources of energy are required for anaerobic metabolism. These produce more $CO_2$ and more lactic acid and thus fetal buffering systems become overloaded. This results in a gradual fall of pH; the fetus demonstrates a metabolic acidosis.

If uterine activity is too frequent or sustained, then blood flow to the fetus may be impaired for a long space of time and this, again, will result in a metabolic acidosis with an increasing base deficit.

Figure 12.21 illustrates the mechanism by which the fetal scalp sample is acquired. The fetal scalp is punctured with a 2 mm guarded blade and the blood is aspirated into a capillary tube.

The pH results are interpreted as follows:
• pH >7.25: normal.
• pH 7.20–7.25: pre-asphyxia.
• pH <7.20: asphyxia.
• Base deficit <6.0 mEq/l: normal.
• Base deficit 6.1–7.9 mEq/l: pre-asphyxia.
• Base deficit >8.0 mEq/l: asphyxia.

In obstetric practice it is common to use the term asphyxia but what is truly meant is a metabolic acidosis.

If a fetus has a pH of <7.20 and a base deficit >8.0 mEq/l he should be considered for delivery by the most appropriate route. Fetuses that demonstrate pre-asphyxia and are in the second stage may be allowed normal delivery but only if this is imminent.

The scalp pH only reflects the state of the fetus at the time of the sample; the base deficit reflects a slower change, and therefore is a longer predictor. If the fetal heart rate trace continues to be abnormal, then the fetal blood sample should be repeated hourly or the baby delivered.

**Figure 12.21** Fetal blood samples can be taken from the scalp through an amnioscope.

# Home deliveries

Until this century, in the UK the place of birth was most usually the home. Hospital deliveries started in the mid-eighteenth century for charitable reasons to help the single mothers and poor women with unsuitable conditions at home. It has grown gradually this century from 2% in 1900 to 98% in 1990.

Home deliveries had reduced to about 1% by 1986, but are slightly increasing to a figure of 2% in 2001 varying around the UK from 0–20% (see Fig. 12.22).

The drift to hospitalization occurred:

• As part of the fashion of using a hospital for more medical managements.

• For safety. In the isolation of the home, it would be difficult to care for an emergency:

   (a) PPH.

   (b) Delayed onset of baby breathing.

   (c) Shoulder dystocia.

Against this, the advantages of home delivery are:

• Familiar surroundings for the woman.

• More relaxation because of confidence at home.

• Would probably know the midwife who was delivering her.

• More family members could attend at the birth and afterwards.

The slight increase in home deliveries means that a community service must be kept going. Two midwives attend each home delivery and these are usually more senior than those working in the hospitals. A general practitioner can be called in an emergency. If the woman has to be transferred to hospital, the use of an ambulance with paramedics, skilled in resuscitation, must be obtained.

The future of the hospital/domiciliary debate could be helped by:

• The use of a birthroom in the hospital, away from the main delivery suite. If delivery is normal and all goes well, they can return home a few hours later and so seem to have never really entered the hospital.

• Use of formal DOMINO (Domestic In and Out) services.

• Reduce the regimentation of hospital.

• Reduce the noise of the wards.

• Provide clean wards, enough linen and lavatories.

• Get the woman back home early on day one or two.

**Figure 12.22** Percentage of home deliveries (England and Wales) 1954–1993.

---

## Self-assessment

**12.1** Put the following sentences into the correct order to describe the passage of the fetus through the birth canal.
   (a) The fetal head engages in a transverse position.
   (b) The fetal head extends round the symphysis pubis.
   (c) The fetal head flexes as it descends into the birth canal.
   (d) The fetal head restitutes to a transverse position.
   (e) The fetal head most commonly rotates through 90° so that the occiput becomes anterior as it reaches the levator ani.

**12.2** Which of the following features of a cardiotocograph (CTG) would be considered non-reassuring in labour?
   (a) Baseline variability of 5–15 beats per minute.
   (b) Early decelerations in the second stage of labour.
   (c) Late decelerations in the second stage of labour.
   (d) A fetal heart rate of 170 beats per minute.
   (e) Accelerations.

**Self-assessment** *Continued*

**12.3** Which of the following are indications for continuous electronic fetal monitoring (EFM)?

(a) A woman at term in spontaneous labour who ruptures her membranes and has meconium stained liquor.

(b) A woman at term in spontaneous labour who ruptures her membranes and has clear liquor.

(c) A woman at term in spontaneous labour who has had a deceleration detected using a sonicaid every 30 minutes.

(d) A woman who ruptured her membranes 6 hours ago, clear liquor and is in spontaneous labour.

(e) A woman at term in spontaneous labour who has had a previous Caesarean section.

**12.4** In normal labour which of the following statements are true?

(a) Uterine contractions are generated in the lower segment of the uterus.

(b) The rate of cervical dilatation should be greater than 1 cm/hour.

(c) The fetal heart should be checked every 15 minutes in the first stage of labour with a sonicaid.

(d) The second stage of labour should not exceed 2 hours in duration in a woman with an epidural.

(e) An episiotomy should be performed in the majority of women.

# Chapter 13

# Abnormal labour

## Dysfunctional uterine action

Prolonged labour is more common in primigravidae and may be due to primary or secondary myometrial dysfunction or to malpresentation of the fetus, e.g. occipitoposterior position. The progress of labour should be monitored on a partogram. Figure 12.4 (p. 159) illustrates the normal rate of cervical dilatation from the start of labour. During the first 8 hours in primiparous women there is minimal change in the cervical dilatation but effacement (shortening and softening) occurs—the latent phase. Effacement is the taking up of the cervix, merging with the lower segment; eventually there is no length to the cervical canal.

Three abnormalities of labour may be recognized.

## Prolonged latent phase (PLP)

This is a rare abnormality and occurs almost exclusively in primigravidae. Figure 13.1 illustrates this together with the possible outcome. Aetiological factors are:
- The wrong diagnosis of labour.
- An abnormal or high presenting part.
- Premature rupture of the membranes.
- Idiopathic: cervical dystocia.
  (a) Primary. Failure of a ground substance of the cervix to soften in late pregnancy.

(b) Secondary. Previous operations on the cervix causing fibrosis.

*Management*
**1** Women who present with regular uterine activity should be assessed by vaginal examination; if the cervix is long and closed, they may be in early labour or not in labour. A short trace cardiotocograph (CTG) should be carried out to ensure fetal well-being and the uterus should be carefully palpated.
**2** The woman should be allowed to walk around or to sit comfortably. She should be re-examined again 4 hours later if the contractions persist.
- If labour has ceased the woman should go home.
- If labour continues and pain relief is required, then it should be given.
- If the cervix continues to efface but not dilate and progress falls more than 2 hours to the right of the partogram the membranes should be ruptured (artificial rupture of membranes, ARM) and labour stimulated by Syntocinon.
- In 85% of cases, labour will progress rapidly and will reach a normal active phase.
- In 15% of cases, adequate uterine activity fails to cause cervical dilatation. If, after 4–8 hours of Syntocinon, the cervix is not further dilated, then a Caesarean section should be performed.

Prolonged latent phase is primarily of primigravidae as the multigravidous cervix tends to efface and dilate at the same time.

**Figure 13.1** Prolonged latent phase in labour and possible outcomes: 1 and 2, vaginal delivery; 3, Caesarean section. ARM, artificial rupture of membranes; Synto, syntocinon infusion.

**Figure 13.2** Secondary arrest of cervical dilatation and outcomes: 1, vaginal delivery; 2, Caesarean section. ARM, artificial rupture of membranes; Synto, syntocinon infusion.

## Secondary arrest of cervical dilatation

The woman enters the active phase of labour, reaches 5–7 cm dilatation and then the cervix stops dilating (Fig. 13.2). Uterine contractions have become less frequent and may even stop.

• The fetal head engages in the occipitotransverse position and, if it is well flexed and asynclitic, will undergo rotation in the mid-cavity to the direct occipitoanterior position. Poor flexion leads to failure of rotation in the mid-cavity; this leads to persistent occipitotransverse position.

• Syntocinon i.v. leads to regular, coordinated uterine contractions that initially cause the fetal head to flex. In most cases (85%) this allows the head to rotate so that a spontaneous vaginal delivery will occur.

• If Syntocinon administration over 4 hours (multigravida) or 8 hours (primigravida) fails to

lead to further cervical dilatation, a Caesarean section should be carried out for relative cephalopelvic disproportion (CPD). This occurs in about 15% of cases.

• This is a benign condition as far as the fetus is concerned and very rarely leads to fetal distress.

## Primary dysfunctional labour

It is defined as slow progress after the onset of established labour and is the most worrying of the abnormalities of labour for it can lead to:

• Fetal distress in a well-grown or a large baby.

• Prolonged labour leading to an increase in maternal fear and anxiety.

• Incoordinate uterine activity which increases maternal pain.

• Maternal dehydration which leads to maternal acidosis.

The release of catecholamines stimulates uterine activity to arise from the lower segment. This means that the fundus and the lower uterine segment contract against each other and the cervix fails to dilate or dilates very slowly.

Maternal dehydration and acidosis lead to hydrogen ions competing with calcium (the final common pathway for smooth muscle contraction) and further dysfunctional uterine activity occurs.

The causes are:

- A malpresentation such as a brow.
- Occipitoposterior position.
- Relative CPD: which means that the fetus is only just small enough to pass through the pelvis but, if all goes well, it will succeed. If there is poor flexion or rotation, delay occurs.
- Macrosomia.

Once diagnosed, the dysfunction is treated with Syntocinon. In very few cases the rate of cervical dilatation returns to normal, but often the rate of dilatation can be increased. The outcome is:

- Spontaneous vaginal delivery (15%).
- Caesarean section for fetal distress (50%).
- A vaginal instrumental delivery (35%). Care should be taken because, even if full dilatation of the cervix is obtained, the fetus may still be high in mid-cavity. This could mean a difficult, rotation forceps delivery.

## Shoulder dystocia

Shoulder dystocia is an obstetric emergency. It occurs when the shoulders do not spontaneously deliver after the head. The anterior shoulder becomes trapped behind or above the symphysis pubis whilst the posterior shoulder may be in the hollow of the sacrum or above the sacral promontory.

*Predisposing factors*
- Previous shoulder dystocia.
- Previous baby >4.5 kg.
- Big baby clinically or on USS (AC >95th centile).
- Diabetic woman.
- Obese woman (BMI >30 kg/m²).
- Secondary arrest in labour augmented by Syntocinon.
- Prolonged second stage.

*Signs*
- Fetal chin pulls back against the perineum.
- No external signs of restitution.
- Anterior shoulder fails to deliver with contraction.

*Management*
- Call for help
- Change the maternal position
  1 McRoberts manoevre—flatten the bed, retract the woman's knees on to her chest as far as possible. This straightens the sacrum and maximizes the pelvic diameter. Apply gentle traction. If not delivered after 30 seconds try the following sequence with 30 seconds to try and deliver the baby with each one.
  2 Place woman on all fours (shoulders move to oblique diameter).
  3 Return to supine. External pressure—place hands, held as for cardiopulmonary resuscitation, on the mother's abdomen just above the symphysis pubis and apply pressure.
- Perform an episiotomy if not already done.
- Internal rotation. Place hand behind the anterior shoulder and bring it forward, rotate the shoulders using the posterior shoulder.
- Deliver the posterior arm.
- Symphysiotomy—division of the symphysis pubis, supporting the hips so they do not separate too quickly.

*Risks*

MATERNAL
- Vaginal trauma.
- Bladder/urethral damage particularly if a symphysiotomy is performed.
- Psychological trauma.

NEONATAL
- Erb's palsy from brachial plexus injury.
- Cerebral palsy from hypoxia.
- Fractured humerus/clavicle.
- Neonatal death.

All parents require sensitive and careful debriefing after shoulder dystocia. It is a frightening experience when a lot of doctors and midwives arrive suddenly, being asked to change positions with minimal explanation yet knowing there is something seriously wrong. They may also have to cope with a baby with physical or mental disability.

## Cephalopelvic disproportion

Classically, CPD is classified as follows:

**1** *Absolute.* There is no possibility of a normal vaginal delivery even if the mechanisms of labour are completely correct. In the Western world, this condition is extremely rare; it may be due to the following:

- Fetal hydrocephalus.
- Congenitally abnormal pelvis (such as Robert's or Naegele's pelvis) in which one or both sacral ala are missing leading to a narrowing of the pelvic inlet.
- A pelvis that has been damaged usually due to a severe roll-over road traffic accident in youth.
- A pelvis that has been grossly distorted from osteomalacia.

**2** *Relative CPD.* This means that the baby is large but would pass through the pelvis if the mechanisms of labour function correctly. If, however, the head is deflexed or fails to rotate in the mid-cavity, then prolonged, abnormal labour will occur.

The above definitions do not include estimates of the weight of the baby or X-ray measurements of the pelvis. CPD can only truly be diagnosed after a trial of labour. This means awaiting the onset of spontaneous labour and, if that labour becomes prolonged and abnormal, stimulating with Syntocinon as described above.

CPD may be suspected antenatally in women who are less than 5′2″ (1.58 m) in height. These women tend to have a small gynaecoid pelvis but they often also have small babies. In a cephalic presentation there is now little evidence that X-ray pelvimetry or a CT scan helps in management. These women should have a trial of labour and in many cases will deliver vaginally.

All women with a high head at term should have an obvious cause excluded by an ultrasound examination. This will diagnose placenta praevia, uterine fibroids, or an ovarian cyst as the cause. In the absence of these findings, one should suspect that the cause is CPD.

Head fitting tests and X-ray pelvimetry have only a small role in the management of women with a cephalic presentation because the correct management is the proper use of a trial of labour.

## Malpresentations and malpositions

### Breech presentation

*Incidence*
At term 2–3%; more in preterm deliveries.

*Aetiology*
- The ratio of amniotic fluid volume to fetal size may be high, allowing freer movement (e.g. polyhydramnios and before 32 weeks).
- Extended legs of the fetus can splint and prevent flexion of the fetal trunk so stopping further turning and causing the fetus to stay as a breech presentation.
- Fetuses in multiple pregnancies may interfere with each other's movements.
- Something might be filling the lower segment (e.g. placenta praevia or fibroids).
- Fetal malformations may prevent cephalic presentation (e.g. hydrocephaly).

*Types* (Fig. 13.3)
Flexed or extended knee joints.

**1** Neither knee joint flexed so that both legs are extended: a frank breech or extended breech. This is the commonest presentation.

**2** Fully flexed fetus with both knees flexed: a flexed breech.

**3** One leg flexed and the other leg extended: an incomplete breech.

**4** Both hips extended; a footling. Often occurs with very small babies.

On vaginal examination, the breech presentation in labour is described according to the relation of the fetal sacrum to the maternal pelvis (Fig. 13.4).

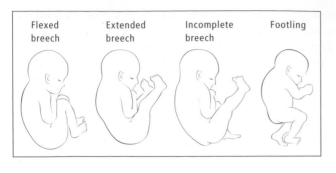

**Figure 13.3** Types of breech presentation.

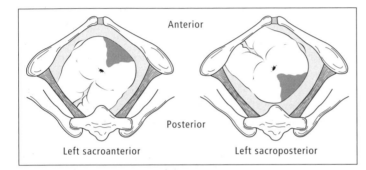

**Figure 13.4** Using the fetal sacrum as the denominator, the position of the breech presentation is described.

*Diagnosis*

ABDOMINAL EXAMINATION
No head is felt at the lower end and a hard, rounded knob is ballottable at the upper end of the uterus.

VAGINAL EXAMINATION
Confirms there is no head in the pelvis.

INVESTIGATIONS
Ultrasound scan confirms the situation.

*Management of a breech presentation in pregnancy*
**1** From about 37 weeks onwards external cephalic version (ECV) is worthwhile trying without general anaesthesia, provided it is easy to perform. If the mother is Rh-negative, anti-*D* immunoglobulin should be given after the first attempt.
  • Listen to the fetal heart immediately before and after the procedure.
  • If it works, the woman should be seen weekly to ensure the fetus stays as a cephalic presentation.

  • If it fails, the woman should be counselled about the route of delivery.
  • Reasons for failure of ECV:
    (a) Breech too deeply engaged in pelvis.
    (b) Too tense a uterus.
    (c) Too tense an abdominal wall.
    (d) Fetal abnormality ⎤ therefore do
    (e) Undiagnosed twins ⎦ an ultrasound.
  • Contraindications to doing ECV.
    (a) Previous uterine scar from Caesarean section (relative).
    (b) Hypertension in the mother.
    (c) Planned delivery by Caesarean section anyway.
    (d) Ruptured membranes.
    (e) Multiple pregnancy.
    (f) Antepartum haemorrhage.
**2** If ECV does not succeed then the woman should be advised about the pros and cons of vaginal breech delivery compared with Caesarean section (Box 13.1).
**3** A standing lateral CT scan of the pelvis should be done for all primiparous patients and any multiparous women who have delivered a baby of

---

**Box 13.1 The pros and cons of vaginal breech delivery**

*Requires*
Pelvic inlet >11 cm (AP)
Pelvic outlet >11 cm (transverse)
Well curved sacrum
Estimated fetal weight <3.5 kg

---

| *Pro* | *Con* |
|---|---|
| ↓ Maternal morbidity | ↑ Risk of fetal intrapartum |
| ↓ Maternal mortality |    hypoxia ×3 |
|   (rare) | ↑ Risk of head entrapment |
| | ↑ Risk of intracranial damage |
| | May lead to emergency CS |
| |    done in less favourable |
| |    circumstances |

---

>3.5 kg in the past. An ultrasound scan of the fetus will establish its estimated weight. In a breech delivery the head (the largest and hardest part of the fetus) is coming last and it is too late to wait and see if this fits the pelvis. Therefore an estimate of the chances of delivery has to be made on these CT and ultrasound measurements. In a cephalic delivery, the descending head acts as a pelvimeter whereas in a breech it does not.

**4** It is wise to deliver most breech presentations by 41 weeks. If the woman has not gone into spontaneous labour before this time then induce or do an elective Caesarean section.

**5** If there is any other variation from normal, many obstetricians will deliver a breech-presenting baby by elective Caesarean section at 38–39 weeks.

A recent randomized trial of vaginal versus elective Caesarean section for breech presentation has suggested that the latter may be safer for the infant if an ECV fails. This is truer for the developed world than the developing world where the perinatal morbidity and mortality for cephalic vaginal deliveries is higher and the risks of Caesarean section for the mother are also higher.

*Management of a breech presentation in labour*

FIRST STAGE

**1** Increased risk of early rupture of the mem-branes. When they do, a vaginal examination should exclude a prolapse of the cord.

**2** An epidural anaesthetic is a good method of pain relief as the normal delivery can rapidly be changed to an operative one if necessary (but is not mandatory).

SECOND STAGE

**1** Delivery is by the most senior obstetrician or midwife available with an anaesthetist and a paediatrician close to the labour ward.

**2** A propped up dorsal position of the mother is the easiest to manage. The labour bed should be capable of breaking in the middle for delivery of the baby's body, so that the mother can assume a lithotomy position.

**3** The buttocks progress down the birth canal and, when on the point of crowning, an episiotomy may be required. The baby is rotated to sacroanterior.

**4** The baby will often progress as far as the umbilicus with the mother's own expulsive efforts. The legs are assisted down, especially if extended.

**5** Commonly, the arms are flexed across the chest and so delivery occurs readily with the next contraction.

**6** If the arms are extended they have to be manipulated down.

**7** After delivery of the body, it is allowed to hang and traction may be gently applied to the legs until the suboccipital region appears under the maternal pubis.

**8** The head is delivered slowly by placing one finger in the baby's mouth or gently flexing the head with forceps, the blades applied to either side of the fetal head from the front of the body which is held up by an assistant. The face is delivered over the mother's perineum and the nose and mouth are cleared of mucus and liquor, allowing the baby to breathe. The rest of the head is slowly delivered, not allowing any sudden decompression which could result in pressure alterations inside the skull and so cause intracerebral venous bleeding.

THIRD STAGE

**1** Syntometrine is given with the delivery of the head for there is an increased risk of PPH.

**2** The placenta is delivered as described in normal labour.

*Caesarean section*
This should be done if vaginal delivery is considered too hazardous because:
- Mild pelvis contraction.
- Fetus thought to be over 3.5 kg.
- Fetus in unfavourable attitude.
- Multiple pregnancy if the first twin is a breech.
- Other complications, e.g. pre-eclampsia or diabetes.
- Non-descent of buttocks in labour.
- Failure of progress in labour.

*Risks to the fetus of breech delivery*
Perinatal mortality in all breech deliveries is two or three times that of cephalic presentations but this is made up mainly of premature births (26–30 weeks). Mature breech deliveries (36+ weeks) in reputable centres have no higher risk than mature cephalic deliveries. Hence the reasons for mortality are:
- Prematurity.
- Intracranial damage: subdural and intracranial haemorrhage often after too rapid delivery of the head.
- Rarely hypoxia. This may be:
  (a) Before delivery (prolapsed cord).
  (b) At the time of delivery (too slow delivery of the head).

## Shoulder presentation (transverse lie)

*Incidence*
0.3% of all deliveries.

*Aetiology*
As for other malpresentation but most commonly:
**1** Polyhydramnios causing an increased ratio of fluid to fetus.
**2** Something preventing the engagement of the head in the pelvis:
- Placenta praevia.
- Fibroids.
- Contracted pelvis.

**3** Abnormal shape of uterus (subseptate or arcuate uterus).
**4** Second twin.
**5** Grand multiparity (5+).

*Diagnosis*
**1** Abdominal examination—the head is in one flank and the buttocks in the other. Commonly, the fetus can be rotated to a cephalic presentation quite readily but reverts back to a transverse position.
**2** Vaginal examination—the pelvis is empty of presenting parts.
**3** Investigation: ultrasound scan confirms diagnosis.

*Management of transverse lie in pregnancy and labour*
**1** Before 36 weeks, ECV may be attempted or the woman referred back to the following week's clinic. The position is usually self-curing.
**2** Past 37 weeks in a multiparous patient, and after 38 weeks in a primiparous one, admission to hospital should be advised, where ECV is attempted each day.
**3** Should the woman go to term with the fetus still in a transverse position, management may be by either of the following:
- A *stabilizing induction*: ECV is done in the labour ward. The fetal head is held over the brim of the mother's pelvis and high membrane rupture is performed. Amniotic fluid escapes and the head often sinks into the pelvis. Labour follows in the normal fashion.
- An *elective Caesarean section*. In the Western world this may be the safer line of treatment for the fetus since it cuts down the risks of prolapsed cord during labour, but it does leave the mother with a scarred uterus for future pregnancies and an increased risk of postpartum problems.

**4** Occasionally a woman is admitted in mid or late labour with a transverse lie. This would lead to an impacted shoulder presentation, the folded fetus having been driven a varying amount down the pelvis, depending on how far labour has gone. Treatment must be by immediate Caesarean section even if the fetus is dead because of the risk of uterine rupture.

## Occipitoposterior positions

The fetal head usually engages in the pelvic brim in the occipitotransverse position (long axis of head fitting into maximum diameter of bean-shaped pelvic brim). When labour starts, the head is driven down the birth canal and rotates.

**1** 80% rotate forward through 90° to an occipitoanterior position.

**2** 15% undergo long internal rotation through 270° to become occipitoanterior having gone through directly occipitoposterior on the way.

**3** 3% rotate back 90° to a directly occipitoposterior position. These may deliver face to pubis.

**4** 2% stay in the transverse and descend in this position. A minority of these might rotate on the perineum but most end up in transverse arrest.

*Aetiology*

*Pelvis.* Flat sacrum with loss of pelvic curve and so loss of room for rotation.

*Uterus.* Poor or disorganized uterine contractions do not push the fetal head down and so there is no impetus to rotate.

*Head.* Poor flexion so that larger diameters present (suboccipitofrontal >10.5 cm).

*Analgesia.* Epidural analgesia causes pelvic floor relaxation. This allows the gutter of the levator ani muscles to become lax so not directing the occiput anteriorly. This is associated with lack of fetal head rotation.

*Diagnosis*

PREGNANCY

Occasionally, by abdominal palpation when in a cephalic presentation, the back cannot be felt in the flank but fetal limbs can be felt all over the front of the uterus. The head is often not engaged after the time it would be expected to be.

LABOUR

• Abdominal palpation as above.

• Vaginal examination feeling the sutures and fontanelles. Both anterior and posterior fontanelles can be felt (deflexion) and the λ-shaped posterior fontanelle is in the posterior quadrant of the pelvis.

*Management in pregnancy*

Leave alone.

*Management in labour*

Laissez-faire. Await events for many will rotate spontaneously. Prepare for a longer labour because:

• Pelvis may be minimally contracted or sacrum slightly flattened.

• Incoordinate uterine contractions.

• Deflexed fetal head.

Therefore:

**1** Watch progress by both:

  • Abdominal assessment of engagement and descent of fetal head.

  • Vaginal assessment:

    (a) Head in relation to ischial spines.

    (b) Rotation of head.

    (c) Dilatation of cervix which is often poorly applied to the head.

    (d) Check no prolapse of cord by vaginal examination straight after membranes rupture.

**2** Women often wish to push before the cervix is fully dilated. If the occiput is posterior there is extra pressure on the sacrum and rectum. Frequent vaginal examinations are needed to make accurate assessments of the real dilatation of the cervix and the progress of labour.

**3** Watch maternal condition. Especially remember:

  • Labour will be long, so maintain morale.

  • Pain relief should be thorough—epidural anaesthesia is good in this situation. If such regional anaesthesia is unavailable many would use morphine or diamorphine for this problem.

  • No food and little fluids by mouth (general anaesthetic may be wanted). Give i.v. fluids.

**4** If head stays directly occipitoposterior, delivery may occur spontaneously but, since larger diameters are passing through the birth canal, the mother will have to work harder and a generous episiotomy may be required. Face-to-pubis delivery will occur.

**5** If head stays in occipitotransverse position it will not deliver spontaneously. It must be rotated to deliver and this will require good analgesia, maybe epidural or general anaesthesia. A rotational delivery is contraindicated if there is fetal distress and a Caesarean section should be performed. Rotation and delivery may be by:

• Manual rotation to the occipitoanterior position and subsequent forceps delivery.

• Kielland's straight forceps rotation and subsequent delivery. These forceps have no pelvic curve.

• Vacuum extraction. This applies only a linear pull on the fetal head so that any rotation can occur as determined by the pelvic muscles and bones.

**6** Give i.v. Syntometrine with the crowning of the head for the risks of PPH are greatly increased. Deliver the placenta promptly after the baby is born.

**7** Be prepared to repair the rather large episiotomy quickly.

**8** If the head does not rotate then a Caesarean section is indicated. This can be difficult as the head is so low in the vagina.

*Results*

MOTHER

Following the operative delivery and the bigger episiotomy, vaginal and vulval oedema and haematomata are more frequent.

BABY

Because of the longer labour and high incidence of operative delivery, perinatal mortality and morbidity are increased. The mortality is due to hypoxia and birth trauma. The morbidity is from these and the results of intracranial haemorrhage.

## Face presentation

As the fetal head gets driven down the birth canal, the front of the head can become extended (Fig. 13.5). Distinguish from face-to-pubis delivery.

**Figure 13.5** Face presentation. Well engaged in the mentolateral position.

*Incidence*

0.3% of all deliveries.

*Aetiology*

**1** Lax uterus, multiple pregnancy, polyhydramnios.

**2** Deflexed fetal head.

**3** Shape of fetal head:

• Dolichocephalic (long head).

• Anencephalic (no cranium).

*Mechanism*

Head descends with face leading. Chin (mentum) used as denominator to determine rotation.

85% engage in the mentotransverse (submento-bregmatic diameter—10 cm). With descent, most rotate to mentoanterior on the pelvic floor, the fetal chin coming behind the maternal pubis. After further descent, the chin can escape from under the lower back of the pubis and the head is then delivered over the vulva by flexion.

Up to this point, the mechanisms of flexion/extension of the fetal head are the reverse of those with a vertex presentation. After delivery of the head, however, the external rotations are the same allowing the fetal shoulders to negotiate the pelvis.

A few face presentations rotate from the transverse to mentoposterior, so that the fetal chin is in the curve of the mother's sacrum; the fetal occiput and back are crushed into each other behind the pubic bone. Further descent is unlikely for the head cannot extend further and so cannot negotiate the forward curve of the birth canal and Caesarean section is needed.

### Diagnosis
Rarely made before labour and of little significance if it is.

### Abdomen
• Longitudinal lie with body nearer to mid-axis of uterus.
• More head felt on the same side as the back.

### Vaginal examination
• Do not expect the face to feel like the newborn baby's face. Oedema always obscures facial parts.
• Supra-orbital ridges lead to the bridge of the nose.
• Mouth has hard gums in it and may suck on the examining finger.

### Management

IN PREGNANCY
• Await events.
• Membranes may rupture early (examine vaginally to exclude prolapsed cord).
• Check that pelvis is adequate and that fetus is not oversized. If either, consider Caesarean section for face presentation in labour has a higher risk.
• Check with ultrasound that the fetus is not an anencephalic for this might alter management.

IN LABOUR
• If anterior rotation to mentoanterior, a longer labour but spontaneous delivery will probably occur (90%).
• If head stays in mentotransverse, either manual rotation to mentoanterior and forceps extraction, or Kielland's forceps rotation and extraction or deliver by Caesarean section.
• If face rotates posteriorly, this is impossible to deliver vaginally. Hence, perform a Caesarean section.

### Results

MOTHER
Higher morbidity associated with operative delivery.

BABY
Higher mortality:
• Abnormalities incompatible with life (anencephaly).
• In the normal, hypoxia and cerebral congestion.

## Brow presentation

A very poorly flexed head may present the largest diameter of the skull: mentovertex (13 cm) (Fig. 13.6).

### Incidence
0.1% of all deliveries.

### Diagnosis
Rarely made before labour and of little significance if it is.

### Abdomen
• Head feels big.
• Not well engaged.
• Groove between occiput and back. Head felt on both sides of fetus.

**Figure 13.6** Brow presentation with mentovertex diameter presenting.

*Vaginal examination*
- Anterior fontanelle presents.
- Supraorbital ridges and base of nose can be felt at edge of field.

*Management*

IN PREGNANCY
- Await events. No point in trying to convert to more favourable presentation.
- Membranes may rupture early (examine vaginally to exclude prolapsed cord).

IN LABOUR
- If diagnosed early, await events for some convert spontaneously to face (by further extension) or vertex (by flexion).
- If presentation persists, it will be impossible to deliver vaginally. Hence deliver by Caesarean section.
- If fetus is dead or there is hydrocephaly, the destructive operation of perforation of head and vaginal extraction is possible provided the operator is skilled in these arts, but in the Western world these are a diminishing number.

*Results*

MOTHER
Higher morbidity associated with operative delivery.

BABY
Because of wider use of Caesarean section, morbidity and mortality rates are low.

## Induction of labour

*Definition*
A planned initiation of labour.

*Incidence*
Varies with the population and the type of obstetric cases seen; in the UK between 5% and 25%.

*Indications*
**1** Maternal disease:

- Existing before pregnancy, e.g. diabetes.
- Occurring in pregnancy, e.g. pre-eclampsia.

**2** Fetal disease, e.g. Rh disease.

**3** Fetuses at risk from reduced placental perfusion, being SGA.

In the UK the most common indications are:
- Post-maturity (or more strictly post-dates), $T^{+10-14}$.
- SGA.
- Maternal disease.
- Rh incompatibility.
- Fetal death or abnormality.

In addition, there are several softer indications which obstetricians commonly employ for which there is little or no scientific basis. These are:
- Poor past obstetric history.
- A pregnancy resulting from infertility treatment.
- Recurrent unexplained APH.
- At the woman's, or her partner's, wish (to be avoided).

Prior to undertaking an induction the woman should be examined vaginally to determine the Bishops score (Table 13.1) and a membrane sweep performed. This can be done if the cervix admits a finger (>1 cm dilated). A circular motion round the edge of the internal os releases prostaglandins. 70% of women at term will go into spontaneous labour within 48 hours so avoiding an induction. The Bishop's score is a weighted means of assessing how likely it is that the woman will go into labour. Women with a Bishop's score of >6 are considered favourable and failed induction rates are usually less than 1%.

The commonest method of induction of labour in the UK is a combination of medical and surgical means. The usual system is:

**Table 13.1** The Bishop's score.

| Cervix | 0 | 1 | 2 |
|---|---|---|---|
| Dilatation (cm) | 0 | 1–2 | 3–4 |
| Consistency | Firm | Medium | Soft |
| Length (cm) | >2 | 1–2 | <1 |
| Position | Posterior | Mid | Anterior |
| Station of head above ischial spines (cm) | 3 | 2 | 1 |

**1** Give prostaglandin (PG) in either vaginal pessaries ($E_2$, 2 mg) or as a gel (1 or 2 mg $E_2$) or orally (200 μg). In up to 40%, this will start labour on its own and no further action is required.

**2** If not, 4 hours later, repeat the PG and wait 4 hours.

**3** If no action after 4 hours, rupture membranes.

**4** Administer Syntocinon if uterine contractions do not follow closely or if labour becomes prolonged and abnormal so that the rate of cervical dilatation is to the right of the cervical partogram.

## Prostaglandins

A ubiquitous group of fatty acids found in many body fluids first described in seminal plasma, hence their name. PGs E and F stimulate uterine activity and are involved in the initiation of normal labour.

*Mode of action*

This is directly on the muscle cells. A secondary effect is that a uterus primed with PGs will respond much better to i.v. Syntocinon.

*Route*

**1** *Intravaginal.* Putting either a gel or a pessary into the vagina—commonest method for induction of labour. A dose of $PGE_2$ in a 2 mg pessary or a 1 or 2 mg gel is placed high in the vagina. If labour is not established and the cervix is not dilating some 4 hours later, then the $PGE_2$ may be repeated. Four hours after this it is usual to do an ARM and then to add Syntocinon if necessary.

**2** *Extra-amniotic.* A fine catheter passed through the cervix comes to lie between the membranes and the uterine sidewall. PGs are then injected through the catheter. This is sometimes used for late therapeutic abortions.

**3** *The oral route.* This is not commonly used because of the side-effects of gastrointestinal colic and diarrhoea.

**4** *Intra-amniotic.* By direct injection of PG into the amniotic sac; may be used for late therapeutic abortions but is not used to induce labour.

## Syntocinon

This is an artificially produced oxytocic agent which mimics the activity of the normally released oxytocin. In normal labour, oxytocin is not detectable until the cervix has reached 7 cm dilatation.

Nowadays labour is not commonly induced with oxytocin alone; it is used:

• When PG pessaries and ARM fail to result in uterine activity and active dilatation of the cervix.

• To augment abnormal labour when the rate of cervical dilatation has fallen to the right of the cervical partogram.

## Artificial rupture of membranes

Figure 13.7 illustrates rupture of the forewaters in order to induce or accelerate labour. This is carried out with an amnihook.

The following conditions should exist before ARM is carried out:

• The fetal head or presenting part should be firmly engaged.

• The woman should be informed of the procedure and the reasons for it; oral consent should be obtained.

**Success of induction of labour**

Even with an unfavourable cervix the use of PGs, ARM and Syntocinon should result in a failed induction rate of no more than 5%.

**Figure 13.7** Artificial rupture of membranes: rupture of the forewaters (arrowed).

Management of women who have a failed induction depends upon the obstetrician's opinion, which may be either of the following:

**1** The need for induction indicated a need for delivery and therefore failure of induction should lead to a Caesarean section.

**2** The indications for induction were borderline and it is therefore reasonable to stop the induction process and attempt it again the next day. This can only be carried out if the membranes have not been ruptured. It is not to be encouraged as it leads to the woman's loss of confidence in the method.

### Risks of induction

- Uterine hyperstimulation may lead to fetal distress and so to a Caesarean section.
- Prolonged rupture of the membranes may increase the risk of intrauterine infection.
- Prolonged labour may lead to a Caesarean section.
- Women whose labours are induced have a higher incidence of Caesarean section (a risk factor of times three). Often this is due to the reason for the induction, e.g. an SGA fetus, but in many cases it is due to prolonged labour.

## Preterm labour

*Definition*
Labour occurring at <37 completed weeks' gestation.

*Incidence*
- 6% of deliveries occur before 37 weeks' gestation.
- 2% of deliveries occur before 34 weeks' gestation.

*Prognosis*
This depends upon:
- The availability of a neonatal intensive care unit. All infants born at <30 weeks' gestation should be transferred to a hospital that contains a neonatal intensive care unit (level 3) if time and maternal/fetal condition allow.

- The gestational age and birth weight. The perinatal team at a typical obstetric and neonatal combined unit usually achieves a 50% survival rate at 26 weeks of gestation.
- The condition of the baby at birth. Asphyxiated infants are more likely to die later from respiratory distress syndrome (RDS).
- Immediate neonatal management.
- The use of antenatal steroids to improve the maturity of the fetal lungs and reduce the risk of intraventricular haemorrhage (IVH) in fetuses of less than 37 weeks' gestation.

*Diagnosis*
Half the women who present with painful contractions before 37 weeks' gestation will stop spontaneously. Conversely preterm labour may be insidious. The following plan is therefore recommended:

**1** Look for a cause for preterm labour (Box 13.2).

**2** If membranes are intact, a vaginal examination should be performed.

**3** The fetal heart rate and uterine activity should be electronically recorded continuously.

**4** Repeat the vaginal examination 2 hours later if there are more than two contractions every 10 minutes. Change in cervical effacement or dilatation confirms preterm labour.

**5** Check fibronectin levels in cervical fluid; elevation may indicate imminent labour.

---

**Box 13.2 Causes of preterm labour**

Previous pre-term labour
Premature rupture of the membranes
Multiple pregnancy
Polyhydramnios
Antepartum haemorrhage
Fetal death
Bacterial vaginosis
Maternal pyrexia (UTI and other infections)
Uterine abnormalities
Cervical incompetence

---

*Principles of management of ongoing labour (intact membranes)*

**1** Full electronic monitoring is mandatory.

**2** Arrange *in utero* transfer if neonatal intensive care facilities are unavailable.

**3** Give tocolytics for 48 hours to allow steroid therapy to mature fetal lungs.

## Tocolysis

There is no convincing statistical evidence that to-colytic agents such as β-agonists or ritodrine use-fully prolong pregnancy. However, at <4 cm dilatation they may delay delivery for 24–48 hours in order to allow time for steroids to act or for the woman to be transferred to a delivery site with a neonatal intensive unit.

*Contraindications*

ABSOLUTE

• Thyroid disease.

• Cardiac disease.

• Severe hypertension (>160/110 mmHg).

• Sickle cell disease.

• Chorioamnionitis.

• Intrauterine death.

RELATIVE

• Advanced labour, more than 4 cm cervical dilatation.

• APH.

• Maternal diabetes mellitus.

*Side effects*

These include

• Tachycardia: treatment should be stopped if the maternal pulse rate exceeds 120/minute.

• Hyperglycaemia: beta agonists are diabetogenic as are steroids. Since steroids are usually given at the same time as tocolytics the maternal blood glucose should be checked 2 hourly and a sliding scale of in-sulin started if the blood sugar exceeds 9 mmol/l.

• Pulmonary oedema: this is due to fluid overload and tachycardia. It can be avoided by giving the to-colytic through a syringe pump to reduce the vol-ume of colloid given as well as ensuring the woman

does not have a prolonged tachycardia of >120/minute.

Recently a new tocolytic—Atosiban—has been introduced. This is an oxytocin antagonist. Other agents that have been used include NSAIDs (in-domethacin) and Glyceryltrinitrite (GTN). NSAIDs may cause oligohydramnios and closure of the patent ductus arteriosus in the fetus if used for more than 48 hours.

## Steroid therapy

Maternal steroids have been shown to reduce the incidence and severity of RDS between the gesta-tions of 26 and 34 weeks.

## Conduct of a preterm delivery

• The fetal heart should be electronically monitored.

• A senior obstetrician should be present.

• A neonatal paediatrician should be present.

• Forceps may be used carefully.

• Ventouse delivery is contraindicated because of the increased risk of bleeding under the scalp (cephalhaematoma).

## Preterm premature rupture of membranes (PPROM)

PROM refers to rupture of the membranes before the onset of labour. At less than 37 weeks' gestation this is referred to as preterm premature rupture of the membranes (PPROM).

*Problems*

Risks of preterm delivery versus risk of intrauterine infection.

*Confirm the diagnosis*

• Avoid vaginal digital examinations.

• Perform a sterile speculum examination.

• If amniotic fluid is seen coming through the cervix, membranes have ruptured.

• The smell of amniotic fluid is characteristic.

• A positive Nitrazine stick test (pH change) is of imprecise help.

*Management*

PPROM AFTER 34 WEEKS' GESTATION

Management is controversial and follows one of two lines:
• Immediate delivery to avoid intrauterine infection. Perinatal mortality because of immaturity is almost identical to that at term. However, these babies do have an increased morbidity.
• Perform an amniocentesis to exclude an infection and if not present then manage the woman conservatively.
• Give steroids.
• Give erythromycin until delivery.

PPROM AT LESS THAN 34 WEEKS' GESTATION

Care must be individualized but the following lines of management are reasonable:
• *In utero* transfer to a hospital with a neonatal intensive care unit for all women <34 weeks' gestation.
• Perform an amniocentesis. If the amniotic fluid shows organisms, this suggests intrauterine infection and the woman should be delivered.
• Conservative management in the absence of an amniocentesis. In this case, women are delivered for the following reasons:
    (a) Evidence of chorioamnionitis.
    (b) Maturity.
    (c) Spontaneous onset of labour.
• Give steroids.
• Give erythromycin until delivery.

## Chorioamnionitis

This is usually diagnosed by one or more of the following:
• Maternal temperature and tachycardia.
• Tender uterus.
• A foul-smelling vaginal discharge.
• Fetal tachycardia.
• Rise in maternal white cell count.
• Organisms in amniotic fluid.

*Management*
**1** Obtain high vaginal swab, a mid-stream urine (MSU) sample and blood culture.

**2** Induce labour. Caesarean section is preferably avoided because of the risk of maternal infection, but it is indicated in the following circumstances:
• Fetal distress.
• Preterm breech or other abnormal lie.
• A failed induction.
**3** Start i.v. broad-spectrum antibiotics such as erythromycin for both mother and baby.

## Presentation and prolapse of the cord

## Presentation of the cord

During labour, loops of cord may be felt ahead of the presenting part; if the membranes are intact this is not dangerous. The cord will probably slip to one side when the presenting part comes down. However, if, in a live fetus, cord presentation is felt at a time of proposed artificial rupture of the membranes, that procedure is better postponed for an hour or so.

## Prolapse of the cord

If the membranes rupture and the presenting part does not fit the pelvis well, the umbilical cord can be carried through the cervix by the flow of amniotic fluid.

*Associated factors*
Badly fitting presenting part:
• Occipitoposterior position.
• Breech.
• Face and brow presentations.
• Transverse lie.
• High head:
    (a) Preterm delivery.
    (b) Small baby.
    (c) Multiparity.

*Incidence*
1 : 300 of all deliveries.

*Findings*
Loops of cord may:

- Pass through cervix and stay in vagina.
- Pass out of vulva.

*Dangers*

Fetus is put at risk of cutting off blood supply.
- Spasm of umbilical arteries from:
  (a) Cooling.
  (b) Drying.
  (c) Altered pH.
  (d) Handling.
- Mechanical compression between presenting part and maternal bony pelvis.

*Diagnosis*

**1** The fetal heart may show a sudden alteration in rate or rhythm soon after membrane rupture.
**2** Loops of cord appear at the vulva or are felt in the vagina at examination. Do *not* handle cord too much. Just determine if the vessels are pulsating.

*Management*

IF FETUS MATURE AND ALIVE
**1** Deliver immediately:
  - If cervix <9 cm dilated—Caesarean section.
  - If cervix >9 cm and favourable cephalic presentation in a multiparous patient—ventouse delivery.
  - If cervix fully dilated—ventouse or forceps delivery.
**2** If immediate delivery impossible (e.g. prolapsed cord occurs outside a properly equipped obstetrical unit):
  - Keep cord moist, warm and do not handle. If outside vulva, return cord to vagina.
  - Prevent compression of cord between the presenting part and the bony pelvis: put mother in lateral position with pelvis raised on pillows; press up presenting part with the fingers in the vagina.

Keep these precautions until delivery about to occur, i.e. if the mother must travel in an ambulance, the doctor or midwife goes with her still doing a vaginal examination to continue to hold up presenting part.

Do not waste time trying to put the cord back into the uterus above the presenting part. Each attempt may allow more loops to come down and the additional handling increases spasm.

IF FETUS DEAD
There is no urgency for there is no increased risk to the mother. Allow events to proceed; the cord will not obstruct labour.

*Prognosis*

MATERNAL
Increased morbidity risks of operative delivery.

FETAL
Depends where the woman is when the prolapse occurs and at what stage of labour. If the mother is in hospital and the prolapse is in the second stage, the fetal loss is <3%. Should she be at home with a first stage prolapse, figures as high as 70% loss occur.

# Postpartum haemorrhage (PPH)

Bleeding from the genital tract after delivery of the fetus.

## Primary PPH

*Definition*

A blood loss in excess of 500 ml from the vagina within 24 hours of birth.

*Incidence*

Varies with use of oxytocic drugs. From 1% to 8% of all deliveries.

*Causes*

**1** Uterus does not contract and so prevent bleeding from placental site.
**2** Partly separated placenta—uterus cannot contract properly and so placental bed bleeds.
**3** Retention of separated placenta—lower areas of the uterus contract so that the placenta is trapped and cannot be expelled.
**4** Tears of the uterus, cervix, vagina or perineum.
**5** A clotting defect of blood.

*Predisposing factors*
- Overstretch of uterus—twins, polyhydramnios.
- Long labour.
- Deep anaesthesia or use of halothane.
- Previous scar on uterus.
- Morbid penetration of placenta.
- Cervical contraction after oxytocic drugs.
- Vaginal operative delivery.
- Hypofibrinogenaemia after abruptio placentae.
- Disseminated intravascular coagulopathy.

*Diagnosis*

Since the definition of a PPH is a loss over 500 ml, an attempt should be made to measure blood loss at delivery. This is rarely accurate since:

1 Not all blood lost is collected:
  - Some on sheets and floor.
  - Some still inside uterus (but lost from intravascular space).
2 Other fluids often included accidentally:
  - Urine.
  - Amniotic fluid.
  - Cleaning-up solutions.

Estimates are made and these are usually smaller in volume than the actual loss, sometimes as much as 50%. Therefore, give treatment on lower estimates of blood loss than would be done at a surgical operation.

**Treatment**

*Prevention*

Give oxytocic drug with delivery of baby, e.g. Syntometrine (ergometrine 0.5 mg and oxytocin 5 i.u.) i.m. This is the best way to prevent PPH. There may be an increased risk of retained placenta but that does not kill, PPH does (0.3/100 000).

*Curative*

1 Give another dose of oxytocic (usually ergometrine 0.5 mg i.v.).
2 Have blood taken for cross-matching and put up i.v. drip of Hartmann's solution.
3 Give blood if loss over 1000 ml or woman was anaemic in pregnancy.
4 Determine cause:
  - If placenta out: examine for completeness.

- If placenta not delivered: make arrangements for removal.

*Uterine atony*

1 Massage uterus to stimulate contraction.
2 Syntocinon i.v. by continuous drip (40 i.u./500 ml fluid).
3 Bimanually compress uterus (Fig. 13.8).
4 Injection of prostaglandin $PGE_{2\alpha}$ or carboprost directly into uterus.
5 Uterine artery embolization.
6 Hysterectomy.

Since the wider use of oxytocics both in prevention and treatment, the last three methods are rarely used. **5** and **6** are exceedingly unusual.

*Partly separated retained placenta*

1 Uterus is often well contracted.
2 Try controlled cord traction again, being careful not to snap cord.
3 Put up i.v. drip with Hartmann's solution while awaiting blood. Give blood if more than 1000 ml loss or patient was anaemic in pregnancy.
4 Empty bladder.
5 If placenta still undelivered 20 minutes after birth of the baby, prepare for manual removal. Try one gentle, sterile vaginal examination; placenta

**Figure 13.8** Bimanual compression of the uterus, wrapping it onto the clenched fist in the vagina.

may be trapped by the closing cervix and an edge can sometimes be hooked down and the placenta gently eased out.

**6** If an epidural is already acting, use this, otherwise a general anaesthetic is needed.

- Try once more to remove placenta by controlled cord traction just before the anaesthetist induces sleep. Sometimes separation has occurred in the meantime.

**7** Give a Syntocinon infusion and prophylactic antibiotics afterwards.

**8** Very rarely, the placenta may be abnormally adherent:

- Placenta accreta: villi just penetrate into myometrium.
- Placenta increta: villi penetrate deeply into myometrium.
- Placenta percreta: villi penetrate through myometrium to peritoneum.

Usually this is not possible to diagnose prospectively. If no plane of separation exists (and often there is little bleeding at the time) placenta accreta, increta or percreta must be thought of. Should the patient wish for no more children, the safest treatment is hysterectomy. If this is not possible, piecemeal removal is very dangerous and it is better to leave the placenta to atrophy with antibiotic control of infection.

*Note:* This is a very rare diagnosis made less often as the observer becomes more experienced.

*Tears of genital tract*

Heavy bleeding may occur from a tear of the cervix despite a well-contracted uterus and a completely expelled placenta.

**1** It is difficult to diagnose certainly and requires:

- Adequate general anaesthesia, unless epidural already acting.
- The woman in lithotomy position on a firm bed.
- Good lights and good assistance.
- Several sponge forceps and retractors (the vagina and cervix are soft just after delivery and tissues flop into the line of sight).

**2** Search cervix systematically using three pairs of ring forceps. If there is a tear:

- Check it does not run up into uterus, especially if at 3 or 9 o'clock.
- Suture with polyglycol absorbable material.

**3** Check lower uterine segment with fingers through the cervix. If a tear is found, either repair through abdominal incision or perform a hysterectomy.

**4** Check top end of episiotomy or tear which may go into posterior or lateral fornix.

- Repair systematically.

**5** Check no actively bleeding vessels in episiotomy or tear.

- Tie them off separately.

*Blood clotting defect*

**1** Check that blood taken from an arm vein clots and stays clotted.

**2** Check:

- Platelets.
- Coagulation studies.

**3** Treat appropriately by fresh frozen plasma (FFP).

- Fibrinogen.

**4** Remember such a state can allow secondary atony of the myometrium, so watch for that too as a cause of bleeding.

**Effects of primary PPH**

Rapid loss leads to hypovolaemic shock. If not corrected, this can cause:

**1** Death—about 8% of direct maternal deaths follow PPH; half of these are avoidable.

**2** Renal shutdown and consequent anuria.

**3** Damage to pituitary portal circulation causing necrosis and subsequent Sheehan's syndrome.

**4** Postpartum anaemia and chronic ill health.

**Secondary PPH**

This is abnormal vaginal bleeding that occurs after 24 hours following delivery. There is no volumetric definition; women usually present:

- With the passage of clots.
- At 7–10 days with a resumption of fresh vaginal bleeding.

*Causes*

- Retained pieces of placenta.
- Retained pieces of membrane.

- Retained blood clot.
- Infection of the residual decidua (endometritis).

*Clinical findings*
- Fresh red vaginal bleeding and clots.
- A large uterus.
- A tender uterus.
- An open cervical internal os.

*Risks*
- Substantial bleeding.
- Infection:
  (a) Septicaemia.
  (b) Blocked fallopian tubes.

*Treatment*
- Admit to hospital.
- Give i.v. broad-spectrum antibiotic cover, 24 hours pre-operatively and continuing for a minimum of 3 days. This combats the bacteraemia that may occur and also reduces the risk of subsequent tubal damage.
- Carry out an evacuation of retained products of conception after 24 hours. This should be performed gently by a senior obstetrician because of the risk of perforation of the very soft uterus.

## Massive blood loss

Rarely, a haemorrhage of 2–3 litres occurs suddenly at delivery. The woman's life will depend on a well-drilled team having a laid-down policy.

*Management*
Massive loss from the woman's circulating blood volume of 2–3 litres in a few minutes. For practical purposes consider it has happened if the woman has required more than 2 units of blood quickly.

   In anticipation of blood loss all women are routinely grouped and screened for antibodies in the antenatal clinics. Furthermore all at high risk of haemorrhage during labour should be cross-matched prospectively.

*Action*
**1** Put in two large-bore (at least 16 gauge) i.v. cannulae.

**2** Contact the duty obstetric registrar, if not already present, and the duty anaesthetic registrar. Call the obstetric consultant.
**3** Use one or more of the following fluids.
  - Up to 2 litres of Hartmann's solution.
  - Up to 1.5 litres of Gelofusin.
  - Uncross-matched blood of the woman's group.
  - Cross-matched blood as soon as available.
  - Give O Rh-negative blood only as a last resort.
  - In an emergency situation the use of blood filters and blood warming devices is not recommended. Pressurized infusion bags should be used.
  - Give I unit of FFP for every 6 units of blood. The haematologist will advise on platelet replacement.
**4** Stop the bleeding. If the bleeding is from the uterus:
  - Give 0.5 mg of ergometrine i.v. and set up 40 units of Syntocinon in 500 ml of Hartmann's solution to run at 40 drops/minute.
  - Commence bimanual compression of the uterus. If trauma, repair uterus/cervix/vagina.
  - Intrauterine injection of $PGE_2$ through abdominal wall.
**5** Contact the blood bank. Send at least 20 ml of blood for further cross-matching. Ask for at least 6 units of cross-matched blood.
**6** Inform the duty haematologist of the clinical situation, the rate of blood loss and the clotting problems.
**7** Insert a central venous line to monitor fluid replacement.
**8** One person should be assigned to record keeping and should record the following:
  - Pulse.
  - Blood pressure.
  - Maternal heart rate, preferably from an ECG.
  - Central venous pressure.
  - Urine output.
  - Amount and type of fluids the woman is given.
  - Drugs the woman has received.
**9** Prepare for theatre if appropriate.
**10** Before proceeding to hysterectomy, the following should be considered:

(a)  Direct i.m. injection of 0.5 mg of PGE$_2$ into the exposed uterus.

(b)  Open the broad ligament and ligate the uterine artery on each side.

(c)  Ligate internal iliac arteries.

## Operative delivery

Before undertaking an operative vaginal delivery the following five conditions should be met:

**1** Adequate analgesia (epidural or pudendal block with infiltration of the perineum with lignocaine).

**2** The fetal head should not be palpable in the abdomen.

**3** Full dilatation.

**4** Presenting part at the spines or below.

**5** Empty bladder via catheter.

## Vacuum extractor

This instrument is used to get a purchase on the smooth fetal head, allowing traction to be applied (Fig. 13.9). The suction raises an edged dome of the soft tissues of the scalp and the pull is on the overhang of this edge.

*Usage*

Used widely in Europe and the UK, least in USA, 5–10% of UK deliveries.

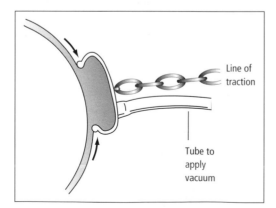

**Figure 13.9** Vacuum cap on fetal head sucks up a chignon of subcutaneous tissues to give a button on which to pull. The tractive efforts are mostly on the overhang (arrowed).

Line of traction

Tube to apply vacuum

Very useful in countries with developing health services (e.g. Africa) for it can be used by less experienced operators than forceps.

*Indications*

FIRST STAGE

**1** Fetal distress after cervix is 8 cm dilated in a multiparous women.

**2** Lack of advance after 8 cm dilated cervix in a multiparous women.

SECOND STAGE

**1** Lack of advance:
- Often with occipitoposterior or transverse position; commonly in association with an epidural.
- Mother is too tired.

**2** Compound presentations—after replacing a presenting hand.

**3** High head of second twin.

(Less use in fetal distress for forceps are swifter but, if the operator is inexperienced, the vacuum extractor is safer.)

*Contraindications*
- Disproportion.
- Malpresentations (face particularly).
- Very immature infants.

*Methods*

This is best learned by watching and helping in the labour ward. Here essentials only are given.

- Apply largest vacuum cap that slips through cervix—60 mm if possible.
- Hold cap flat against fetal head just anterior to the occiput and start to build up vacuum.
- With just enough vacuum to hold cap on head, check around the whole perimeter that maternal soft tissues have not been sucked under the cap's rim.
- Increase vacuum to 0.4 kg/cm$^2$ and then slowly to 0.8 kg/cm$^2$; again check full circumference of cap.
- Pull on handle, apply traction to fetal head in line with the curve of the pelvis (Fig. 13.10).
- Press cap onto head at right angles to line of traction with fingers of other hand.

• Remove cap by reducing vacuum suction.
• As well as the metal caps, there are softer rubber and Silastic caps and hand-held disposable caps which cause fewer fetal abrasions.

*Complications*

MATERNAL
• Cervical damage.
• Vaginal wall damage; reduced if application of cap checked so as not to suck in walls when vacuum is being established.
• Possible urinary retention later.

FETAL
• Cephalhaematoma.
• Skin abrasions.
Both are usually minor.

## Forceps

The function of forceps is to get purchase on a rounded object (the fetal head) and to apply traction. This is usually needed to hasten delivery, but it can control the speed of descent, e.g. slow down the aftercoming head in breech delivery.

*Usage*
Depends on availability of obstetricians. In UK 5–10% of all deliveries.

*Mechanism*
There are many types of forceps. Basically all have:
• Curved blades to fit around the head (Fig. 13.11).
• Handles to apply traction.
 Some have also:
1 A curve to allow for the curve of the pelvis (Fig. 13.12).
2 If they do not have a pelvic curve, they may be straight-handled to allow rotation manoeuvres.
3 Some have a sliding lock to allow for an asymmetrically aligned head.

**Figure 13.11** Cephalic curve of a pair of forceps to embrace a fetal head.

Line of pull at this level of pelvis

**Figure 13.10** Line of traction with vacuum extractor.

Angles of traction
2 Delivery of head
1 Descent to perineum

**Figure 13.12** The pelvic curve of the forceps to fit the curved line of advance of a fetus through the pelvis.

Thus there are two basic types. All have curved blades and handles for traction. In addition:
- Traction forceps incorporate **1**.
- Rotation and traction forceps incorporate **2** and usually **3**.

*Indications for use*

**1** Poor progress in the second stage. No exact time limits but most would consider the longer limits as 2 hours in a primigravida and half that in a multigravida. If an epidural anaesthetic is being used, these time limits are usually extended.

**2** Clinical fetal distress.
- Alterations of fetal heart rate and rhythm.
- Passage of meconium.

**3** Biophysical or biochemical signs of fetal hypoxia.
- On the fetal heart rate trace:
  (a) Tachycardia or bradycardia.
  (b) Loss of baseline variability.
  (c) Late decelerations.
- On fetal blood sampling, scalp capillary blood: base deficit greater than 10mEq/l; pH below 7.15 in second stage.

**4** Maternal distress.
- A tired woman after a long first stage.
- One who is frightened or has not had proper analgesia.

**5** To prevent fetal morbidity.
- Very immature babies.
- Delivering the head of a breech presentation.

**6** To prevent maternal morbidity.
- Women with cardiac or respiratory disease.
- Following a dural tap at attempted epidural injection.

*Method*

These methods are best learned by watching and helping in the labour ward. Here essentials only are given.

**1** Each blade of the forceps is slipped in turn along the obstetrician's cupped hand holding back the vaginal walls in turn.

**2** The blades are locked together.

**3** Traction is applied in a downwards and backwards direction to follow the line of the curve of the birth canal (Fig. 13.13).

**4** For a rotation, forceps are applied on the sides of the baby's face and then rotated through 90° occipitoanterior and delivered by traction.

*Complications*

MATERNAL
- Perineal tear: avoid by a properly sited episiotomy done at the right time; often an episiotomy will extend at a forceps delivery. Check for this at the apex of the episiotomy cut.
- Damage to vagina: occasional split of vagina where caught between descending head and ischial spines.
- Retention of urine: possibly due to oedema at bladder neck. Responds to continuous drainage.

FETAL
- Bruising to head: may go on to cephalhaematoma.
- Facial palsy: facial nerve in front of ear unprotected in fetus. May be compressed by forceps blade. Usually only temporary effect.
- Intracranial haemorrhage: if blades incorrectly applied or excessive traction used.

Push down with left hand

Pull on handles with right hand

Resultant of two lines of forces draws fetal head down in line with this part of the birth canal

**Figure 13.13** Correct line of pull is achieved by use of two hands working in cooperation, thus performing the task more simply than a pair of axis traction forceps.

*Failed forceps*
An attempt to deliver with forceps which is unsuccessful.

REASONS
**1** Cervix not fully dilated.
**2** Misdiagnosis of position of head. Thought to be occipitoanterior when it is occipitotransverse or occipitoposterior.
**3** Unsuspected disproportion.

TREATMENT
Get senior help in hospital. Then:
If **1**, with mother and fetus well, await full dilatation.
If **2**, rotate head and deliver.
If **3**, Caesarean section.

## Caesarean section (CS)

Delivery of the fetus by surgical means through the abdominal wall.

*Usage*
Depends on availability of obstetricians and on the population served. In UK 25% of all deliveries.

The Caesarean section rate has risen rapidly in the last 25 years. There are several reasons for this:
• The introduction of epidural anaesthesia has reduced the anaesthetic risks of the procedure. This has led to a lower threshold for doing a Caesarean section in the second stage of labour rather than performing rotational/high cavity forceps deliveries which led to maternal and neonatal morbidity.
• The increased use of electronic fetal monitoring has increased our awareness of fetal distress although the majority of babies are born in good condition despite an abnormal CTG and/or low pH at fetal blood sampling.
• The reduction in the number of rotational forceps deliveries has led to a deskilling of obstetricians who do not feel confident to carry out these procedures.
• The evidence that breech presentation babies have a reduced morbidity and mortality if delivered by elective Caesarean section
• An increasing demand from women for elective Caesarean sections with no medical reason.

The latter group are difficult to deal with, as a first elective Caesarean section does have a lower maternal morbidity than an emergency Caesarean section but it is still higher than a normal vaginal delivery. In first pregnancies we do not have a reliable indicator for the outcome of labour and so we cannot guarantee that a woman will not end up with a Caesarean section. Seventy per cent of women who go into spontaneous labour at term can expect to have a normal vaginal delivery. Many of the women who request Caesarean section have a genuine fear of labour and/or motherhood which may be based on past experiences of sexual abuse, poor mothering or other psychological problems. It is wise to refer them to a psychologist or midwife trained in these areas before agreeing to perform a Caesarean section. All subsequent Caesarean sections carry an increased morbidity.

*Indications*
Few are absolute, most are relative to the individual patient, the obstetrician and the obstetrical environment. Generally when the risks of vaginal delivery to the mother or baby are greater than those of abdominal delivery in any given circumstance, a CS should be done.
• CPD.
• Fetal distress in first stage of labour or a prolapsed cord.
• Failure of labour to progress despite adequate stimulation.
• To avoid fetal hypoxia of labour: pre-eclampsia; intrauterine growth restriction.
• Antepartum bleeding: placenta praevia; abruptio placentae.
• Poor past obstetric history.
• Malpresentations: brow.
• Malpositions: transverse lie, breech.
• Death of mother in late pregnancy, a live fetus removed *peri mortem*.

The only absolute ones are gross disproportion, the higher grades of placenta praevia.

In a UK population, a hospital in this decade would have the following indications in differing proportions for operations:
• Fetal distress.
• Pre-eclampsia.

- Poor fetal growth.
- Disorderly uterine action.
- Breech, face and brow.
- Previous CS.

*Types of approach*

**1** Lower segment operation: transverse approach through lower segment. In the UK, over 99% of operations are lower segment because:
- Wound is extraperitoneal so less risk of intra-peritoneal infection.
- Fewer post-operative complications.
- Healing of scar is better for lower segment is relatively at rest in puerperium.
- Risk of rupture less in subsequent pregnancies.

**2** Classical operation: vertical approach through upper segment, performed:
- If lower segment unapproachable, e.g. fibroids.
- If transverse lie.
- If very small baby expected (24–28 weeks), lower vertical incision (De Lee's incision).

*Anaesthesia*

The operation requires an anaesthetic. The alternatives are:
**1** General anaesthetic.
**2** Epidural block.
**3** Spinal block.
**4** Infiltration of local anaesthetic agents.

*Surgical technique*

These surgical operations are best learned by watching and helping in theatre.

*Complications*

**1** Haemorrhage
- Worst if angles of transverse uterine incision extend into uterine vessels.
- Always have 2 units of cross-matched blood available.

**2** Infection
- Watch asepsis and antisepsis.
- Give prophylactic antibiotics to all women.

**3** Abdominal distension
- Common for a day or so.
- Await events.

**4** Ileus
- Mild regional ileus may last 24 hours.

- Await events and avoid overloading the gut (keep on i.v. fluid for 24 hours).

Longer ileus may follow if there was a lot of handling and packing of the gut. Treat with stomach aspiration and i.v. fluids.

**5** Thromboembolism
- Much higher risk after CS than after vaginal delivery.
- Avoid thrombosis by:
  - TED stockings intraoperatively until woman fully mobilized.
  - Intraoperative compression stockings.
  - Intraoperative subcutaneous heparin continued daily until woman fully mobilized.
  - Early mobilization and leg exercises.
  - Keep woman well hydrated post-operatively.
- Avoid embolism by taking leg and pelvic signs seriously and anticoagulating early.
- Prevent thrombosis with prophylactic anticoagulation (subcutaneous heparin) in all women and particularly those women at higher risk:
  - (a) Aged over 35.
  - (b) Obese.
  - (c) Past history of thrombosis, particularly if oestrogen associated (e.g. oral contraception).
  - (d) Anaemia.

*Prognosis*

MATERNAL
- *Mortality.* 1:3000 CS with causes mostly in the above complications group.
- *Morbidity.* Subsequent pregnancies following a CS may be affected.
  **1** If non-recurrent indication (e.g. fetal distress), two-thirds deliver vaginally.
  **2** If recurrent indication (e.g. disproportion), only one-eighth deliver vaginally.

Hence patients who have had a CS must have all subsequent pregnancies properly conducted in a hospital. Watch for dehiscence of uterine scar in late pregnancy next time. Take extra care if giving oxytocic stimulation.

FETAL
- *Mortality.* Depends on indication; CS reduces risk, but, if done for progressive fetal condition, it

may be indicated only in the women with worst degrees of that condition and so fetal prognosis is worse, not from the operative delivery but the condition which indicated it.

• *Morbidity.* Higher risk of retained lung fluid if delivered by CS especially before 32 weeks' gestation.

## The flying squad

Every major hospital doing obstetrics in the UK used to have available obstetricians and midwives who could be taken urgently to any patient who presented with an obstetric emergency outside the hospital environment. In some teams, which covered a larger area, an anaesthetist was included. The squad used to represent the patching up of a domiciliary and GP unit service.

Much of the real service has become a resuscitation one, the woman being brought to a state suitable for transfer back to the hospital where definitive treatment takes place. Problems at delivery have almost disappeared and the squad was being called inappropriately. One-quarter of patients are given i.v. therapy but <1% had uncrossmatched blood. Many of the calls related to normal women who had just delivered. The ambulance service transports such women but no flying squad is needed, rather a community midwife or a paramedic.

The flying squad was introduced because private transport was rare, telephones were unusual and it was hard to get to the hospital. All that has changed and now, every time obstetricians, midwives and anaesthetists have to leave the centre to look after an individual, it leaves the larger number of women at that hospital with a diminished service.

Now paramedics in the ambulance services are trained in advanced resuscitation. They go to the home or GP unit and bring the woman safely into hospital.

A few flying squads persist in rural areas, but by 2004 virtually all have been closed down for the reasons discussed above.

## Multiple pregnancies and deliveries

The commonest litter size in the human species is one. Other multiples are rare (Table 13.2) and vary with racial characteristics inside the species (e.g. there is a higher incidence in West Africa than in Europe).

The differences between actual and theoretical figures are probably due to the reducing birth rate, more births to older women and fewer to those of higher parity; (both having increased multiple pregnancy rates). Higher rates in the UK are now due to ovarian stimulation and assisted conception with a trebling of triplets in IVF.

**Table 13.2** Rates of multiple pregnancies per 1000 deliveries in England and Wales in 1995 compared with the biologically expected rate.

|  | Actual | Theoretical |
|---|---|---|
| Twins | 13.6 | 12.5 (1 : 80) |
| Triplets | 0.44 | 0.16 (1 : 80$^2$) |
| Quadruplets and higher orders | 0.014 | 0.02 (1 : 80$^3$) |

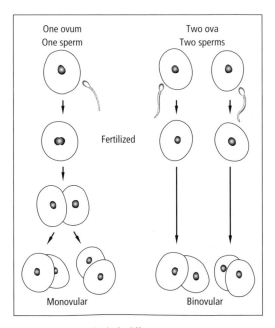

**Figure 13.14** Biological differences in monovular and binovular twins.

# Twins

## Types (Fig. 13.14)

### Monovular twins

Monovular twins are produced from one ovum fertilized by one sperm. After the two-cell division instead of going into the four-cell stage, the blastomere divides into two separate cell bodies which go on to two individuals. Thus there is common chromatin material; sex and physical characteristics will be the same, producing identical twins.

### Binovular twins

Binovular twins are from two separate ova fertilized by two different sperms. These ova are shed in one menstrual cycle and most likely to be fertilized after one intercourse although they can be at separate times with different fathers. The two blastomeres develop separately and have different chromatin material. They can, therefore, be of different sexes having no more in common than any other members of the same family. They are non-identical twins. Early ultrasound can help differentiation.

*Incidence*
Monovular twins have an incidence of 3 or 4 : 1000 worldwide and there is only a slight familial tendency. Binovular twins may have a family history on the maternal side. It is these that account for racial and maternal age variations. Binovular twins are more common than monovular ones (4 : 1). Binovular twins are commoner if:

• Maternal family history of non-identical twins.
• Over 35 years.
• After replacement of two, three or more fertilized ova at *in vitro* fertilization.

*Differentiation of twins*
**1** *Sex*. If of different sexes, obviously binovular. If of one sex, may be either.
**2** *Placenta*. If two separated placentae, will be binovular; if one placenta, may be monovular or binovular (Fig. 13.15). Check septum between sacs by peeling amnions from each other (Table 13.3).

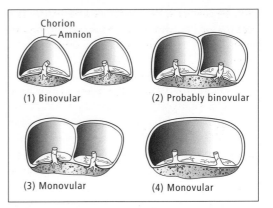

(1) Binovular      (2) Probably binovular
(3) Monovular      (4) Monovular

**Figure 13.15** Placental types in twinning. Often the intervening membranes can be seen in early pregnancy on ultrasound and the two types of twins differentiated.

**Table 13.3** Differentiation of twins by checking placentae.

| Septum | Placenta type | Twin type |
|---|---|---|
| (4) None | Monoamniotic Monochorionic | Monovular |
| (3) Amnion only | Diamniotic Monochorionic | Monovular |
| (2) Amnion and chorion | Diamniotic Dichorionic | Binovular or monovular |
| (1) No common septum | Diamniotic Dichorionic | Binovular |

**3** *Blood groups*. If doubt in dichorionic types, check the ABO, Rh, Duffy, Kell and MNS.
**4** *Fingerprints*. If different, binovular.
**5** *DNA fingerprinting* with probes identifying about 60 dispersed sequences of variable size.

## Diagnosis of twins

*History*
• Suspicion on family history especially maternal non-identical twins.
• Suspicion on past obstetric history of twins.
• Suspicion from excessive vomiting in early pregnancy.

*Examination*
Examination from 20 weeks onwards shows uterus bigger than expected. At first a lot of limbs are felt

and later, about 30–32 weeks, more than two separate poles determined (e.g. two heads and one breech).

*Investigation*

Ultrasound at 6–7 weeks may show two or more sacs. The embryos can be seen in these at 7–8 weeks. The differentiation of mono from binovular can often be made by expert examination of the dividing membranes.

Commonly one of a pair of twins diagnosed early does not develop and is absorbed: the vanishing twin syndrome.

Without ultrasound, twins may not be diagnosed until delivery on rare occasions. While embarrassing to the attendants, this usually does not affect the second twin unless Syntometrine was given inadvertently at the birth of the first baby. This could jeopardize the $O_2$ supply to the second twin and so his or her delivery should be expedited.

## Management of twins

*Complications in pregnancy*

**1** Miscarriage is more frequent.
**2** Preterm labour commoner (50% before 37 weeks).
**3** Pre-eclampsia commoner (×3).
**4** Risk of anaemia increased.
  • Iron deficiency.
  • Folic acid deficiency.
**5** Polyhydramnios commoner (×10 with monovular twins).
**6** Risk of APH increased.
  • Abruptio placentae.
  • Placenta praevia.

*Management in pregnancy*

**1** Diagnose early by bearing it in mind (one only diagnoses what one thinks about); often ultrasound will give the result before clinical suspicion.
**2** Give extra iron and folic acid supplements and see that the woman takes them.
  • Check blood more often for haemoglobin levels.

*Complications in labour*

**1** Delay in delivery of the second twin is associated with a higher mortality.
**2** PPH is more common.
**3** Prolapse of umbilical cord is more common.
**4** Mechanical collision of leading parts (or locking of a breech–cephalic) as they both enter the pelvis. This is very rare.

*Management in labour*

**1** Always plan for hospital delivery.
**2** Ensure the first twin is longitudinal. Commonest combinations of presentations show that both twins lie longitudinally 90% of the time and the first twin is a cephalic presentation in 80% (Fig. 13.16). Non-cephalic presentations are common if early preterm labour.

If the first twin is transverse, do a Caesarean section.

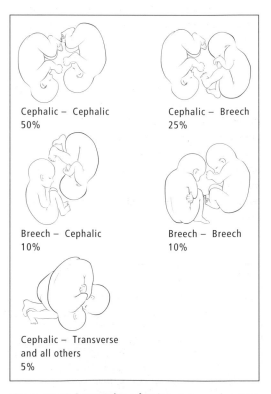

Cephalic – Cephalic
50%

Cephalic – Breech
25%

Breech – Cephalic
10%

Breech – Breech
10%

Cephalic – Transverse
and all others
5%

**Figure 13.16** Presentation of twins at time of mature delivery (after 36 weeks).

**3** Check for cord prolapse when membranes rupture (often early in labour).

**4** Progress is usually uneventful. Monitor both fetal hearts and have an i.v. drip running.

**5** An epidural anaesthetic is useful for it allows rapid anaesthesia for any manoeuvres that may be required for the second twin in the second stage.

**6** Deliver the first twin appropriately. Have an anaesthetist and a paediatrician in the labour ward. Make sure that nobody inadvertently gives Syntometrine to the mother at this point.

**7** Clamp cord of the first twin and divide. Hand baby to competent assistant or paediatrician in case resuscitation is required.

**8** Immediately check the lie of the second twin. If longitudinal, check presenting part. If oblique or transverse, convert to longitudinal.

- External version—usually easy for uterus is lax, *or*
- Combined external and internal version—rupture membranes and bring a leg of the fetus down through the cervix. This produces an incomplete breech presentation but it is at least longitudinal.

**9** The second twin is best delivered within 20 minutes of the first. Usually uterus starts contracting again about 5 minutes after first delivery. If it does not do so spontaneously, use i.v. oxytocin augmentation. Very little is needed. Rupture membranes of second sac and deliver appropriately.

**10** Give Syntometrine with delivery of the second twin and continue oxytocin infusion for another hour.

**11** Deliver placentae as soon as uterus is contracted after delivery of the second twin, for retained placentae and PPH are common.

*Outcome*

MATERNAL
Higher risk:
- The complications of pregnancy, e.g. pre-eclampsia.
- The complications of delivery, e.g. anaesthesia and PPH.

FETAL
- Risks to the first twin are twice, and to the second twin, about three times those of single births.

Causes of death:
(a) Immaturity. ⎫ Especially
(b) Hypoxia. ⎬ the second
(c) Risks of operative delivery. ⎭ twin.

- Neonatal risks are jaundice or anaemia following intrauterine shunting of blood inside the placenta leading to twin-to-twin transfusion in monovular twins.

## Triplets

Rarely due to tri-ovulation:
- Usually binovular twins with one fertilized egg dividing into two individuals or assisted conception.
- Usually born at an even more immature stage than twins and have double the risks.
- The complications and management are as for twins. Because of the immaturity of the fetuses, delivery is commonly by Caesarean section.

---

**Self-assessment**

**13.1** A woman in her first pregnancy is admitted in spontaneous labour at 39 weeks. On examination the presentation is cephalic, 2/5 palpable. The cervix is 1 cm long and firm, 1 cm dilated posterior to the head and the head is 2 cm above the spines. Which of the following statements are true?
(a) She is in the active phase of the first stage of labour.
(b) Her Bishop's score is <4.
(c) She is in the latent phase of the first phase of labour.
(d) Her Bishop's score is >4.
(e) She should be encouraged to mobilize and re-examined in 4 hours time.

*Continued on p. 202.*

**Self-assessment** *Continued*

**13.2** Which of the following presenting positions can be delivered spontaneously vaginally?
- (a) Face presentation.
- (b) Brow presentation.
- (c) Occipitotransverse.
- (d) Occipitoposterior.
- (e) Vertex presentation.

**13.3** Which of the following statements are true?
- (a) Breech presentation is more common in premature babies.
- (b) All women with a breech presentation should be offered external cephalic version at 37–38 weeks.
- (c) Breech presentation is more common at term than at 34 weeks.
- (d) Breech presentation is associated with a higher perinatal mortality regardless of the mode of delivery.
- (e) Caesarean section should be offered to all women with twins where the presentation is cephalic in the first twin and breech in the second twin.

**13.4** List the five conditions that should be met before undertaking an operative vaginal delivery for a cephalic presentation.

**13.5** Which of the following are true about primary postpartum haemorrhage (PPH)?
- (a) It is defined as a loss of blood of >500 ml.
- (b) It is more common following a spontaneous vaginal delivery.
- (c) The commonest cause is uterine atony.
- (d) It can be prevented by giving syntometrine with the birth of the anterior shoulder.
- (e) It is more common in women with pre-eclampsia.

# Chapter 14

# Puerperium

In the puerperium the mother is returning to her pre-pregnant state. The various organ systems take different times but most physical restoration has occurred by 6 weeks. During this time, one should aim at:

- Restoring maternal health and preventing illness.
- Maintaining infant health and preventing illness.
- Establishing infant feeding.
- Educating the mother about her child's and her own future health.

## Physiological changes in genital tract

### Uterus

Uterine bulk reduces by involution following withdrawal of oestrogens so that the organ is back in the pelvis by 10–12 days.

- Thrombosis of blood vessels.
- Autolysis of cellular cytoplasm of myometrium.
- Regeneration of endometrium within 6 weeks.
- The uterus never returns quite to nulliparous size but close to it.
- The cervix is normally stretched at delivery and the external os is split after a delivery.

### Vulva

After stretching, tissues revert to non-pregnant state with the following differences:
- Less fatty tissue in the labia.
- Hymen is wrecked leaving skin tags only.
- Episiotomy or tear area leaves a scar which might be tender.

## Management of first week

### Observations

- Temperature: watch for pyrexia.
- Pulse rate: watch for transient tachycardia associated with thrombosis.
- Blood pressure: check especially if pre-eclampsia occurred in pregnancy.
- Uterine size: check daily reduction by abdominal palpation.
- Lochia: loss from vagina in the first days is the shedding of the decidua. Starts red with fresh blood but pales over 2 weeks to yellow-white. This may last for weeks.
- Urine output: normal diuresis starts within 24 hours and lasts about 3 days.
- Bowels: often constipation. Avoid too long a gap for a very hard stool is painful. Provide fibre and extra fluids to give bulk to stools.
- Haemoglobin: check level about day two even if

blood loss at delivery is recorded as minimal. Give oral iron if below 11 g/dl. Readvise on diet.

## Pain relief

*Uterine contractions*
• After-pains (contractions) are variable, painful and need analgesia.
• Warn the woman that they are coming so that she is prepared.
• Often felt more in multigravida, worse after successive deliveries.

*Perineal*
• After the local anaesthetic wears off, the episiotomy will hurt. Further, oedema and burning may make sitting uncomfortable. Give analgesics, local heat and, if oedematous, ice packs.
• Check sutures are not cutting in.

## Bed rest

A balance must be struck between resting in bed to recover from the work of labour and resting so much that stagnation of blood leads to deep vein thrombosis.

## Exercises

In association with bed rest, graduated exercises restore muscle tone to stretched areas and maintain venous flow in limbs and pelvis. They are aimed at:
**1** Breathing exercises.
**2** Legs to prevent stagnation of blood in veins.
**3** Abdominal wall to restore tone of rectus muscles.
**4** Pelvic floor to restore levator ani.

Exercises are best taught by a physiotherapist in hospital teaching women what to do after leaving. Fifteen minutes twice a day should be set aside for these for some weeks.

## Psychological support

Producing a baby is a psychological stress. Women with different emotional backgrounds respond variously. Most women find a balance between the excitement and pleasure of the event on the one hand and the worry and responsibility of looking after the baby on the other. Watch for this and prevent excessive worry by:
• Adequate explanation of any baby problems.
• Ensuring good sleep.
• Pain relief.

## Discharge to home

The length of postnatal stay in hospital is determined by social and financial factors as well as by medical ones. The length of stay is reducing and the community services are supposed to take up their share of looking after those who the hospital discharges.

Many Trusts now run planned, very early DOMINO discharge schemes (Domestic in and out) where a woman comes into hospital with her community midwife, delivers and goes home a few hours later. In some instances a *birthroom* is used, geographically apart but close to the labour suite; here the woman can be delivered by her midwife in less hospitalized surroundings. If an emergency arises, obstetric, anaesthetic or paediatric care is immediately available.

Fifty percent of women now leave the hospital by day two under planned discharge schemes evolved between the hospital and the local community midwives and general practitioners. Those who had uncomplicated Caesarean sections go home at 3–5 days.

*Advantages of earlier discharge*
**1** Satisfaction. By planning and letting the woman know she will return home in a short time, she is happier and more willing to come into hospital for the time of maximum risk: labour.
**2** Leaves more beds available for those with antenatal/pastnatal complications allowing intensive care for the fetus or mother.
**3** Reduces the risks of hospital cross-infection. This is a rapidly diminishing factor in the UK but outbreaks of gastroenteritis and haemolytic streptococcal infection do still occasionally happen.

*Disadvantages of earlier discharge*

**1** *Lack of rest.* Household duties soon demand the woman's attention.

**2** *Poor housing conditions.* If the woman is unsupported or from the lower income groups, she may be better kept in hospital for a little longer. This is a diminishing problem in the UK but a small proportion of homes (5–10%) are still considered to be unsuitable for early discharge.

**3** *Medical problems* after delivery may be missed. This is unlikely if proper community cover is given so that women who go home are visited by midwives and GPs by arrangement. In fact less than 2% of early discharged women are re-admitted for medical problems.

## Problems in the puerperium

Over half of maternal deaths associated with pregnancy and childbirth occur in the first few days following delivery. Although rare, it is a measure of the need for vigilance; postnatal women should be seen each day for the first 10 days by a qualified doctor or midwife. Ideally a postnatal visit should be at about 6 weeks; this should be by the family practitioner if the delivery was straightforward or at the hospital if there were complications.

## Psychological problems

### The baby blues

Many women feel weepy and depressed 3–5 days after delivery but this is usually short-lived. Factors that prolong the baby blues are:
• Postpartum pyrexia.
• Anaemia of <8 g/dl.
• Inadequate sleep.
• Delayed healing of the episiotomy or Caesarean section wound.
• Delay in establishing breast feeding.
• Decline in sympathy, congratulations and attention of friends and family as the time from childbirth increases.

### Depression

Baby blues merge with serious depression. There is not a specific form of depression that is related solely to pregnancy and childbirth. The factors that aggravate depression are:
• A background predisposition due to previous history or family history.
• A conflict in the responsibilities of looking after a new baby.
• Hormone changes acting on predisposition to depression.
• Fantasies.
• Anxiety and guilt.
• Residual pain.
• Sleeplessness.

*Treatment*
• Involve a psychiatrist.
• If no psychotic delusions, can be managed as an outpatient.
• Oral antidepressants.

### Postpartum psychosis

This is a rare condition which affects less than 1 in 500 women. It is potentially life-threatening to both the mother and the baby.

*Symptoms*
• Rejection of the baby.
• Delusion.
• Confusion.
• Agitation.

*Management*
**1** Admit the mother and baby to a special ward in the psychiatric unit.
**2** Ensure 24 hour supervision.
**3** Give appropriate psychotherapy drugs. Some use electroconvulsive therapy.

Postpartum psychosis is recurrent (about 20%) but chances are decreased by a 2-year or more gap between pregnancies.

### Infections

The common infections of the puerperium are:

**1** Infections of the genital tract.
**2** Urinary tract infection.
**3** Breast infections.

## Genital tract infection

An ascending infection which largely involves the placental bed. Unlike pelvic inflammatory disease (PID) it spreads directly through the uterus to the parametrial tissues.

The commonest organisms are *E. coli* and *Streptococcus faecalis*.

*Diagnosis*

HISTORY
• Puerperal pyrexia—temperature above 38°C twice.
• Offensive discharge.
• Low abdominal pain.
• Passage of clots and a return of red lochia.
• Systemic symptoms associated with the pyrexia.

EXAMINATION
• Raised temperature and pulse.
• Bulky uterus.
• Tender uterus.
• Offensive lochia (often bleeding with clots).
• An open internal cervical os.

INVESTIGATIONS
• Hb—may be reduced.
• White cell count—raised with a neutrophilia.
• High vaginal or endocervical swab—may grow the organisms.

*Management*
**1** Admit to hospital.
**2** Evacuation of retained products of conception under antibiotic cover.

Broad-spectrum antibiotics should be used to cover the bacteraemia and subsequently for 5 days.

*Complications*

ACUTE
• Parametritis.

• Salpingitis.
• Broad ligament abscess.
• Peritonitis
• Septic thromboembolism.

LONGER-TERM
• Infertility.
• Menstrual irregularities and pelvic pain.

## Urinary tract infections

These are common in the puerperium because of:
**1** Bladder stasis.
**2** Oedema of the bladder base.
**3** Diminished bladder sensation.
**4** Catheterization in labour.

The commonest organisms are *E. coli* and *Proteus* spp.

*Diagnosis*

HISTORY
• Dysuria.
• Frequency of micturition.
• Loin pain if pyelonephritis supercedes.
• Systemic symptoms such as pyrexia and tachycardia.
• May be asymptomatic and recognized on routine mid-stream urine (MSU) sample. This should be performed on all patients who have been catheterized in labour.

EXAMINATION
• Raised temperature.
• Tender suprapubically or in the renal angle.

INVESTIGATIONS
• MSU.
• White cell count.
• Nitrites and leucocytes on dipstick.

*Management*
• Bed rest.
• High fluid, light solid diet.
• Broad-spectrum antibiotics until the results of culture and sensitivity are known, then be specific.

*Complications*
- Pyelonephritis.
- Exacerbation of the baby blues.

## Breast infection

This usually enters through a break in the skin (cracked nipple). It is usually confined to one quadrant of the breast. Most commonly it is due to *Staphylococcus aureus*.

*Diagnosis*

HISTORY
Painful area of one breast.

EXAMINATION
- Raised temperature.
- Erythematous segment of the breast.
- If an abscess, brawny swelling or even fluctuation.

INVESTIGATION
Bacteriology of expressed breastmilk from the affected side.

*Management*
**1** *Without abscess*
- Supportive brassiere.
- Continue breast feeding on other breast and empty the affected breast with a breast pump.
- Give broad-spectrum antibiotic such as flucloxacillin orally.
**2** *With abscess*
- Incise under a general anaesthetic.
- Circumareola incision.
- Break down septa and leave a drain through dependent part.
- Adequate supportive brassiere.
- Appropriate i.v. antibiotics.

## Thromboembolism

The postpartum period is the commonest time in pregnancy for a thromboembolism because:

**1** *Increased coagulation.* The increase in clotting factors from pregnancy remains although plasma volume reduces to normal within a few hours of delivery.
**2** *Stasis.* Many women have been immobilized in pregnancy, during labour or the immediate puerperium.
**3** *Damage to venous endothelium.*
- Uterine veins—following uterine sepsis.
- Deep leg veins—weight of legs compresses veins if immobilized.

*Diagnosis*

HISTORY
- Calf pain.
- Unilateral leg oedema.

EXAMINATION
- A low-grade postpartum pyrexia.
- An unexplained maternal tachycardia.
- Tenderness over the deep veins of the calf.
- A positive Holman's sign (calf tenderness on dorsiflexion of the foot).

INVESTIGATIONS
**1** *Doppler ultrasound.*
- Simple continuous wave Doppler ultrasound will fail to show flow in the femoral vein.
- Colour flow Doppler may demonstrate the clot in the veins.
**2** *Venography.*
- This is the definitive test using image intensifiers and low-viscosity contrast medium.

*Management*

PREVENTION
**1** Early mobilization—all women are encouraged to be up as soon as they wish. Non-weight-bearing exercises used for postoperative mothers.
**2** Prophylaxis is usually given to women who have had a previous history of thromboembolism or are at moderate to high risk.
- Compression (TED) stockings worn during labour or Caesarean section.
- Subcutaneous low molecular weight heparin.

TREATMENT

**1** Anticoagulate immediately with full dose i.v. heparin to prevent further extension of the thrombosis with the risk of pulmonary embolism and allows earlier recanalization of the clotted veins.

**2** Long-term anticoagulation with warfarin for 12 weeks.

## Pulmonary embolism

The most dangerous destination of a clot embolus from the leg or pelvic veins is in the pulmonary circulation.

**1** *Mild cases* follow microemboli. Dyspnoea and slight, poorly defined pleural pain. The condition resolves in a few days with no specific treatment and may not even be diagnosed.

**2** *Severe cases* arise from clot from the:
• Soleal veins—clot extends to popliteal vein and breaks off (30%).
• Uterine and ovarian veins—a thrombophlebitis with a friable clot following mid-pelvic sepsis (20%).

In 50%, no clinical signs of the origin exist before the pulmonary embolism.

*Diagnosis*

HISTORY

Pre-existing deep vein thrombosis (in half the cases only).

Early:
• Acute dyspnoea.
• Faintness.

Later:
• Chest pain.
• Haemoptysis.

EXAMINATION

Early:
• No physical signs beyond dyspnoea.

Later:
• May be cyanosis.
• Local signs of pulmonary underperfusion.
• Right heart failure.

Later still:
• Pleural signs.
• Collapse of a pulmonary lobe.

INVESTIGATIONS

Often no positive tests early. Next day:

**1** X-ray:
• Raised diaphragm on affected side.
• Consolidation and infiltration of lung(s).

**2** ECG—rhythm disturbance.
• Lead I—S wave inversion.
• Lead III—T wave inversion and deep Q wave.
• Leads VI, 2, 3, 4—T wave inversion.
• Excludes cardiac infarction.

**3** Lung ventilation–perfusion studies with radioactive albumin to show ischaemic areas.

**4** Pulmonary angiography to show clot.

**5** Left and right heart catheterization to show reversal of pressures.

The last two are used in specialist thoracic units.

*Management*

Two-thirds of those dying do so within 2 hours, so act quickly on suspicion, not awaiting the sophisticated tests even if they are available.

IMMEDIATE TREATMENT

**1** External cardiac massage if required.

**2** Positive pressure $O_2$ by intubation if necessary.

**3** Heparin (see below).

**4** Emergency embolectomy is only performed in hospitals with their own thoracic units with bypass facilities and rarely used.

DEFINITIVE TREATMENT

If resuscitation is successful, give:

**1** Anticoagulants (more i.v. heparin):
• 25000 units immediately.
• 25000 units 6-hourly for 24 hours.

This is to prevent further emboli.

At the same time start warfarin oral therapy controlled by prothrombin time.

**2** Thrombolytics (streptokinase). Actively accelerate lysis of existing clot:
• 500000 units immediately.
• 100000 units hourly for 72 hours.

**3** Embolectomy (mortality rate 25%). Useful if:
- Thoracic unit in the same hospital.
- No response to streptokinase.
- Too ill for streptokinase.
- Contraindication to streptokinase, e.g. recent surgery, peptic ulcer or hypertension.

Both high-dose heparin and streptokinase have high risk of starting bleeding. Not indicated unless embolus is thought to be life-threatening. If started, reduce to conservative dosage in 2–3 days and continue for 4–6 weeks.

## Secondary postpartum haemorrhage

Any considerable fresh bleeding occurring in the puerperium after 24 hours. This is dealt with in Chapter 13.

## Previous diseases continuing into the puerperium

### Pre-eclampsia and eclampsia

When these conditions occur before delivery, their ultimate treatment is delivery of the baby. Usually the woman gets better rapidly after the placenta is delivered and the normal diuresis starts to remove the water/salt overload. A few women stay as bad or worsen in the first few days of the puerperium. Management is the same as in pregnancy (see pp. 123–6). Postpartum eclampsia has a high mortality rate.

### Diabetes

Delivery may have been operative and for a day immediately after the woman may be on i.v. therapy. Remember that insulin requirements drop very sharply in the puerperium so that many diabetics are at their pre-pregnant levels of insulin by 2 days into the puerperium. Infection of any wounds is more likely and breast feeding may be an irregular drain of carbohydrates, making insulin balance more difficult.

### Heart disease

The first 24 hours of the puerperium are dangerous, for the post-delivery shunting of blood from the uterine vessels may lead to pulmonary oedema and subsequent right-sided cardiac failure. After that the risk is reduced.

Puerperal infection could release bacteria that might colonize on any damaged endothelium in the heart (acute bacterial endocarditis). This is more likely to follow a congenital heart disease than rheumatic conditions, but antibiotic cover is often provided for either into the puerperium.

### Ovarian tumours

These are more likely to undergo torsion in the puerperium because of the lax abdominal wall and the diminishing uterus. Surgery is recommended for any ovarian masses above 10 cm diameter.

---

**Self-assessment**

**14.1** A woman on the postnatal ward bursts into tears when you go and see her 48 hours after the birth of her baby. Which of the following might indicate that she is at high risk of developing postnatal depression?
(a) She does not show any interest in her infant who is crying insistently.
(b) She is bottle feeding the baby.
(c) She is unable to sleep.
(d) Her mother had severe postnatal depression.
(e) Her partner has recently left her and was not present at the birth of the baby.

**14.2** A woman presents 10 days after a normal vaginal delivery with a raised temperature of 38.4°C. Match the additional information given in 1–5 to the five most likely of the diagnoses (a)–(j)
**1** She has passed several clots and is in pain. Her uterus is 16 weeks size and tender.
**2** She complains of pain on passing urine. Her left loin is tender.

*Continued on p. 210.*

**Self-assessment** *Continued*

    **3** She complains of right breast tenderness and has a fluctuant mass in the upper quadrant.

    **4** She complains of a productive cough with chest pain particularly on inspiration.

    **5** Her left leg is swollen and tender with erythema particularly over the inner aspect of her calf where she has varicose veins.

    (a) Breast engorgement.

    (b) Salpingitis.

    (c) Pyelonephritis.

    (d) Bronchitis.

    (e) Deep vein thrombosis.

    (f) Retained products of conception.

    (g) Pulmonary embolism.

    (h) Thrombophlebitis.

    (i) Cystitis.

    (j) Breast abscess.

**14.3** Which of the following would be appropriate management/treatment of the conditions in question 14.2(1)–(5)?

    (a) Increased fluid intake and antibiotics.

    (b) Broad spectrum antibiotics with physiotherapy.

    (c) Heparin i.v. followed by 6 months anticoagulation.

    (d) Oral flucloxacillin with good breast support.

    (e) Broad spectrum antibiotics i.v. alone.

    (f) Flucloxacillin i.v. with support stockings.

    (g) Heparin i.v. followed by 3 months anticoagulation.

    (h) Broad spectrum antibiotics and surgical incision and drainage.

    (i) Broad spectrum antibiotics i.v. with evacuation of retained products.

    (j) Oral broad spectrum antibiotics alone.

# Chapter 15

# The newborn

## Evaluation at birth

The most usual assessment of the newborn recorded is the Apgar score (Table 15.1) which mixes two precise observations (heart rate and respiration) with three more subjective ones.

It is not a guide to prognosis but a description of the baby's condition at birth and response to resuscitation.

If there are any problems of respiration, a sample of cord blood is taken for pH and base deficit estimation.

## Immediate management

*Temperature*
Newborn babies cool rapidly and need to be kept warm.
• Dry and wrap in a warmed, sterile, cotton blanket.
• Room temperature after birth should be 23–25°C.

*Infection*
All babies are at a higher risk of infection.
• Wipe baby clean of vernix, blood, meconium after birth.
• Wash eyes, face, skin, flexures and genitals at each nappy change.
• Regular cleaning of umbilical cord stump until separation.

*Examination*
All newborn babies should be examined soon after delivery and a detailed examination repeated within the first 24 hours of life. The first examination is often done by the doctor or midwife in charge of the delivery, the second by a paediatrician. See Box 15.1.

*Cord care*
• Reclamp cord with plastic clip.
• Keep dry after washing.
• No dressings, for the stump dries quicker if exposed to air.
• It should separate on about the 8th–10th day.

*Blood glucose*
Small-for-dates, preterm and infants of diabetic mothers are at risk of hypoglycaemia. BM Stix should be checked regularly in these babies and any others at risk. If 2 mmol/l or less, a paediatrician should be informed.

*Screening tests*
• Two blood spots on 6th day:
   (a) Guthrie test, to detect raised level of phenylalanine indicating phenylketonuria;
   (b) Thyroid stimulating hormone (TSH) assay. Raised level indicates hypothyroidism.
If either test is positive, paediatric evaluation is needed.
• Babies of Rh-negative mothers should have

**Table 15.1** Apgar score performed at 1, 5 and 10 minutes after birth.

| Sign | Score 0 | Score 1 | Score 2 |
|---|---|---|---|
| Heart rate | Absent | <100 | >100 |
| Respiratory effort | Absent | Irregular | Good, crying |
| Muscle tone | Flaccid | Some limb tone | Active |
| Reflex irritability | None | Cry or grimace | Vigorous cry |
| Colour | White | Blue | Pink |

**Box 15.1  Suggested items to be checked at first examination**

*General observations*
- Breathing pattern and rate.
- Neurological behaviour, cry and movements.
- Skin pallor and cyanosis.

*Head*
- Anterior fontanelle: tenslon.
- Eyes: check epicanthic folds and for subconjunctival haemorrhages.
- Lip and palate: check for cleft.

*Upper limbs*
- Count digits and note interdigital webing.
- Paimar creases.

*Chest*
- Auscultate for:
  - (a) Respiratory sounds.
  - (b) Heart sounds: a faint heart mumur heard during the initial examination is usually innocent. Check daily if mumur heard.

*Abdomen*
- Umbilicus: check two arteries and one vein.
- Umbilical hemia.
- Palpate abdomen for masses.
- Groins:
  - (a) Femoral pulses.
  - (b) Hemiae.
- Anus: check patency.

*Genitalia*
- Female: clitoris size.
- Male: hypospadias, undescended testes and hydrocele.

*Back*
- Myelomeningocele.
- Mid-line hairy patch, suggesting spina bifida occulta.
- Stralghtspine: any kyphosis or scoliosis.

*Lower limbs*
- Examine hips for congenital dislocation.
- Number of digits.
- Talipes deformities of ankles and feet.

*Measurements of body size*
- Weight.
- Occipitofrontal head circumference.
- Crown-heel length.

blood group, haemoglobin, Coombs' test and bilirubin on umbilical cord blood at delivery.
- Babies at high risk for inherited disorders from a positive family history should be seen by paediatricians early and necessary treatment undertaken, e.g. cystic fibrosis, clotting disorders, inborn errors of metabolism.

## The newborn after delivery

If a preterm or at-risk infant is to be delivered, an experienced paediatrician should be on hand.

As soon as the infant is born, assess its condition. A shorthand analysis is in the Apgar score.

The three essential states may be:

- *Healthy*: pink; effective regular respiration.
- *Inadequate breathing*: irregular, shallow or gasping respiration.
- *Terminal apnoea*: white; floppy; no attempt to breathe.

  Care of the second and third stages is in the hands of the paediatrician (see Meadow R. & Newell S. (2001) *Lecture Notes on Paediatrics*, Blackwell Publishing, Oxford.).

*Healthy*
- If upper airway contains meconium, blood or mucus, then laryngoscope and aspirate trachea and larynx under direct vision.
- Wrap in a blanket and hand to mother.

*Inadequate breathing*
**1** If not already present, call paediatrician urgently. Carry out the following:
  - Face mask $O_2$.
  - Gentle peripheral stimulation.
  - Oropharyngeal suction.
  - Dry and cover the body with warm towels.

**2** If the infant does not respond to this by 1–1.5 minutes (i.e. respiration not established and heart rate falling below 80 beats/minute) extend neck, hold jaw forward and apply face mask closely to face to obtain a tight seal and give intermittent positive-pressure ventilation (IPPV) through the mask, at about 30 breaths/minute, 100% $O_2$, 30 cm of water pressure.

**3** If the infant still remains blue with inadequate respiration and a falling heart rate at 2–2.5 minutes, laryngoscope, aspirate any mucus or meconium under direct vision and intubate. Give IPPV at pressures of 20 cmH$_2$O (a little more if lungs are stiff) and a rate of 30/minute.

**4** As soon as the infant improves with any of the above (i.e. heart rate 140 beats/minute, spontaneous respiration and pink in colour) remove endotracheal tube, watch for respiration to be established.

**5** Analgesics such as pethidine or morphine given to the mother late in labour depress respiration in the infant. Naloxone can be given (10 μg/kg estimated weight i.v. or i.m.). Do not give naloxone to the baby of a drug-dependent mother as this may cause withdrawal, fits or death.

**6** There is no indication for analeptic drugs in the management of birth asphyxia.

**7** Preterm babies need intubation earlier than term babies.

**8** Do not perform IPPV with a mask on very small babies.

*Terminal apnoea*
**1** Do not delay resuscitation if, at this stage, the infant is pale, limp and apnoeic with a heart rate of less than 100.

**2** If not there, call paediatrician urgently.

**3** Laryngoscope, aspirate under direct vision and intubate. Give IPPV: rate 30/minute, 20–30 cmH$_2$O with 100% $O_2$.
  - May require naloxone if mother given pethidine.

**4** If still apnoeic—assume birth asphyxia likely and give sodium bicarbonate i.v. and adrenaline via endotracheal tube under supervision of paediatrician.

**5** Cord blood at birth to estimate pH and base deficit.

**6** Admit to neonatal unit if:
  - Poor response to resuscitation.
  - Base deficit >15 mEq/l.

**7** Let mother hold baby before transfer to neonatal unit, if possible.

## Feeding

Babies are best breast fed; in the UK 60% of mothers do at first and 30% are still breast feeding at 16 weeks. Mothers should be given advice in the antenatal period when breast feeding should be encouraged.

## Breast

Mothers who wish to breast feed put the baby to the breast for a few minutes at each side in the labour ward or certainly within 4 hours of birth.

**1** The infant will initially obtain only a small amount of colostrum when he sucks but this contains anti-infective substances. By sucking, the infant stimulates the production of more colostrum and then milk.

**2** Most of the feed is obtained within the first 3–5 minutes. The time the baby is on the breast is not proportional to the amount of milk received.

**3** Baby takes the nipple towards the back of his mouth, not just between the gums.

**4** The most satisfactory method of breast feeding is on demand. A rigid regimen of feeding is not to be encouraged. Infants who are initially fed on demand usually settle down within a few weeks to a regular pattern of feeding every 3–4 hours. In general, hungry babies cry and it is difficult to overfeed a breast-fed baby.

**5** If lactation is insufficient in the first few days, breast feeding should not be abandoned. Help and guidance should be given to the mother by one midwife, as often breast feeding is not established until mother and baby are at home and in the second week.

*Factors which help breast feeding*
• Motivation: encouragement at antenatal classes.
• Good midwife or health visitor with plenty of time to advise.
• Adequate fluid in mother's diet.
• Baby awake and mother comfortable.
• Change nappy before feeding to have a contented baby.
• Proper brassiere to hold breasts correctly.

*Factors which hinder breast feeding*
• Mother does not really wish to feed.
• Inverted, retracted nipples.
• Poor fixation on the nipple.
• Child with deformity of palate, tongue or lips.

*Advantages of breast feeding*
**1** Breastmilk protein, fat and solute content designed for human babies.
**2** Promotes infant–mother bonding.
**3** Contains anti-infective agents: active white cells, macrophages, IgA, IgG and lactoferrin.
**4** Eliminates risk of infection from dirty bottles.
**5** Cheap and always available on demand.

*Problems in first week*
**1** Engorged breasts. Days 5–10 when breast feeding is uncomfortable.
**2** Cracked nipples.
**3** Excessive air swallowing during first morning feed:
• Too rapid flow of milk.

## Formula or bottle milk

All cow's milk preparations in the UK are low solute milks. They have sodium and protein concentrations similar to those in human milk and most have added vitamins. Only these preparations should be used in newborn infants.

**1** A normal full-term infant receives about 60 ml/kg on the first day of bottle feeding. This should then be increased to 150 ml/kg/day by the end of the first week. This is usually divided into 6 feeds/24 hours, e.g. 75 ml in each feed for a 3 kg baby.

**2** Make up feeds according to instructions. If feeds are made up for 24 hours, keep in refrigerator.

**3** Wash bottles and teats, then sterilize with dilute hypochloride solution.

**4** When feed is due, place bottle in pan of hot water or microwave and warm milk to temperature acceptable to back of hand. However, feeding at room temperature does not cause any problems.

**5** Solids should start around 4 months or earlier if the baby can take them and weighs more than 6.5 kg.

*Problems*
**1** Protein, fat and solute load not exactly the same as human breastmilk.
**2** Lacks anti-infective properties of breastmilk.
**3** Teat hole is too large (too much milk) or too small (too little milk).
**4** Dirty bottles may lead to infections.
**5** Cost of formula milks.

## Neonatal jaundice

Nearly all babies become mildly jaundiced after 3–5 days. This is due to the breakdown of red blood cells with haemoglobin F whilst they are replaced with red blood calls with haemoglobin A. For the majority of babies this is a self-limiting condition which requires no treatment. If the jaundice persists or the baby becomes deeply jaundiced, sleepy and refuses to feed then the bilirubin level should be checked. Using a neonatal bilirubin chart the value is plotted and the baby may require phototherapy for a few days.

Rhesus negative babies or babies born with an ABO/other RBC antibody incompatibility with their mother may become severely jaundiced within 24–48 hours of birth. If the bilirubin levels reach very high levels then they may require an exchange transfusion to prevent bilirubin being deposited in the supraventricular nuclei of the brain causing kernicterus. Kernicterus is associated with deafness, delay in development and sometimes fitting.

## Statutory duties of the health professionals after birth

As well as the moral obligations of doctors, midwives and health visitors, the statutory duties are laid down of each in relation to a woman who is pregnant, in labour or recently delivered. The woman may book for her delivery at a variety of sites; basically they are in an institution or at home. The woman has a legal right to choose either and the midwifery services have to back this up. The supervisor of midwives in the health district has a duty to provide a midwife wheresoever a woman wishes to deliver and however inadvisable this might be on medical or midwifery grounds.

General practitioners have no such obligation. They may not wish to cover the obstetrical adventures of the woman who does not take advice and they have no obligation to do so. If a midwife looking after a pregnant or labouring woman runs into difficulty, she calls upon the emergency duty general practitioner who then has an obligation to attend and help. Perhaps that help will be passed on swiftly to the nearest hospital, but the doctor on duty must advise if called, although he or she may disapprove of the proceedings.

After the delivery there is an obligation for the woman to be under the care of a midwife for ten days although visiting may not be daily. At this point there is a handover to the health visitor who takes on the care of the mother and the child. The health visitors are first rate community workers but they have to look after the whole spectrum of life and, with an increasing load of older people, it is difficult for some health visitors to fit in all they would wish to do for the recently delivered woman and her baby.

---

**Self-assessment**

**15.1** List the five elements of the Apgar score.

**15.2** A baby is born in the following condition at 1 minute. She is pink with a heart rate of 120 bpm. She is not moving or crying and has taken a few irregular gasps. Her limbs are flaccid but she is moving her facial muscles. What is her Apgar score?

(a) 9

(b) 8

(c) 7

(d) 6

(e) 5

**15.3** OSCE question.

**Candidate's instructions:** During an antenatal visit at 32 weeks, Jane Wooller says that she is unsure whether she wants to breastfeed her baby and wishes to discuss this with you. You are expected to discuss the advantages and disadvantages of breastfeeding versus bottle feeding.

*Continued on p. 216.*

**Self-assessment** *Continued*

**Role-player's instructions:** You are Mrs Jane Wooller, a 34-year-old woman in her first pregnancy. You are now 32 weeks. The midwife discussed breastfeeding with you at the booking visit but you didn't take much in because it seemed so far away then as an issue. You have been to two antenatal classes where breastfeeding has been discussed amongst the mother's to be. You thought you would definitely breastfeed but found that during the discussion you felt rather revolted by the idea, particularly feeding in public. You are a very private person who, prior to pregnancy, took a great pride in your appearance and figure and you want to get back to your original clothes size as soon as possible after the birth. Breastfeeding sounds rather invasive of your privacy and you do not relish leaking breast milk onto your clothes. However, you do want to do the best for your baby. The rest is up to the role-player's imagination.

**15.4** Which of the following babies are at increased risk of developing significant neonatal jaundice?

(a) Group A negative baby born to a group A positive mother.

(b) Group A negative baby born to a group A negative mother.

(c) Group A positive baby born to a group A negative mother.

(d) Group A positive baby born to a group B positive mother.

(e) Group A positive baby born to a group A positive mother.

# Part 4

# The mature woman

# Chapter 16

# Abnormal vaginal blood loss

## Regular bleeding

There are many Latin words to describe abnormal vaginal bleeding. It is better to use Anglo-Saxon and describe the symptoms as *heavy periods* or *prolonged periods* but the classic terms are still in use and need definition.

- *Menorrhagia* is an excessive loss of blood (>80 ml) with regular menstruation.
- *Metrorrhagia* is prolonged bleeding from the uterus.
- *Metro-menorrhagia* is heavy and prolonged periods.
- *Polymenorrhoea* is frequent menstruation.

These may be associated with

1 *Complications of early and undiagnosed pregnancy.*
   - Miscarriage.
   - Ectopic pregnancy.
   - Hydatidiform mole.
2 *Foreign bodies in the uterus*—intrauterine contraceptives.
3 *Treatment with hormones* especially in menopausal and postmenopausal women. Breakthrough bleeding may occur with synthetic progestogens given for oral contraception or for treatment of pelvic disorders.
4 *Psychosomatic causes*, for example a severe emotional shock, may induce irregular bleeding.
5 *An abnormal bleeding tendency* may be present such as leukaemia or Hodgkin's disease.
6 *Hyper- or hypothyroidism* may be associated with menorrhagia or irregular bleeding.

## Intermittent bleeding

The causes of non-cyclical abnormal vaginal bleeding not associated with menstruation include:
- *lesions of the cervix*—polypi, carcinoma, ectropion;
- *lesions of the body of the uterus*—endometritis, fibroids, polypi, adenomyosis, carcinoma, sarcoma.

The level of haemoglobin is generally lower in women between the ages of 15 and 50 than in men; this difference is accounted for by blood loss and the consequent iron deficiency associated with menstruation and childbearing. Menorrhagia or metrorrhagia can lead to anaemia but many women with true heavy loss are able to respond to the chronic repeated demand on their bone marrow, but may require iron therapy.

## Menorrhagia

The range of menstrual loss is 10–80 ml per cycle. If above 80 ml, this is considered excessive. More commonly, diagnosis is made on the woman's history:
- increase in the number of pads or tampons used to more than 10 per day;
- starting to pass clots in the menstrual flow;
- use of a pictorial blood loss assessment chart which gives a semi-quantitative measure of loss.

Up to 30% of women in the later part of menstrual life complain of heavy periods. Only a half of these actually lose more than 80 ml of blood per period. The diagnosis, however, rests on the woman's history rather than scientific measurement.

## Aetiology

Menorrhagia commonly is a presenting symptom in:
• fibroids if increase uterine mucosal area;
• adenomyosis (endometrium within the uterine muscle wall);
• endometritis;
• incorrectly controlled hormone therapy (including oral contraception).
    Less commonly, it is associated with:
• endometrial polypi;
• an intrauterine device (IUD);
• recent tubal ligation (usually secondary to stopping the contraceptive pill which keeps periods artificially light);
• functional ovarian tumours;
• disorders of clotting (e.g. von Willebrand's disease).
    Menorrhagia is not caused by idiopathic thrombocytopenic purpura.
    After full examination and investigation (ultrasound scan, full blood count (FBC), endometrial biopsy in women over 40) in about 50% of women with true menorrhagia, no obvious pathology is found. This is *dysfunctional uterine bleeding* (DUB) implicating a malfunction of the endocrine controlling systems. A better name would be *menorrhagia of unknown origin*.

## Clinical course

While menorrhagia is most commonly found in the over 35-year-old, it can occur at any stage in female life up to the menopause. The causes and management may be classified according to age group.

### Birth to 18 years of age

See Chapter 4.

## Women aged 18–40 years

In this group true dysfunctional bleeding is uncommon and the most likely cause of abnormal bleeding is some complication of pregnancy or polycystic ovary syndrome (PCOS) (Chapter 4). Occasionally heavier periods follow tubal ligation for sterilization. Endometrial biopsy is rarely needed in this group for the possibility of malignant disease is unusual.

*Women aged over 40*
All the organic causes of bleeding, including malignant disease, may occur and it is essential to exclude them.
    Among women without organic disease, three main patterns of the endometrium are seen on histological examination.
• *Atrophic* (postmenopausal).
• A *mixed pattern* with proliferative and secretory endometrium with possibly endometrial polypi. This is associated with irregular shedding of the endometrium for the normal mechanism of ovulation is disordered so the endometrium is irregularly or excessively shed.
• *Hyperplasia* of the endometrium may involve the glands or the stroma or both. *Cystic hyperplasia* is common in perimenopausal women. There is usually amenorrhoea followed by prolonged bleeding from the hyper-oestrogenized endometrium. A similar pattern is seen with an oestrogen secreting tumour of the ovary. There is no great risk of cystic hyperplasia going on to carcinoma of the endometrium. Atypical hyperplasia, however, is more likely to be associated with endometrial carcinoma, the risk depending on the degree of atypia.

## Treatment of dysfunctional uterine bleeding

Treatment should never be given without accurate diagnosis except perhaps in girls under 18 with puberty bleeding. Blind hormone treatment is particularly dangerous as malignant disease may be masked.

## Diagnosis

Ultrasound shows:

- Endometrial thickness should be less than 12 mm in perimenopausal women.
- 5 mm in postmenopausal women.
- Endometrial polyps.
- Fibroids.
- Ovarian pathology in women with PCOS. Investigations should include:
- Endometrial biopsy in:
  (a) Women over 40.
  (b) Those with abnormal endometrial thickness.
  (c) Those with endometrial polyps.

This may be done in the out-patient department by suction curettage. With appropriate skills, passing these causes little discomfort, about the same as fitting an IUCD. This avoids admission and the general anaesthetic for dilation and curettage (D&C). However, a fuller curettage is indicated if:

- it is impossible to pass the curette because of a tight cervix;
- the woman is anxious and cannot relax;
- there is a high risk of malignancy of the endometrium.

  Hysteroscopy may accompany the curettage in the out-patients department if the gynaecologist is skilled and properly equipped. It is excellent at showing endometrial polyps and submucous fibroids which could be missed by blind curettage. In many cases an organic diagnosis will be made and appropriate treatment be given.

- Cervical smear to exclude carcinoma, *in situ* or cervical intraepithelial neoplasia (CIN) (see Chapter 19).

### Drug therapy

This is the first line of treatment because it:

- retains the uterus, a major factor for most women;
- avoids surgery with general anaesthesia;
- is more convenient, being administered in the outpatients department or GP surgery;
- is much cheaper:
  (a) to the Health Service;
  (b) to the woman.

  Drug treatment may be non-hormonal (first line) or hormonal (second line) (see Boxes 16.1 and 16.2).

> **Box 16.1 Non-hormonal treatment**
>
> Taken during menses hence no problem if accidental pregnancy is present
>
> *Prostaglandin synthetase inhibitors*
> Reduce uterine prostaglandins
>
> *Fenamates*
> Mefenamic acid, 500 mg six-hourly during menstruation
> Avoid if peptic ulceration
>
> *Antifibrinolytic agents*
> Reduce abnormal fibrinolysis
> Avoid if history of thrombosis
> Tranexamic acid, 1 g six-hourly during menstruation
> Ethamsylate, 500 mg four-hourly during menstruation

## Surgical therapy

Based on removal of the endometrium or the uterus with its endometrium.

### Curettage

- Removes outer layers of endometrium but leaves the basal layers from which new tissue arises in a month or so.
- Ineffective as a treatment—one or two menses may be less heavy but are soon back to previous levels or heavier.

### Local ablation

- Balloons, heated with 80°C water.
- Microwave local destruction.
- Free flowing heated water to 98°C.

### Transcervical ablation

- Under vision through a hysteroscope, endometrium is destroyed:
  (a) with electrocoagulating loops;
  (b) with a laser.
- At present, uses general anaesthesia but needs only one day in hospital:
  (a) uterus retained although lining (mostly) gone;
  (b) after a year, 30% have amenorrhoea and another 60% report lighter blood loss;
  (c) if it fails (10–20%), can proceed to either repeat ablation or to hysterectomy.

---

**Box 16.2 Hormonal treatment**

This aims at imitating or restoring the normal endocine cycle

| | |
|---|---|
| Norethisterone | • 5 mg three times a day for six to nine months |
| Medroxyprogesterone acetate | • Best for those with anovular cycles |
| | • Cheap and good for emergency treatment: 10 mg three times a day for very heavy bleeding |
| Danazol | • 200 mg daily continuously for three to six months |
| | • Derivative of testosterone so anti-oestrogenic at hypothalamus and at endometrium |
| | • Expensive. May be weight gain and androgenization |
| Oral contraceptive | • Dose according to brand but probably best to use cyclical combined oestrogen (30 μg) and progestogen (0.25 mg) |
| | • Praetical, cheap and easily available |
| Mirena IUS | • Progestogen IUS 75 μg/day to uterine lining only |

---

• It is not a minor operation:
   (a) requires manipulative skills;
   (b) requires expensive equipment;
   (c) risks of perforating uterus (1%);
   (d) risks of artery damage and bleeding (less than 1%);
   (e) risks of damaging bowel (less than 1%).
• However, saves time and hospital stay:
   (a) early return to normal activity;
   (b) keeping uterus makes it popular;
   (c) contraception is still required unless there is complete amenorrhoea.

*Hysterectomy*
• Removal of the uterus stops periods.

*Abdominal hysterectomy*
• Major procedure with general anaesthesia.
• Abdominal scar to heal.
• Hospital stay 4–6 days.
• Risks of damage to ureters <1%.
• Risks of damage to the bladder <1%.
• Risks of damage to the bowel <1%.

*Vaginal hysterectomy*
• Needs to be a mobile, adhesion-free uterus.
• Uterus not greatly enlarged.
• Helps if there is some prolapse.

*Laparoscopy assisted hysterectomy*
• Smaller abdominal incision.
• Needs skilled laparoscopic surgeon.
• Does the difficult part of a vaginal hysterectomy from above ligating tubes, ovarian suspensory ligament and round ligament via laparoscopy. Then an easy vaginal removal.
• Has all the complications of laparoscopic surgery.
Hysterectomy does not have to be accompanied by removal of ovaries.

*Indications for oophorectomy*
• If ovaries abnormal.
• If family history of ovarian cancer.
• Consider if over 45 years old and post-menopausal. Full informed consent is essential.
   Retain:
• if menses cycling regularly;
• if ovaries healthy at surgery;
• if patient's wish.

## Atrophic vaginitis

Secondary to a lack of oestrogens postmenopausally, the epithelium becomes thin, smooth and shiny with subepithelial haemorrhages. Low-grade infection from pathogens, which can more easily penetrate the surface, may occur.

*Symptoms*
- Vulval soreness.
- Superficial dyspareunia.
- Pink discharge.
- Introital shrinking.

*Physical signs*
Red shiny epithelium with skin cracking and sub-cuticular haemorrhages. Occasionally causes post-menopausal bleeding. It is important to exclude other causes such as carcinoma.

*Treatment*
If there is secondary infection, antibiotics to which the organism is sensitive may be given. Topical oestrogen creams or pessaries can be used, e.g. dienoestrol or Premarin once or twice a week. This is enough to thicken the epithelium and reduce the pH, but insufficient to produce excessive endometrial stimulation or other causes of bleeding.

## Endometrial polypi

If the endometrium hypertrophies under oestrogen stimulation, areas of it may protrude above the surface producing a sessile or eventually a pedunculated polyp. This may not be shed at the time of menstruation, but forms a site for persistent symptoms and signs.

*Symptoms*
There may be intermenstrual spotting or postmenstrual spotting.

*Signs*
There would be no signs, but a hysteroscopy would show the polyp.

*Management*
Endometrial polypi should be removed. Those inside the uterus will require an anaesthetic and have to be twisted off with a polypi forceps diathermy loop. Should the endometrial polyp stalk be long and the polyp present at the cervix, it is probably

wise not to remove it in the out-patients department, because this could lead to heavy bleeding. A D&C with hysteroscopy should be performed at the same time to allow removal of any other polypi that are higher up.

## Pre- and postoperative care

Gynaecological operations are best learnt in the operating theatre, preferably acting as a scrubbed assistant, but the pre- and postoperative care must be understood by a wider range of medical personnel than just the surgeon.

## Preoperative care

*History*
A complete history is taken with special attention to any recent illness. The date of the last period should be noted, to ensure the patient is not pregnant. Drugs and medicines recently taken should be noted—these may include hormones, especially oral contraceptives, antibiotics and tranquillizers.

*Examination*
A general examination is made. The heart and lungs are examined and blood pressure measured. Examination of the abdomen and pelvis follows. The legs are inspected for varicosities.

*Investigations*
Investigations include an examination of haemoglobin. Except in an emergency, it is unwise to carry out major surgery with a haemoglobin level below 10.5 g/dl, or minor surgery below 8.5 g/dl. In women of Negro or Asian origin, a test for haemoglobinopathies is essential.

The blood group and rhesus factor are determined and serum saved in the laboratory. If there is a probability that transfusion will be needed during the operation, blood is cross-matched in readiness.

The urine is tested for albumin, bacteria and sugar. If there is a suspicion of a urinary infection, a mid-stream sample is sent for bacteriological examination. Renal function tests are advisable if there is a suspicion of abnormal kidney function.

An X-ray of the chest may be taken if indicated. Urography and magnetic resonance imaging (MRI) are done before operations when the ureters may be involved, as in Wertheim's hysterectomy. An electrocardiogram is advisable in patients with any suggestion of heart disease. Other investigations may be suggested by the examination or the nature of the case.

A pregnancy test should be performed prior to surgery.

*Preparation*

The patient should be weighed on admission or in the out-patient clinic. Shaving of the vulva has now generally been abandoned for minor cases although most surgeons prefer it for major vulval and vaginal surgery. Postmenopausal women with prolapse may be helped by preoperative treatment with oestrogen, given before admission in the form of oestrogen by mouth or vaginal cream. Antibiotics, e.g. Flagyl or Augmentin, are usually given before major elective surgery.

*Thromboprophylaxis*: TED stockings should be worn intraoperatively and until the woman is fully mobilized. During major surgery flowtron boots which inflate and deflate regularly should be used during the operation. Daily prophylactic doses of low-molecular-weight heparin should be considered for all women at moderate to high risk undergoing major surgery, during and after surgery.

The patient should have nothing by mouth for at least 6 hours before the operation. If the operation may involve the intestines or rectum, the bowel is emptied and prepared by the use of succinyl sulphathiazole, neomycin or another suitable preparation.

A physiotherapist should visit every patient ideally before the operation and certainly everyone for major surgery. He or she can teach breathing and leg movements for the postoperative period.

Valid consent must be given in writing for the operation by the patient herself. This must be clearly and legibly countersigned by a doctor, who should have explained the operation and its possible sequelae. Girls aged 16 or over sign consent for the operation on their own behalf; for those under

that age, the consent of a parent or legal guardian is usually necessary except in an emergency. There may be difficulty in the case of a girl under 16 requesting a termination of pregnancy and insisting that her parents are not to be informed. In such a case, the doctor will have to exercise discretion and act in what he or she considers to be the girl's best interest.

At the time that consent for the operation is obtained, an explanation should be given of the procedure which is contemplated, its nature and effects, including possible complications. These should be written on the consent form. In the case of a married woman, her husband's consent is not legally necessary in the UK for operations which lead to sterility such as hysterectomy or sterilization, but it is important that counselling of the couple takes place. It should be made clear in the case of operations for sterilization or vasectomy that the operation should be considered irreversible; on the other hand it must be emphasized that a few failures occur with sterilizations. This advice should be recorded in the case notes.

Counselling in general is important since many women do not understand the anatomy of their pelvic organs and have unnecessary fears concerning the effects of operations, in particular their effects on sexual function. Explanation, if necessary illustrated by a model or diagram, will help to dispel these fears.

## Postoperative care

A period of recovery is required after any surgical operation. After *minor operations,* such as hysteroscopy, the patient can go home on the same day. She should not drive or operate machinery for two days after general anaesthetic. She must be warned to expect some bleeding for up to 14 days after the operation. More profuse bleeding can follow deep cauterization or conization of the cervix; this may on some occasions be enough to require readmission and possible suture of the cervix. These women should be advised to refrain from intercourse for 6 weeks.

After *major surgery* such as uncomplicated hysterectomy or prolapse repair, patients are encouraged to get up from bed and move about on the day following the operation. Breathing exercises and leg movements are begun from the day after the operation. The length of stay in hospital varies but many can leave after 3–6 days. Before departure a clear explanation of the operation and the prognosis must be given by a doctor. An adequate period of convalescence at home is necessary before returning to work and normal activity.

The patient may be examined six weeks after the operation. She must be encouraged to return to normal life. Intercourse may be resumed as soon as the vagina is healed. If the ovaries have been removed premenopausally, the woman should be offered oestrogens by tablet, patch or implant. Patients treated for carcinoma must be followed up carefully by gynaecological oncologists.

## Postoperative complications

During the first 12 hours after an operation, the patient must be carefully observed for the following:
• respiratory failure or obstruction to the airways;
• shock;
• haemorrhage;
• cardiac failure.

She should be nursed in a recovery unit until she has recovered consciousness and only then returned to a general ward. The pulse rate and blood pressure should be taken and charted every quarter of an hour for the first two hours and thereafter every few hours for the first 12 hours, longer if there is any anxiety.

Pain must be relieved by adequate doses of analgesics such as morphine or pethidine. Patient-controlled analgesia, with the woman controlling the flow of weak solutions of analgesia intravenously, is very useful for recovery from elective gynaecological surgery. Addition of promazine or chlorpromazine increases the effect of analgesics and helps to prevent postoperative vomiting.

### Haemorrhage

**1** *Primary*, occurring during the operation and requiring immediate transfusion.
**2** *Delayed*, occurring during the immediate postoperative period, is generally due to a slipped ligature or a bleeding vessel in the vagina or cervix. Blood transfusion is given and the patient returned to the operating theatre to deal with the haemorrhage.
**3** *Secondary*, occurring up to 14 days after operations and generally from the vagina or cervix, but occasionally from the abdominal wound. Infection is commonly associated, but suture of the bleeding area and blood transfusion still may be needed in all but the slightest cases. After cauterization of the cervix there is generally some bleeding about the 10th and 12th day and patients should be warned to expect this.
**4** Anaemia is common after gynaecological operations and should be prevented with a correct diet and iron therapy.

### Respiratory tract

Complications of a general anaesthetic include sore throat, tracheitis, bronchitis, bronchopneumonia and massive collapse of the lungs. Breathing exercises should be given after general anaesthetics. Pulmonary infection should be treated with antibiotics. Chest symptoms after the first week sometimes indicate pulmonary embolism.

### Urinary tract

Retention of urine is common after gynaecological operations and it may be complete or partial. Complete retention of urine often occurs after hysterectomy or repair of prolapse. Rarely unexplained retention occurs after a minor operation such as hysteroscopy.

Treatment is by immediate catheterization usually emptying the bladder once. If it must be repeated, an indwelling catheter has to be put in for a few days. Some surgeons prefer suprapubic catheterization.

Partial retention of urine is common after operations for prolapse and a catheter should be passed for residual urine five days after operation. Catheter drainage should continue until the residual urine is below 200 ml.

Cystitis and pyelonephritis are very common after gynaecological operations. A catheter specimen or a mid-stream specimen should be examined for evidence of infection after all major operations and suitable treatment given.

Poor or absent urine output may be due to obstruction to the ureters which may be accidentally injured, ligated or obstructed by a haematoma; it may also be reflex blockage. Warning is often given by unilateral loin ache and a slight temperature. It is a very serious complication and must be dealt with urgently if necessary with relieving surgery by a urologist.

Incontinence of urine through the urethra sometimes occurs after catheterization and in elderly women; it is usually transient. Persistent incontinence suggests a fistula. Urinary fistulae may be vesico-vaginal or uretero-vaginal. These may be caused by trauma at operation, by haematoma formation or by difficult obstetric delivery. They also result from malignant disease.

An uretero-vaginal fistula may follow operations, especially Wertheim's hysterectomy if the ureters are extensively dissected so that their blood supply is imperilled and they become devascularized.

### Venous thrombosis

Two types can occur after surgery.

*Phlebothrombosis* is primary venous thrombosis and generally begins in the deep veins of the calf; predisposing causes are:

- trauma;
- anaemia;
- stasis;
- high oestrogen levels.

*Thrombophlebitis* is caused by infection, generally in the pelvic veins initially and spreading to involve the iliac veins.

*Pulmonary embolism* can follow thrombosis and if massive is rapidly fatal. Small emboli cause pulmonary infarction.

Prevention of thrombosis and embolism consists of:

- the use of pneumatic boots and leggings during the surgery;
- elasticated stockings worn before, during and after operation;
- early movement;
- avoidance of anaemia;
- prompt treatment of infection;
- prophylactic low-dose heparin before and just after surgery.

The contraceptive pill should ideally be stopped four to six weeks before major elective surgery.

In established thrombosis, heparin is given initially intravenously in a continuous dose of 1000–1500 iu per hour or by separate intravenous injections of 10000 iu every six or eight hours. Calcium heparin can be given subcutaneously. Warfarin is started with a loading dose of 10 mg for two days followed by a daily dose which is determined by the clotting time. In proven DVT this should be continued for three months and, if there was a pulmonary embolism, for six months.

---

### Self-assessment

**16.1** OSCE question.

**Candidate's instructions:** A 37-year-old woman, Elizabeth Parker, has come to see you in your GP surgery. She has only recently moved to your area. She is complaining of heavy periods. Please take a history. You have 7 minutes.

**Role-player's instructions:** You are Mrs Elizabeth Parker, a 37-year old. Over the last 2 years your periods have become increasingly heavy. They are regular every 28 days and last for 7 to 10 days. They used to last only 5 days. You have noticed that the first 4 days are particularly heavy with clots the size of 50p pieces. On the first day you can bleed so heavily that you have to change every 30 minutes to 1 hour. At night you wear two pads, a tampon and an incontinence pad and still have to change in the middle of the night. You have painful periods but this has not changed. You have three children and you were sterilized when you were 35. Prior to this you had been on the combined oral contraceptive pill. You smoke 25 cigarettes a day so you had stopped the pill. Your last smear test was 2 years ago and was normal. You are otherwise fit and well. All other details are up to the role-player.

**Self-assessment** *Continued*

**16.2** From the list below select the three most relevant investigations for Mrs Parker.
 (a) Endometrial biopsy.
 (b) Transvaginal ultrasound scan.
 (c) Hormone profile.
 (d) High vaginal swab.
 (e) Cervical smear.
 (f) Hysteroscopy.
 (g) Full blood count.
 (h) Thyroid function tests.

**16.3** The investigations are all normal. What is the most appropriate first line treatment?
 (a) Mirena IUS.
 (b) Norethisterone from day 15–26 of the cycle.
 (c) Antifibrinolytic therapy during menses.
 (d) Paracetamol during menses.
 (e) Endometrial ablation.

**16.4** A woman is admitted for a total abdominal hysterectomy. Which of the following are routine prophylactic measures for all women undergoing this procedure?
 (a) Augmentin 1.2 g i.v. intraoperatively.
 (b) Subcutaneous low-molecular-weight (LMW) heparin intraoperatively.
 (c) Flowtron boots intraoperatively.
 (d) TED stockings.
 (e) Penicillin V 1 g i.v. intraoperatively.

**16.5** When consenting a woman for a total abdominal hysterectomy which of the following should be included on the consent form as possible complications?
 (a) Infection.
 (b) Haemorrhage.
 (c) Removal of the ovaries.
 (d) Damage to the ureters.
 (e) Damage to the bladder.

# Chapter 17

# Pelvic pain

Many diseases causing lower abdominal symptoms are gynaecological in origin. The general surgeon and gynaecologist must both be trained to recognize and deal with them. When available, consultation will take place, but delay and mortality are linked and acute abdominal conditions do not leave time for leisurely consultations. If the condition is obviously gynaecological in origin, it is best dealt with by gynaecologists as they are more used to conservation of genital tract tissue, particularly the ovaries.

Acute intra-abdominal emergencies present with pain, shock, vomiting or abdominal distension. The first of these is the most common in gynaecological conditions.

## Pain

Pain in pelvic organs may arise from:
• inside the organ with irritation of its lining or stretch of its walls;
• stretch of the visceral peritoneum over the organ;
• involvement of the parietal peritoneum in proximity.

For example, an ectopic pregnancy can cause pain from:
• damage to the muscle of the oviduct by trophoblast invasion and bleeding;
• stretch of the peritoneum from the broad ligament over the fallopian tube at the site of the pregnancy;

• blood spilt onto the peritoneum by the rupture of the tube (acute) or trickling from the outer end of the tube (chronic).

The first two origins of stimuli are mediated by the autonomic nervous system with poor localization; hence non-specific pain in the pelvis results.

The parietal peritoneum is innervated by the somatic nervous system and localization may be more specific. The peritoneum of the pouch of Douglas, however, has a poor nerve supply and is often undemonstrative. Since this is the area in which the tubes and ovaries spend much of their time, it makes pain localization in the abdominal wall difficult in pelvic conditions in the earlier stages, but signs are easier to detect on pelvic and rectal examination.

## Shock

A sudden deterioration in a woman's vital state may be characterized by:
• a rise followed by a fall in pulse rate;
• a fall in arterial blood pressure;
• pallor;
• faintness and later unconsciousness.
This may be due to either:
• true hypovolaemia, e.g. a ruptured ectopic pregnancy with two litres of blood in the peritoneal cavity;
• relative hypovolaemia, e.g. excess of autonomic

stimulation after peritoneal irritation with a sudden release of pus or blood.

Pallor, sweating, agitation and restlessness are traditional indications of shock, of which pallor is the most important for prognosis in the gynaecological field. Fainting and unconsciousness come later in shock and may be considered as signs of more extensive involvement.

## Nausea and vomiting

These happen rarely in non-pregnant gynaecological conditions but have a number of causes.
• Stimulation of a large number of nerve endings of the peritoneum overlying an affected pelvic organ, e.g. torted ovarian cyst.
• The direct action of toxins on the central nervous system from infective organisms. Pelvic inflammation often becomes localized early and toxins are released intermittently into the general bloodstream.
• Vomiting is a common accompaniment of early pregnancy. Many gynaecological conditions happen in early gestation so vomiting might be nothing to do with the acute condition in the pelvis but more with the human chorionic gonadotrophin (hCG) produced by the pregnancy trophoblast.

## Distension

Distension is unusual in gynaecological conditions but common in alimentary tract ones, particularly those of the large bowel. In consequence, if distension is present, it is probably due to an associated bowel problem rather than a gynaecological one.

## Diagnosis

The triad of history, examination and investigations applies here as anywhere else in medicine. This section is to be read in conjunction with the account of gynaecological diagnosis making in Chapter 2.

## History

Women in severe acute abdominal pain do not like having long histories taken. Hence, the questions must be tailored to the situation.

*Pain*
• Characteristics of the pain site, time and nature.
• Relationship of pain to various body functions, e.g. vaginal bleeding or micturition.
• Past gynaecological or obstetrical events.
• Menstrual history, i.e. details of last menstrual period.
• Symptoms of a possible pregnancy, e.g. breast changes and the woman's own impressions.

## Examination

A general examination must cover a number of points.
• Paleness (conjunctival assessment).
• Pulse rate.
• Arterial blood pressure.
• Temperature.
• Abdominal examination helps to localize pelvic causes.
• *Observation* will show old scars and the degree of distension; the site of the pain can be elicited from the woman at this point.
• *Gentle palpation* of the abdomen leading to the lower pelvic zones may help localization further.
• *Firmer examination*—if tenderness allows; this will reveal guarding or any rebound tenderness.
• Many pelvic abdominal conditions do not have specific localizing signs in the abdomen and so, therefore, any opinion should await the performing of a bimanual vaginal examination.
• At *bimanual vaginal assessment* tenderness from a pelvic organ will obviously limit the thoroughness of the examination because the woman will guard if there is pain on moving the cervix. This is called cervical excitation (Fig. 17.1); moving the cervix to the side of an ovarian or tubal mass will cause intense pain by a further stretch of the overlying peritoneum. Moving the cervix towards the opposite side will decrease the pain by releasing the tension of the peritoneum.
• *Rectal examination* may be needed but usually one can assess acute pouch of Douglas problems at a vaginal assessment. If structural changes are

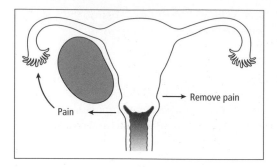

**Figure 17.1** Moving the cervix pushes the uterus, so altering the tension on the overlying peritoneum and causing pain.

sought in the back of the pelvic cavity, the rectal examination is useful, e.g. endometriotic lesions on the uterosacral ligaments, or to differentiate from appendicitis.

## Investigations

There are a few investigations that help.
- Haemoglobin to check on chronic bleeding.
- Differential white cell count to assess inflammation.
- Urine cells and organisms to diagnose urinary infection.
- hCG levels to check for pregnancy.
- High vaginal swab and cervical swab to test for genital tract infection.
- X-rays may be used to check for bowel obstruction.
- Ultrasound is extremely useful to check the pelvic organs, particularly using a vaginal probe. Then the transmitter and receiver are within a centimetre or two of the affected organs.

The vaginal ultrasound examination gives far more precise images of pelvic organs and tissues.
- Changes in ovarian morphology and size:
  (a) cysts;
  (b) polycystic ovary syndrome (not a cause of pelvic pain *per se*);
  (c) irregular masses.
- Fallopian tube:
  (a) occasionally a swollen tube from a pyo- or hydrosalpinx is identified;
  (b) ectopic pregnancies may be diagnosed (Chapter 8).
- Uterine size can be detected:
  (a) the thickness of the endometrium is shown;
  (b) the presence of a pregnancy sac can be detected as early as five weeks, embryonic parts and fetal heart beats by six weeks from the last menstrual period.
- Fibroids of the uterus.
- Pouch of Douglas fluid can often be detected in as low a volume as 7 ml. This might indicate blood loss from an ectopic pregnancy.

Often a combination of ultrasound with other tests is helpful. For example, in the UK now, many unruptured ectopic pregnancies are diagnosed at ultrasound in symptomatic women who have an empty uterus but a thickened endometrium and fluid in the pouch of Douglas in the presence of raised urinary hCG levels.

## Conditions to be considered

We diagnose what we are thinking of and it is helpful to have a check list (see Table 17.3, on pp. 244–245).

### Pelvic organs (Table 17.1)

## Vagina

**Vaginal trauma**
Intercourse occurring forcibly or after a long interval of abstinence can cause damage to the vaginal tube.
- Lower end—usually obvious but may be labial or fourchette.
- Upper end—vaginal guarding to prevent the easy passage of the speculum. Hence, hard to see.
- Haematoma—paravaginal or paracervical haematoma.

The obvious point needed in the history may not be volunteered readily. Treatment is by vaginal repair under anaesthesia.

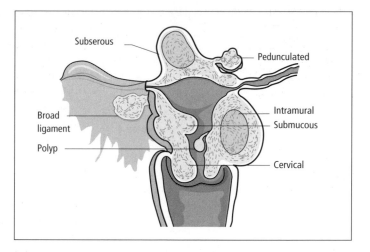

**Figure 17.2** Uterus with fibroids.

## Uterus

### Uterine fibroids

Alternatively named myomata or leiomyomata, uterine fibroids are the commonest of all pelvic tumours. They are benign fibromuscular swellings, arising in the muscle wall of the uterus. Fibroids are oestrogen sensitive.

• *Submucous*—lying immediately below the endometrium and enlarging the surface of the uterine cavity often leading to menorrhagia. Fibroids may become pedunculated forming polypi which can extrude through the cervix.

• *Intramural*—the commonest site for fibroids, surrounded by smooth muscle, enlarging the uterine wall and distorting venous drainage.

• *Subserous*—fibroids just beneath the peritoneum on the outer uterine surface (Fig. 17.2). May be on an elongated stalk (pedunculated) with a risk of torsion; may grow into the broad ligament.

*Degeneration*

Uterine fibroids frequently outgrow their blood supply and degenerate.

• *Hyaline*—an aseptic necrosis with loss of muscle cell structure. This may lead to calcification.

• *Cystic*—a sequel to hyaline change with subsequent breakdown and cyst formation giving a honeycomb appearance.

• *Fatty*—in which partial necrosis results in the development of fatty substances which may sub-sequently undergo calcification (visible on X-rays and ultrasound).

• *Red*—necrobiosis, particularly encountered in the mid-trimester of pregnancy or the early puerperium. This breakdown of blood supply by thrombosis leads to necrosis and suffusion with red blood cells.

• *Sarcomatous*—rare malignant change reported in 0.2–0.4% of fibroids examined in asymptomatic older women at autopsy.

*Symptoms*

• *None*—a pelvic swelling is found incidentally on examination.

• Occasional *tightness* of waistband of clothes.

• *Pressure*—bladder compression causing daytime frequency and occasionally impaired urinary stream. In the supporting ligaments it causes backache and overall sensation of pelvic heaviness.

• *Pain*—associated with red degeneration or torsion of subserous pedicles. Dysmenorrhoea may indicate the presence of a submucous fibroid.

• *Menstrual disturbances*:
   (a) menorrhagia—heavy bleeding;
   (b) metrorrhagia—prolonged menses;
   (c) irregular, intermittent bleeding—often associated with polyps and other surface lesions.

*Investigations*

• Ultrasound—to define the location, the dimensions and the consistency.

**Table 17.1** Pelvic diseases which may present as acute abdominal emergencies.

|  | Organ | Condition |
|---|---|---|
| *Non-pregnant* | Vagina | Trauma |
|  | Uterus | Fibroid |
|  |  | Torsion |
|  |  | Degeneration |
|  |  | Adenomyosis |
|  |  | Endometritis |
|  |  | Pyometra |
|  | Fallopian tubes | Salpingitis |
|  |  | Pyosalpinx |
|  |  | Torsion |
|  | Ovaries | Tumours |
|  |  | Simple cyst |
|  |  | Torsion |
|  |  | Bleeding |
|  |  | Rupture |
|  | Peritoneum | Endometriosis |
| *Early pregnancy* | Uterus | Abortion |
|  |  | Impacted retroversion |
|  |  | Red degeneration of fibroids |
|  | Fallopian tubes | Ectopic pregnancy |
|  |  | Torsion |
|  | Ligaments | Round ligament Stretch |
|  | Extra-pelvic | Vomiting in pregnancy |
|  |  | Pyelonephritis |
|  |  | Appendicitis |
|  |  | Rectus haematoma |

*Diagnosis*

Bimanual palpation reveals hard rounded non-tender often bosselated mass, moving when the cervix is displaced.

• Grow fast in pregnancy.
• Shrink:
  (a) at the menopause;
  (b) with antigonadotrophic hormone therapy.

*Pathology*

Fibroids may be single or multiple (occasionally numbering greater than 100) and vary in size from a seedling to a football. They form a pseudocapsule by compressing surrounding uterine muscle, a process helpful to the surgeon at myomectomy.

*Aetiology*

Cause is unknown:
• rarely found under the age of 30 years;
• commoner in Afro-Caribbean populations;
• commoner in the nulliparous and women with low fertility;
• often a family history.

*Differential diagnosis*

• Pregnancy—particularly if fibroids have been softened by cystic degeneration.
• Ovarian tumour—often cystic, unilateral and does not move with cervical displacement.
• Adenomyosis—more commonly causes uniform diffuse and tender uterine enlargement.

*Treatment*

• If small and asymptomatic, conservative management with annual examination and ultrasound monitoring of size is sufficient. This is especially used in women over 40 because fibroids do not grow after menopause and may shrink.
• Menstrual or pressure symptoms may dictate surgery.
• Pain—requires analgesia.
• Heavier and longer periods with anaemia are the commonest indication for proceeding to surgery.
• Embolization under radiological control: a cannula is passed into the uterine arteries via the femoral artery. The uterine arteries are embolized by injecting tiny silicon particles causing the fibroids to degenerate. Pain relief is essential for 48 hours. In women with large/multiple fibroids there is an increased risk of hysterectomy compared to surgical treatment. Pyrexia and abscess formation can occur. It is not recommended for women who wish to preserve their fertility, although live births have been reported following the procedure.

*Surgery*

• Abdominal hysterectomy—suitable when family is complete with women over the age of 40 or when the uterus is grossly enlarged and distorted by multiple fibroids.

• Vaginal hysterectomy—when fibroids are small and few in number and there is an associated prolapse of the uterus.

• Myomectomy—in young women whose families are incomplete or when there is a personal desire to retain the uterus. The procedure is often vascular and may cause scarring, with adhesion formation impairing fertility. If the fibroids are numerous it may be impossible to remove them all, and growth of the remainder may cause problems in the future. Women undergoing this procedure should be warned that the surgeon may have to proceed to a hysterectomy and consent to the possibility of this (1% risk).

• Submucous fibroids may be resected with laser or diathermy through a hysteroscope.

### Effects on childbearing

• Implantation over a fibroid may lead to spontaneous miscarriage.

• Pain may develop from red degeneration.

• Premature labour may develop if the fibroids are large, multiple and/or undergo red degeneration.

• Dysfunctional uterine contractions may follow the interruption of smooth waves of electrical stimulation by masses of inert, non-myometrial tissue.

• The pelvis may be obstructed causing malpresentation or even obstructed labour. This is unusual because most fibroids usually move up as the uterus grows in pregnancy.

• Postpartum haemorrhage and retained placenta are more common.

• Management in pregnancy is conservative.

The aim should be to secure a vaginal delivery. If a Caesarean section becomes necessary, the incision in the uterus should be manoeuvred around the fibroids. They should not be removed or incised as severe haemorrhage may develop leading to the need for a hysterectomy.

### Uterine adenomyosis

Adenomyosis is a condition where endometrial glands of stroma are found within the uterine musculature. If localized to one site, it is called an ad-

enomyoma. It is like diffuse endometriosis in the muscle of the uterus.

### Pathology

The uterus is enlarged and thick-walled with no pseudocapsule formation, as in fibroids. The endometrial glands sometimes do not all menstruate, as they derive from the basal layer of the endometrium.

### Symptoms

This condition is most frequent in women aged 35–40, with reduced fertility. The symptoms usually are:

• dysmenorrhoea;
• menorrhagia;
• dyspareunia.

### Signs

A uniformly enlarged uterus which is rarely larger than 12 cm. It is tender on palpation, particularly premenstrually.

### Differential diagnosis

• Uterine fibroids.
• Early pregnancy.
• Uterine infection.

### Treatment

• Conservative use of progestational therapy, e.g. norethisterone 10–20 mg daily.

• Danazol 200–400 mg daily.

• Gonadotrophin analogues: buserelin or goserelin.

All hormone regimes aim to suppress menstruation, but each carries side-effects and usually cannot be used for more than some months at a time.

### Surgery

Abdominal hysterectomy is the treatment of choice, although occasionally resection of the affected area can be considered.

### Endometritis

The condition is usually acute and associated with ascending infection. The disease may result from:

• post-abortal infection;
• criminal abortion;

- excessive curettage;
- intrauterine device infection;
- postpartum, particularly after Caesarean section. It rarely results from blood-borne tuberculosis.

*Findings*
*Acute infection:*
- irregular bleeding;
- uterine tenderness.
*Chronic infection:*
- occasionally secondary amenorrhoea and secondary infertility, caused by the development of intrauterine adhesions leading to partial or complete occlusion of the uterine cavity (Asherman's syndrome).

### Pyometra
- Infection leading to pus formation may be associated with blocking of the fallopian tubes and the cervix.
- Pyometra are commoner in older women.
- A bag of pus builds up pressure and distends the uterus causing:
    (a) pain from the stretch of the muscle wall;
    (b) occasional acute bursts of toxaemia as a bolus of pus is forced into a vein and so to the vascular network;
    (c) chronic infection with low-grade temperature and malaise;
    (d) occasionally pus is forced through the cervix to produce a purulent or bloodstained discharge.
- Many pyometra are associated with cancer of the endometrium (Chapter 20).
    Any woman with such symptoms should have a hysteroscopy and a D&C under appropriate antibiotic cover to exclude endometrial malignancy.

## Fallopian tubes

### Torsion of the fallopian tube
This rare cause of lower abdominal pain is usually associated with ovarian torsion on a long pedicle. Treatment is by laparotomy or laparoscopy and depends upon the degree of devascularization of the tube and ovary:

- if on unwinding the tissues are healthy, they are best conserved with a securing suture to the side wall of the pelvis to prevent retorsion;
- if the tissues are devitalized, the ovary and tube must be removed.

### Salpingitis
An ascending infection from the vagina through the cervix is the usual cause of salpingitis. It is often associated with:
- intercourse;
- transcervical surgery (D&C or evacuation);
- intrauterine foreign bodies such as an intrauterine device (IUCD);
- retained products of conception;
- very rarely, blood-borne infection.

### Acute salpingitis
The fallopian tubes become red, swollen and distorted, often obstructed at the abdominal end so a pyosalpinx forms later becoming a hydrosalpinx. Peritoneal inflammation with adhesions to the serosal surface occurs, leading to pelvic abscess and, if severe, to septicaemia. The condition is usually bilateral. The destruction of the cilia later leads to infertility. Chronic hydrosalpinges may become reinfected.

*Clinical features*
- Pyrexia, often with a temperature higher than 39°C.
- Tachycardia.
- Dehydration.

*Abdominal examination*
- Lower abdominal pain with guarding.
- If parietal peritoneum is involved, rebound tenderness.
- Distension.

*Vaginal examination*
- Cervical excitation pain (bilateral).
- Tender, normal sized uterus.
- Fullness in the fornices and tenderness over the tubes.
- Vaginal discharge.

*Investigations*
- Organisms may be isolated from cervical discharge.
- Gonorrhoea (see Chapter 6).
- *Escherichia coli*, haemolytic streptococcus and staphylococcus are often found in the puerperium and post-abortion.
- *Clostridium welchii* may thrive on dead tissue, e.g. placental products.
- Chlamydia is a common secondary organism.
- Leucocytosis (in excess of $20 \times 10^9$/l).
- Laparoscopy is the only certain way of making a true diagnosis. Remember to take serosal swabs.

*Differential diagnosis*
- *Appendicitis*—pain is usually central then radiating to the right iliac fossa; the fever is lower.
- *Ruptured ectopic pregnancy*—if there is intraperitoneal bleeding, symptoms such as faintness and shoulder tip pain. Tenderness tends to be unilateral and a pregnancy test is usually positive. There is no pyrexia.
- *Ovarian tumour torsion*—the pain is localized and unilateral. Pregnancy test is negative and there is no pyrexia. Ultrasound will confirm.
- *Pyelonephritis*—the pain is usually associated with loin tenderness and there are pus cells in the urine.
- *Intestinal obstruction*—usually associated with colicky pain and abdominal distension. X-rays show fluid levels.

*Treatment*

CONSERVATIVE
- Sit the patient upright in bed.
- Set up intravenous infusion.
- Administer broad-spectrum antibiotics until the high vaginal swab (HVS) microbiology and sensitivity reports have been returned.
- Drugs such as Clindamycin, Augmentin, cephradoxyl or Flagyl are suitable. Continue the antibiotics after the acute phase for 2–3 weeks with doxycycline.
- Provide analgesia and fluids.
- Refer to GU clinic with partner for treatment and contact tracing (see Chapter 6).

RADICAL
- Exploratory surgery should be contemplated if diagnosis is in doubt.
- Use only minimal interference, e.g. drainage under antibiotic cover.

## Chronic salpingitis

Chronic salpingitis is usually a sequel to acute or subacute infections, but is often associated with a lower grade purulent organism, e.g. chlamydia.

*Pathology*
- Thickened fallopian tubes.
- Fibrosis.
- Hydrosalpinges.
- Pelvic floor peritoneal adhesions.

*Symptoms*
- Persistent recurrent episodes of low abdominal pain.
- Deep dyspareunia.
- Congestive dysmenorrhoea.
- Heavy periods.
- Subfertility.

*Investigations*
- Ultrasound scan of pelvis.
- Laparoscopy. If there is no recent acute episode, dye installation with antibiotic cover.

*Long-term sequelae*
- Subfertility.
- Ectopic pregnancy.

## Ovaries

### Infections
Pure oophoritis is rare. However, the ovary is often involved in general pelvic infection. The condition of salpingo-parametro-oophoritis is probably a better description of what is usually called pelvic abscess.

Certain viral conditions such as mumps can affect the ovary, and can cause ovarian swelling and some upset in ovulation, although this is very rare. Unlike such infections in the male, this is usually temporary.

**Tumours**

*History*
Enlargement of the ovary often occurs without any symptoms, for the ovaries are tucked away in the pelvis and can expand without causing very much pressure on surrounding organs until they get quite large. Pain is not a usual association nor is vaginal bleeding, except with the few hormone manufacturing ovarian tumours.

*Symptoms*
When ovarian tumours do produce symptoms they are varied.
• *Abdominal distension*—this is usually noticed by the woman herself with an increase of waist size or when washing in the bath. Usually the tumour has to be greater than 14 cm in diameter before she notices it and often, in the mildly plump, it could be missed until 20 cm.
• *Pressure* on the rectum, bladder or lymphatic system producing appropriate pressure or back symptoms.
• *Pain*—this is usually associated with complications of tumours:
  (a) torsion;
  (b) rupture;
  (c) haemorrhage.
There is peritoneal irritation leading to a degree of shock and a tendency to abdominal muscle guarding. Torsion is usually accompanied by vomiting.
After resuscitation, a laparoscopy is usually required. In skilled hands, minimal access surgery through a laparoscope can deal with an obviously simple ovarian cyst, which has either undergone torsion or has bled. If there is doubt about whether the tumour is malignant, most surgeons prefer to open the abdomen at laparotomy and perform a formal removal.
• *Hormone secretion*—this only happens with a few rare tumours. They may synthesize either:
  (a) oestrogens—leading to menstrual upset (e.g.

granulosa cell tumours);
  (b) androgens—leading to masculinization including amenorrhoea (e.g. arrhenoblastoma).

*Examination*
The woman may look cachectic and show signs of weight loss if presenting with malignant tumours of the ovary. Otherwise, there are few general signs.
• The *abdomen* may appear enlarged. If there is gross stretch of the abdominal wall, there may be shiny skin with possible oedema and *peau d'orange*.
• *Palpation* may allow a firm ovarian cyst to be felt. If there is ascites or the cyst is lax, it might be difficult to delineate it.
• *Percussion* may demonstrate central dullness with resonance of the flanks. However, if ascites is present, this sign is lost and shifting dullness may replace it.
• *Auscultation* is usually not helpful.
• *Pelvic examination* may reveal a tumour or pain.
If benign, the mass can be felt separate from the uterine body and may be freely mobile. If it is fixed, infection, endometriosis or malignancy should be suspected.

*Investigations*
Ultrasound of the abdomen can detect masses and ascites; with smaller masses, a vaginal probe approach is even better at delineation. X-rays are not very helpful unless calcification is present (e.g. dermoids).
Some tumour marker blood concentrations are raised, e.g. $CA_{125}$. However, they are probably of more use in screening tests than confirming a clinical diagnosis which is best done by ultrasound.

*Features of common tumours*
It is difficult to classify ovarian masses precisely, for the ovary has several histological tissues in it and each can contribute to ovarian tumours. Many are simple variations of normal physiology.

**Cysts**

*Follicular cysts*
These consist of unruptured and enlarged Graafian

follicles and a normal ovary commonly contains one or more small cysts (less than 5 cm in diameter). They are not neoplastic and tend to disappear by resorption of fluid. These cysts rarely exceed 15 cm in diameter and are lined with one or more layers of granulosa cells which degenerate in long-standing cysts. There may be difficulty clinically in distinguishing a follicular cyst from a small serous cystadenoma.

### Corpus luteum cysts

These are lined with luteal cells derived from the granulosa layer. The corpus luteum of pregnancy may reach 3 cm or more in diameter and appear cystic. Sometimes, apart from pregnancy, the corpus luteum persists, becoming cystic and causing amenorrhoea followed by bleeding. Haemorrhage into a corpus luteum can cause pain and the symptoms and signs may resemble those of ectopic pregnancy.

### Haemorrhagic cysts

A haemorrhagic cyst may result from bleeding into a Graafian follicle or corpus luteum. Sometimes acute symptoms result, leading to laparotomy. Removal of the ovary may be performed unnecessarily in young women. All that is required is haemostasis of the affected area after shelling out the haematoma.

### Theca luteal cysts

Theca luteal cysts are found in association with raised hCG levels:
- hydatidiform mole;
- choriocarcinoma;
- gonadotrophin therapy.

Both ovaries are enlarged (10 cm or more) with multiple cysts lined by luteal cells. The ovaries return to normal when hCG levels reduce.

## New growths

### Serous cystadenoma

This benign tumour contains fluid which is rich in protein, resembling blood serum. It often contains papillary growths each with a connective tissue core with a covering of cubical cells, similar to those which line the cyst. In larger cysts, papillae are always present and in some cases grow rapidly, almost filling the cyst and giving the appearance of a solid tumour.

Bilateral tumours are often seen and malignant change is frequent. The histological diagnosis of malignancy is occasionally not easy and may have to be made on the clinical features.

### Mucinous cystadenoma

The commonest of the benign new growths, it contains viscous mucin, the secretion of the lining of the tumour. The cyst grows slowly and may reach a very large size, so as to fill the abdominal cavity. Tumours over 100 kg have been reported (i.e. heavier than the woman from whom they are taken).

It is multilocular, each loculus being lined with tall columnar epithelium which may be ciliated and can proliferate to form papillary folds. Goblet cells are found among the epithelial cells.

Malignant change occurs in about 5%.

### Pseudomyxoma peritonei

This is a rare condition whereas mucinous tumours are common; it may occur if the contents of a cyst leak or are spilled into the peritoneal cavity. Epithelial cells lining the cyst proliferate and produce a mucinous ascites, the whole peritoneal cavity becoming filled with viscid mucinous material. The condition arises also from a mucocoele of the appendix and thus may be found in males as well as females.

### Fibroadenoma

A benign tumour that occurs in about 3% of women with an ovarian tumour. It arises from connective tissue as a solid non-encapsulated tumour which may be bilateral and can grow to 20 cm. The normal ovary is compressed but not invaded. The histological appearance is that of a benign tumour composed of whorls of fibrous connective tissue resembling the ovarian stroma. These tumours are associated with:
- ascites;
- hydrothorax—only occasionally;
- hydropericardium.

This association is Meigs' syndrome and is also found with a Brenner tumour, granulosa cell or theca cell tumours. The effusions into the serous cavities disappear when the tumour is removed.

*Brenner tumour*

A rare tumour found mostly in postmenopausal women, often discovered accidentally at autopsy since it remains small and symptomless. It is a mostly solid tumour with nests of epithelial cells resembling transitional epithelium enclosed in dense fibrous tissue. Cavities arising in the epithelial nests contain mucin like mucinous cystadenoma. A Brenner tumour is sometimes found in a mucinous cystadenoma. Meigs' syndrome may occur.

*Germ cell tumours*

This is a group of primitive germ cell tumours. The best known is the *dysgerminoma*. This rare tumour arises from primitive undifferentiated sex cells; histologically identical tumours are found in the ovary (dysgerminoma) and in the testicle (seminoma). It consists of epithelial cells arranged in alveoli separated by septa of fibrous tissue infiltrated with round cells, resembling lymphocytes. The epithelial cells are large and round or polygonal, like spermatocytes. It may happen in young patients and is liable to malignant change in both sexes. Dysgerminoma is more common in individuals with infantile genitalia and in males with undescended testicles, but it also occurs in normal individuals. It secretes gonadotrophin so that a positive pregnancy test may be obtained.

*Endodermal sinus tumour* or *embryonal carcinoma* may occur with dysgerminoma.

*Dermoid or benign teratoma*

This common tumour of the ovary makes up 15% of all ovarian tumours. It occurs mainly between 15 and 30 years and is the commonest tumour in this age group because it develops from an unfertilized ovum by parthenogenesis and thus occurs mostly in the reproductive period. These tumours are often multiple and bilateral (10%).

A dermoid is a thick-walled cyst with solid parts, rarely exceeding 20 cm in diameter. It does not

adhere to surrounding structures so torsion is common. The cyst is lined by squamous epithelium and contains:

- a fatty sebaceous secretion resembling sebum;
- hairs;
- sebaceous glands;
- hair follicles;
- teeth;
- cartilage;
- gastrointestinal epithelium;
- nervous tissue;
- thyroid tissue.

Malignant change sometimes occurs in the form of squamous epithelioma or embryonal carcinoma in one of the elements of the tumour.

Hyperthyroidism can follow in a benign teratoma consisting mainly of thyroid tissue.

*Solid teratoma*

This is a very rare tumour. It has a variety of primitive tissues with ectoderm, mesoderm and endoderm all represented so that the tumour consists of masses of embryonic cells of all varieties in a bizarre histological pattern. It is highly malignant.

*Gonadoblastoma*

This tumour occurs in abnormal gonads and in individuals who are sex chromatin negative. It consists of large germ cells like those of a dysgerminoma and small cells like granulosa cells. It may show hormonal activity and may become malignant.

*Granulosa cell tumour*

The cells resemble granulosa cells, being polygonal with deeply staining nuclei. They tend to be arranged in rosettes; clear space may be seen between them and strands of connective tissue run between the granulosa cells. Malignant change may occur and they secrete oestrogens.

Granulosa cell tumours may occur at any age. In infants and young children they are a rare cause of precocious puberty with uterine bleeding. In adult women, granulosa cell tumours cause profuse and irregular uterine bleeding from a hyperoestrogenized endometrium, often of metropathic type. An ovarian tumour must not be overlooked when considering these symptoms. In postmenopausal women irregular uterine bleeding is caused, with oestrogenization of the uterus, vulva and vagina. A hyperoestrogenized endometrium is found and there may be malignancy with associated carcinoma of the uterus.

### Thecoma

This is a solid tumour which is usually 5 cm in diameter but may grow to 15 cm although this is rare. It resembles a fibroma and Meigs' syndrome can occur. Yellowish fatty areas which show up in sections stained for fat are scattered among the fibrous tissue cells. These are theca lutein cells. A mixed granulosa cell tumour and thecoma also occurs.

Thecoma occurs mainly in women over 30. It may present with a pelvic mass or with uterine haemorrhage or both; ascites and pleural effusions may be seen. There is a high incidence of carcinoma of the endometrium in association with thecoma.

### Sertoli–Leydig cell tumour

Often called androblastoma or arrhenoblastoma, this tumour causes virilism from its testosterone metabolism, but it is rare. The tumour may be cystic or solid and is potentially malignant. The cells consist of undifferentiated mesenchyme, and may be arranged in tubules as in the testicle.

## Dysmenorrhoea

Dysmenorrhoea or pain associated with menstruation occurs in two main forms:
- primary spasmodic;
- secondary, congestive or acquired.

## Spasmodic dysmenorrhoea

This is very common; most normal women have some discomfort at the onset of menstruation. In dysmenorrhoea, pain is severe during the first hours or days of the period. It may be:
- continuous or spasmodic like colic;
- accompanied by vomiting and fainting;
- felt in the pelvis and lower back;

- radiating into the legs;
- diarrhoea.

### Cause

The pain is probably caused by excessive prostaglandin production producing contractions of the uterine muscle in the first days of menstruation. There is rarely any pathological cause found.

It is associated with adenomyosis (p. 233).

### Management

- Simple analgesics. Aspirin, paracetamol and codeine or a combination of these may be used. Mefenamic acid (500 mg three timesa day) gives good relief of pain in many cases.
- Hormone treatment includes oral contraception to inhibit ovulation and thus cause painless bleeding. One of the low-dose oral contraceptives may be preferred though women sometimes object to contraceptives being given. The best effect follows hormones that inhibit ovulation. Given for a few months at a time they cause no ill effects and improvement may continue when treatment is stopped.

## Secondary, congestive or acquired dysmenorrhoea

This is rare before 25 years and uncommon before 30.

### Symptoms

Pain begins before menstruation and may be relieved when bleeding starts. It is felt in the pelvis and back and made worse with exertion. Other symptoms such as menorrhagia and dyspareunia may be present.

This type of dysmenorrhoea usually occurs with a physical cause.
- Chronic pelvic sepsis (p. 235).
- Endometriosis.
- Acquired fixed retroversion of the uterus.
- Fibroids.

# Endometriosis

Endometriosis is the presence of endometrium outside the uterus. This tissue responds to the hormone variations in the cycle as does normally sited endometrium.

Endometriosis is most commonly a disease of women in the second half of their reproductive life, between 30 and 45 years, and tends to regress at the menopause or even before. The greatest incidence is in women who are childless or have few children; full-term pregnancy leads to regression of the growth, though abortion does not. Endometriosis is commonest in women of European origin.

## Pathology

Deposits of endometriosis consist of endometrial glands and stroma. The tissue bleeds in response to hormone cyclical changes, but there is no escape for the blood, which becomes encysted; infiltration of surrounding structures such as bowel occurs with subsequent fibrosis. These endometriotic areas vary in size from a pinhead to a large cyst with tarry material—the chocolate cyst. Perforation and leakage from chocolate cysts in the ovaries is very irritant and leads to dense adhesions.

The cause of endometriosis is unknown, but hypotheses are:
• Retrograde spread of collections of endometrial cells shed from the uterus at menstruation passing along the fallopian tube to the peritoneal cavity. This would account for by far the highest incidence of endometriosis occurring in the pelvis.
• Blood or lymph borne embolization.
• Metaplasia of islands of totipotential coelomic epithelium.
• Altered immunological recognition of endometrial tissue allowing acceptance of emboli of endometrium in these.

Probably a combination of the first and last theories is the most likely.

## Sites

Endometriosis is commonest in the pelvis. It is very occasionally found in bizarre sites such as the pleura, umbilicus, Caesarean section scars, diaphragm, arm, leg or kidney, but these cases are rare.

### Ovaries

The ovaries are a very common site for the disease which may take the form of:
• numerous endometrial cysts containing blood;
• a large chocolate or tarry cyst, densely adherent to the surrounding tissues.

Histological examination does not always reveal typical endometrial glands as these may have been destroyed in large cysts.

### Pelvic peritoneum

The pelvic peritoneum is very often affected over the back of the uterus, the fallopian tubes, the uterosacral ligaments and the pouch of Douglas. Peritoneal deposits often present as widespread black nodules with scarring and puckering of the peritoneal surface. Adhesions may form between these and the back of the uterus, causing fixed retroversion.

### Uterine ligaments

The uterosacral ligaments and the rectovaginal septum are commonly involved. Endometriosis in the round ligament may be found inside the abdominal cavity or may present as a tumour in the groin if the inguinal end of the ligament is involved.

### Bowel

The intestines and rectum may all become infiltrated with endometriosis. The commonest result is that fibrosis in the wall of the bowel leads to stricture formation and thus to obstruction. Bleeding into the bowel lumen is uncommon.

### Urinary tract

Endometriosis may occur in the bladder leading to haematuria and painful micturition. Fibrosis around the ureters can follow longstanding endometriosis leading to obstruction of renal flow.

## Abdominal wall

Endometriosis may occur as an isolated lesion at the umbilicus probably by travelling up a patent urachus; this presents as cyclical bleeding. It occurs in scars following operations on the uterus, particularly where the cavity of the uterus is opened, such as myomectomy or Caesarean section.

## Perineum and vagina

Deposits of endometriosis may be seen in perineal scars and in the vaginal wall, though these are surprisingly uncommon.

## Classification

Endometriosis is classified into stages to allow comparison between clusters and grade response to treatment (Table 17.2).

## Clinical features

*Symptoms*
The symptoms of pelvic endometriosis depend on the site and the activity of the disease.
- *Pain*—three main types of pain are found:
  (a) *congestive dysmenorrhoea* begins with menstruation. It is felt in the pelvis and lower back;
  (b) *ovulation* pain is sometimes severe in mid-cycle;
  (c) *dyspareunia* is felt deep in the pelvis due to pressing on the uterosacral ligaments and recto-vaginal septum during coitus.
- *Infertility* may be the main complaint. This may be due to:
  (a) ovulation occurring into closed off areas of fibrosis;
  (b) damage to tubal fimbria;
  (c) kinking of tubes by adhesions;
  (d) blockage of tube by deposits of endometriosis in the wall.
- *Disturbances of menstruation.* Menorrhagia may occur if deposits are in the myometrium. Shorter cycles and episodes of prolonged bleeding may occur (adenomyosis).

Other symptoms from endometriosis may be:
- haematuria;
- dysuria;
- intestinal obstruction;
- pain on defaecation;
- occasionally a chocolate cyst may rupture, causing symptoms and signs of an acute abdomen.

*Physical signs*
The most typical clinical picture is that of fixed retroversion of the uterus with enlarged, tender ovaries adherent behind it. Deposits in the uterosacral ligaments may be palpable as tender nodules. Laparoscopy is essential to establish the diagnosis.

**Table 17.2** Classification of endometriosis from The American Fertility Society. Reproduced with permission of the publisher.

| Size of deposits | <1 cm | 1–3 cm | >3 cm |
|---|---|---|---|
| *Peritoneum* | | | |
| Superficial | 1 | 2 | 4 |
| Deep | 2 | 4 | 6 |
| | | | |
| *Ovary* | | | |
| Right superficial | 1 | 2 | 4 |
| Deep | 4 | 16 | 20 |
| Left superficial | 1 | 2 | 4 |
| Deep | 4 | 16 | 20 |
| | | | |
| **Adhesions** | | | |
| *Ovary* | | | |
| Right film | 1 | 2 | 4 |
| Dense | 4 | 8 | 16 |
| Left film | 1 | 2 | 4 |
| Dense | 4 | 8 | 16 |
| | | | |
| *Tube* | | | |
| Right film | 1 | 2 | 4 |
| Dense | 4 | 8 | 16 |
| Left film | 1 | 2 | 4 |
| Dense | 4 | 8 | 16 |
| | | | |
| *Pouch of Douglas* | | | |
| Partly obliterated | 4→ | | |
| Completely obliterated | 40→ | | |
| | | | |
| *Score* | | | |
| 1–5 Minimal | | | |
| 6–15 Mild | | | |
| 16–40 Moderate | | | |
| >40 Severe | | | |

*Differential diagnosis*
• *Chronic pelvic infection* most closely resembles pelvic endometriosis, with dysmenorrhoea, menorrhagia, sterility and dyspareunia being identical, but the history and laparoscopy findings are different and pelvic inflammatory disease (PID) pain is rarely cyclical.
• *Fibroids* of the uterus are often associated with endometriosis, and the differential diagnosis may be difficult.

## Treatment

Treatment of pelvic endometriosis is essentially conservative because the condition:
• tends to occur during the reproductive period;
• does not become malignant;
• tends to regress at the menopause.

### Hormone therapy
This is successful in many cases. The diagnosis must first be made at laparoscopy and if there are large chocolate cysts these should be drained; local areas of endometriosis can be coagulated with laser/diathermy through the laparoscope.

*Danazol* inhibits pituitary gonadotrophin secretion and in adequate doses will suppress menstruation. The initial dose is 200 mg daily in divided doses, increasing up to 600 mg daily as required. Treatment should be given initially for six months. There may be androgenic effects:
• acne;
• hirsutes;
• weight gain due to fluid retention.

It is important to be sure that the woman is not pregnant and it must be stressed that danazol is not a contraceptive.

*Progesterone* used to be the major therapy, using norethisterone starting on the fifth day of menstruation with 10 mg daily and increasing up to 40 mg daily. Nausea, vomiting, weight gain and fluid retention occur, while a cure is unusual.

An alternative progestogen, medroxyprogesterone acetate (10–30 mg daily by mouth), can suppress menstruation for six months. If breakthrough bleeding is troublesome, the dose should be increased.

Side-effects are common with hormone treatments, but in patients who persist, regression of the endometriotic lesions occurs and pregnancy may become possible, though ovulation may be delayed for several months after treatment.

Synthetic substitutes of *gonadotrophin releasing hormone* (GnRH) and their agonists are inhibitors of ovarian function. Two weeks' treatment (subcutaneously or nasal spray) reduces FSH and LH concentrations and leads to lower oestrogen levels. Treatment for 3–6 months gives relief. Side-effects may be:
• headaches;
• hot flushes;
• depression;
• loss of bone density if treatment is over 6 months.

### Surgery
Very small lesions may be treated at laparoscopy by diathermy or laser. Laparotomy is indicated in:
• pelvic masses over 5 cm;
• acute rupture of a cyst;
• intestinal obstruction.

Conservative surgery is always performed if possible, aiming to leave the uterus and normal ovarian tissue.

In intractable cases, and especially among women who do not want children, wider surgery may be needed. Hysterectomy with bilateral salpingo-oophorectomy may be performed for intractable menorrhagia and dysmenorrhoea or when there are fibroids or adenomyosis. Some ovarian tissue may be left if not actually involved in the destructive process.

## Premenstrual tension

Premenstrual tension occurs most usually in the second half of the menstrual cycle. It consists of a cluster of behavioural symptoms and physical signs which come in the second half of the cycle with abolition immediately after menstruation.

*Symptoms and signs*
• Irritability.

- Depression.
- Lassitude.
- Insomnia.
- Lack of concentration.
- Oedema with fluid retention.
- Abdominal swelling.
- Swollen fingers and ankles.
- Weight gain.

Migraine can occur during this phase or at the onset of menstruation. The symptoms tend to come on 7–10 days premenstrually, after the luteal phase is established. Women may become more accident prone and there is an increased prevalence of suicide. Some women who suffer from premenstrual tension have endogenous depression exacerbated at this time.

*Aetiology*

HORMONAL
- Timing in cycle in luteal phase.
- Improved in absence of cyclical ovarian activity.
- Renin–angiotensin system.
- Reduction of endogenous opioids.
- Changes in mono-amine neurotransmitters.

Probably a combination of the second and third factors.

*Treatment*
- Explanation and reassurance.
- Progestogens—may be deficient in second half of cycle so replace them.
- Oestrogens—to suppress ovulation.
- Oral contraceptive—combined preparation of both of the above; works for some.
- Danazol—stops ovulation; beware unwanted androgenic side-effects.
- Evening primrose oil—may effect essential fatty acid metabolism.
- Pyridoxine (B$_6$)—may affect dopamine and serotonin metabolism. Benefit weak—beware overdosage and neuropathy with long-term treatment.
- Antidepressants—during the premenstrual phase may help. More severe cases need psychiatric treatment. Fluoxetine has been shown to be the most effective.

The variety of medication emphasizes how little the cause of this syndrome is understood. Treatments may be a matter of trial and error.

## Abdominal organs

### Pyelonephritis

The woman presents with ill-defined abdominal pain, pyrexia and shivering. The diagnosis differs from an acute abdominal problem for the pain is often round the side in the loin and tenderness is then high up in the costal angles.

Examination of the urine for pus cells and organisms reveals the diagnosis. Treatment is conservative with bedrest, fluids and appropriate antibiotics.

Very rarely a ureteric stone may present in pregnancy. If this sticks in the ureter, it causes pain by stretch of the ureter from dammed-back urine. Pethidine is helpful both for its analgesic properties and because it is an antispasmodic.

### Appendicitis

This occurs equally commonly in early pregnancy as during any other nine months of a young woman's life. It is a young person's disease.

Diagnosis can be difficult for the appendix rises up from its usual position in the right iliac fossa. The typical history of peri-umbilical pain moving to the right iliac fossa may not be given in pregnancy; the signs are confusing as the caecum with its attached appendix is pushed up the right paracolic gutter by the enlarging uterus. Remembering this, the examiner must seek the point of maximum tenderness higher in the abdomen.

Treatment should be by surgery and the surgeon in later pregnancy would do well to mark the site of maximum tenderness before the anaesthetic and incise there rather than over McBurney's point.

There used to be a higher mortality of appendicitis in pregnancy because of the reluctance of people to operate for fear of miscarriage. However, it must be realized that a progressing appendicitis carries a much higher risk to the fetus and mother than the problems of carrying out a surgical procedure under controlled anaesthesia.

## Rectus haematoma

The deep epigastric arteries with their concomitant epigastric veins may be stretched by the growing uterus and occasionally, after a severe attack of coughing, one of these veins under tension may rupture. This leads to a haematoma that is very difficult to diagnose. If seen early, the pain is localized under one segment of one rectus muscle, but after a few hours this sign spreads. If seen very late, there may be anaemia due to loss of blood into the haematoma.

If diagnosed competently, surgical treatment is not needed. Occasionally, a laparotomy is performed and the diagnosis becomes obvious when the rectus muscles are separated before opening the peritoneum. Usually it is too late to ligate any of the veins. The operator need proceed no further.

## Bowel problems

Should a gynaecologist open the abdomen and find a bowel or peritoneal problem, he would be wise to consult with a surgical colleague urgently. Although gynaecologists may have been trained once to do general surgery they do not practise such operations daily. Combined surgical and gynaecological operating would probably be better for the woman.

**Table 17.3** Differential diagnosis of acute abdominal/pelvic pain.

| Condition | History | Examination | Investigation | Ultrasound scan |
|---|---|---|---|---|
| *Ectopic pregnancy* | • Pain—sudden onset, constant, shoulder tip <br> • Other—sudden collapse, period of amenorrhoea, minivaginal bleeding | Rebound, guarding BP↓, P↑, T < 37°C VE—unilateral Cx excitation, uterus small for dates, os closed | Hb = or ↓ WBC = hCG +ve | Empty uterus Free fluid in POD ?Adnexal mass |
| *Acute salpingitis* | • Pain—gradual onset, constant, generalized, bilateral <br> • Other—vaginal discharge, irregular menses | Guarding? rebound T > 37.5°C, BP =, P ↑ VE—bilateral Cx excitation | Hb = WBC ↑ hCG –ve +ve HVS | NAD ?? Free fluid |
| *Fibroid degeneration* | • Pain—gradual onset, constant, generalized <br> • Other—? menorrhagia | Tender over fibroid T 37–37.5°C, VE—no Cx excitation, enlarged uterus | Hb = WBC = or ↑ hCG –ve | Fibroid seen in uterine wall with cystic areas |
| *Ovarian cyst accident:* <br> Torsion | • Pain—sudden onset, constant, may be getting less <br> • Other—vomiting | Rebound, guarding T 37–37.5°C, BP =, P ↑ VE—unilateral Cx excitation, adnexal mass | Hb = or WBC = or ↑ hCG –ve | Echogenic mass seen separate from uterus ?Free fluid |

**Table 17.1** *Continued*

| Condition | History | Examination | Investigation | Ultrasound scan |
|---|---|---|---|---|
| Rupture | • Pain—sudden onset, constant, getting less<br>• Other—? irregular menses | Rebound, guarding<br>T 37°C, P, BP =,<br>VE—generalized tenderness only | Hb =<br>WBC =<br>hCG –ve | Free fluid in POD<br>No cyst seen |
| Haemorrhage | • Pain—sudden onset, constant, becoming less | Rebound, guarding<br>T 37°C, BP =, P ↑<br>VE—unilateral Cx excitation, adnexal mass | Hb = or ↑<br>WBC =<br>hCG –ve | Echogenic cyst<br>Free fluid if ruptured |
| *Appendicitis* | • Pain—gradual onset, right-sided<br>• Other—anorexia, no BO, nausea/vomiting | Rebound, guarding, right-sided tenderness<br>T 37–37.5°C,<br>BP =, P ↑<br>VE—NAD<br>PR—empty rectum, right-sided tenderness | Hb =<br>WBC ↑<br>hCG –ve | NAD |
| *Pyelonephritis* | • Pain—loin pain, colicky<br>• Other—nausea, vomiting, rigors, dysuria | Loin tenderness<br>T > 37.5°C,<br>VE—NAD | Hb =<br>WBC ↑<br>hCG –ve<br>MSU +ve | Renal pelvicalyceal dilatation<br>Pelvis—NAD |
| *Obstruction* | • Pain—intermittent, generalized, colicky<br>• Other—nausea, vomiting, anorexia, bowels not open | Rebound, guarding, distension<br>No BS. T 37°C,<br>VE—NAD<br>PR—empty rectum | Hb =<br>WBC = or ↑<br>hCG –ve | Pelvis—NAD<br>AXR—dilated loops with fluid levels |

BP = blood pressure; T = temperature; P = pulse; VE = vaginal examination; PR = rectal examination; NAD = no abnormality detected; AXR = abdominal X-ray; Hb = haemoglobin; WBC = white blood count; hCG = pregnancy test; MSU = mid-stream urine; HVS = high vaginal swab; POD = pouch of Douglas; Cx = cervical; BS.= bowel sounds.

**Self-assessment**

**17.1** OSCE question.

**Candidate's instructions:** Rosemary Beckett, a woman of 32 is referred to the gynaecology clinic by her GP. She gives a 2 year history of increasingly severe period pains. You are expected to take a history and outline your initial management of Mrs Beckett.

**Role-player's instructions:** You are Rosemary Beckett, a 32 year old primary school teacher. You have been married for 3 years. You have never been pregnant and use condoms for contraception. You tried the pill in your early 20s but found that it made you feel depressed. Your periods are regular but are becoming increasingly painful over the last 2 years. The pain starts as a low constant ache in your back radiating to the front. It starts 3–4 days before your period, is worst on the first 2 days of your period and then subsides. Sex is uncomfortable in some positions particularly before your period. The pain can be acute and is deep inside especially when your husband is particularly vigorous. He is sympathetic but you feel that it is beginning to affect your relationship as your libido is less than when you first married. You and your husband are planning to have a baby within the next 2 years and are worried that the pain may prevent pregnancy. You have no past medical or surgical history of relevance, no allergies and take Neurofen for the pain but no regular medication. All other details are up to the role-player.

**17.2** Submucous fibroids are commonly associated with which of the following?
(a) Constant lower abdominal pain.
(b) Menorrhagia.
(c) Vomiting.
(d) Secondary dysmenorrhoea.
(e) Ectopic pregnancy.

**17.3** A 24-year-old woman presents with unilateral abdominal pain, vomiting, abdominal rebound and guarding. She is apyrexial and her LMP was one week ago. Which of the following is the most likely diagnosis?
(a) Pelvic inflammatory disease.
(b) Bleeding into a corpus luteal cyst.
(c) Ruptured corpus luteal cyst.
(d) Torted dermoid cyst.
(e) Ruptured mucinous cystadenoma.

**17.4** Which of the following is true of benign ovarian cysts?
(a) May undergo degeneration.
(b) May rupture causing acute abdominal pain.
(c) May contain well differentiated tissues.
(d) May contain altered blood.
(e) May secrete testosterone.

**17.5** A 19-year-old woman presents with right iliac fossa pain. The pain came on gradually and was associated with nausea and vomiting. She has not opened her bowels for 36 hours. On examination she has a temperature of 37.6°C. Abdominal examination reveals tenderness in the right iliac fossa (RIF) with guarding and rebound. Vaginal examination reveals mild tenderness on the right with no cervical excitation. What is the most likely diagnosis?
(a) Appendicitis.
(b) Pyelonephritis.
(c) Torted right ovarian cyst.
(d) Small bowel obstruction.
(e) Ruptured right ovarian cyst.

# Chapter 18

# Breast disease

In the UK, gynaecologists do not usually deal with breast problems. Breast disease is managed by specialist breast surgeons or general surgeons with an interest in breast surgery. This is partly a consequence of the work of Sir Hedley Atkins who set up the first specialist breast surgical unit in the world at Guy's Hospital.

Breast problems are extremely common comprising one in six of all general surgery referrals. This is partly the result of a heightened awareness of breast cancer, which is the commonest malignancy in the UK among men and women.

## Breast history

The most frequent breast symptom is a lump. The particular features of a breast lump are usually ascertained during clinical examination but it is important to find out:

• *Time*—how long the lump has been there.
• *Pain*—whether it is painful. Breast pain is rarely associated with malignancy but may be severe and may interfere significantly with a patient's lifestyle. Its site, distribution, severity, radiation, precipitating factors and relieving factors should all be asked about, but the affect that it has on a patient's lifestyle is the most relevant question.
• *Size*—whether it has changed in size. In particular, areas of benign breast thickening and nodularity may become more pronounced and more tender prior to each menstrual period.

• *Nipple discharge*—a common symptom which can be a sign of malignancy. It should be noted whether this is unilateral or bilateral, occurs spontaneously or only on expression from a single or multiple ducts, its colour and whether there is blood staining.
• *Nipple inversion*—can also be a sign of malignancy. The salient points are whether is it unilateral or bilateral and how long it has been present.
• *Nipple eczema*—should be distinguished from Paget's disease of the nipple. This often requires a skin biopsy.

## Breast examination

Examination is carried out with the patient seated in good light and in a warm room. She should be stripped to the waist.

## Inspection

Inspection involves comparing one breast with the other, particularly with regard to:
• symmetry;
• preservation of the natural curved contour of the breast;
• position and appearance of the nipples;
• scars;
• changes in the skin (erythema, peau d'orange, ulceration) and skin dimpling. It is quite common for one breast to be a little larger than the other but

be sure to find out whether this is a recent change. Always look underneath the breast in the infra-mammary fold. Skin dimpling is a very significant sign as it is associated with malignancy in more than 95% of cases.

## Palpation

Each breast should be palpated in turn starting with the normal breast. Palpation is carried out with the palmer aspect of the index, middle and ring fingers. It is usually more sensitive to use the dominant hand. The impression of a breast lump is obtained by moving the examining fingers in a circular motion. The fingers should be pressed down gently but firmly and moved in a circular manner so that any underlying mass will be felt as something slipping under the fingers. The examining fingers and the patient's skin move more freely than a mass within the breast tissue, and the latter is therefore felt to slip under the fingers but over the stationary chest wall. A mass in the breast can be felt to move relative to the fixed structures of the underlying chest wall and ribs.

In the relatively uncommon instance where the breast mass is tethered to the underlying muscle there is significantly less mobility, and virtually no mobility when the underlying muscle is tensed (by pressing the hand onto the hip).

A mass within the skin, such as a sebaceous cyst, does not slip under the fingers and is only felt by direct pressure that particularly identifies the edge of the lesion. Palpation of breast lumps is easier with the patient lying absolutely flat with the bed high enough so that the elbow of the examiner is at least flexed to 90°. It is important to examine the breast systematically so that none of the breast is missed. It is usually best to develop your own method for this. One way is to examine the breast a quadrant at a time and then to specifically feel the retro-areola area and the axillary tail. During examination the non-dominant hand can be used to stretch out the breast tissue, particularly the tissues in the lateral aspect of the breast.

Axillary nodes can be examined with either the patient sitting up (hands on hips) or lying supine (with the arm abducted to 45° and supported by the examiner). The boundaries of the axilla should be examined in turn:

- the medial boundary (lateral chest wall);
- the anterior boundary (the anterior axillary fold);
- the posterior boundary (latissimus dorsi);
- lateral boundary (the upper aspect of the arm);
- the apex.

Lymph nodes draining the breast are usually situated in the medial, posterior or apical parts of the axilla. Sometimes a pathological axillary node lies particularly low in the axilla or in the axillary tail of the breast.

Lastly, the supra- and infra-clavicular fossae should be palpated with the patient sitting up (preferably from behind). If metastatic disease is suspected the lower lung field should be percussed for the presence of pleural effusion and the liver palpated.

## Benign breast disease

### Breast cysts

*Aetiology*
All women will develop cysts in their breasts at one time or another. Usually they are too small to feel. They develop under the influence of oestrogen and are therefore usually only found during the reproductive years or in women on hormone replacement therapy (HRT). They are not common between the ages of puberty and 25. Breast cysts develop by the dilation of a breast duct.

*Symptoms*
Breast lump (sometimes of considerable size) which is frequently painful or tender.

*Signs*
Smooth, round, circular mass which may be visible. Breast cysts are usually tense and can feel remarkably hard.

*Investigations*
Breast cysts are best investigated with ultrasound which can show any irregularity in the wall of the

cyst. Mammography is generally not able to differentiate between a solid and a cystic mass.

*Natural history*

Breast cysts often appear suddenly and equally may disappear relatively quickly. Some cysts, however, remain for a number of years. Breast cysts practically never become malignant. Rarely, they can develop *in-situ* malignancy (intracystic papillary carcinoma).

*Treatment*

Breast cysts do not need any treatment unless they are uncomfortable in which case they can be aspirated with a needle and syringe.

## Fibrocystic change

*Aetiology*

Fibrocystic change, previously termed fibroadenosis, is a normal way that the breast develops with time and under the influence of the normal menstrual cycle. It involves an increase in the fibrous tissue of the breast stroma, together with the formation of multiple small and large cysts. It occurs to a greater or lesser extent in every woman and may be responsible for breast lumps.

*Symptoms*

Tender breast lump that varies with the menstrual cycle and becomes more prominent prior to each period.

*Signs*

A diffuse area of tender thickening or nodularity, only rarely amounting to a discrete mass with definable edges. The thickening may be approximately symmetrical with the same site in the opposite breast.

*Investigations*

Fibrocystic change shows as a diffuse increase in the density of the breast parenchyma on a mammogram. If the associated cysts are large enough these will appear as discrete, rounded masses. An ultrasound shows small and large cysts.

*Natural history*

Some women have more fibrocystic change than others resulting in permanently lumpy breasts. This is more apparent in slim women. The changes generally resolve after the menopause.

*Treatment*

Reassurance only is required.

## Breast pain (mastalgia)

*Aetiology*

The vast majority of breast pain is caused by either hormonal changes in the breast tissue or a chronic inflammatory condition of the major breast ducts close to the nipple—periductal mastitis. Breast pain is only very rarely associated with malignancy and then only when it is unilateral and localized to a specific site.

*Symptoms*

The pain is usually described as an aching, particularly in the lateral aspects of the breasts, radiating into the axilla and sometimes into the upper arm. The pain may be unilateral. It is often worse in the second half of each menstrual cycle although mastalgia relating to hormonal changes can also frequently be non-cyclical. Hormonal breast pain does not respond significantly to standard analgesics. It is usually associated with marked tenderness and is helped by wearing a supportive brassiere. The breast pain relating to periductal mastitis is non-cyclical, sharper, more transient and frequently radiates through the nipple.

*Signs*

Breast tenderness. Patients with hormonal mastalgia often have denser and more nodular breast tissue.

*Investigations*

No investigations are necessary except in the case of unilateral and focal breast pain.

*Treatment*

Simple measures such as reducing the amount of dietary caffeine and taking regular Starflower or

Evening Primrose Oil. Drugs that are helpful include Tamoxifen (10 mgs, daily), Danazol (100 mgs, daily) and Bromocriptine (1 mg, daily).

## Nipple discharge

*Aetiology*
Nipple discharge may be caused by malignancy but is more frequently the result of either periductal mastitis (chronic inflammation involving a number of breast ducts) or a duct papilloma (usually involving a single duct). Periductal mastitis is much more common in smokers.

*Symptoms*
Periductal mastitis causes discharge of any colour (brown, green, clear, milky). It is often bilateral. A duct papilloma causes clear discharge which is usually unilateral. Breast cancer causes unilateral discharge. All three causes can be associated with blood staining.

*Signs*
- *Periductal mastitis*: multiduct, multicoloured discharge, usually bilateral.
- *Papilloma*: single duct, crystal clear discharge.
- *Carcinoma*: unilateral discharge, often with blood staining and associated underlying breast lump and/or nipple distortion.

*Investigations*
Mammography and ultrasound should be carried out to exclude malignancy. An ultrasound scan may demonstrate a large papilloma. Nipple discharge fluid can be sent for cytological examination.

*Natural history*
- *Periductal mastitis*: this is a chronic condition.
- *Duct papilloma*: a duct papilloma can cause profuse discharge which is inconvenient for the patient.

*Treatment*
- *Periductal mastitis*: no treatment is available except for surgical total duct excision.

- *Duct papilloma*: breast duct microendoscopy and microdochectomy.

## Fibroadenoma

*Aetiology*
A fibroadenoma is a solid mass arising in the breast of young women, particularly from the age of puberty to the mid 30s. It is also more common in post menopausal women who take HRT. The aetiology is unknown although there is undoubtedly a hormonal influence.

*Symptoms*
Painless lump. Some patients have multiple lesions.

*Signs*
Firm to hard, rounded or elliptical mass which is characterized by unusual mobility underneath the palpating fingers (colloquially known as a breast mouse).

*Investigations*
A well defined mass with discrete clear margins on both mammography and ultrasound.

*Natural history*
Fibroadenomas do not become malignant. They may gradually increase in size and in this case they should be removed to definitely exclude a malignant mass that may have the same clinical features as a fibroadenoma.

*Treatment*
It is important to differentiate this solid mass from other solid masses in the breast such as a carcinoma. This should always involve at least needle aspiration cytology and over the age of 30 preferably a core needle biopsy. If there is any doubt about the diagnosis the lesion should be removed surgically by excision biopsy. This latter operation can often be carried out under a local anaesthetic.

## Breast abscess

*Aetiology*
A breast abscess can either be associated with lactation or periductal mastitis.

*Symptoms*
Painful, rapidly enlarging mass in the breast with associated pyrexia.

*Signs*
Lactational abscess may be very large and the borders may be quite indistinct so that the mass forms a prominent area of hardening of the breast tissue. Abscesses associated with periductal mastitis are found either in the retroareolar region or just around the areola. Breast abscesses are always associated with overlying breast erythema. There may be peau d'orange. This latter scenario mimics inflammatory breast cancer and this differential diagnosis should always be entertained.

*Investigations*
Breast abscesses are best shown by ultrasonography.

*Treatment*
Early in the development of a breast infection (whatever the aetiology) treatment with antibiotics may be successful in averting a frank abscess. Use either Augmentin or Flucloxacillin and Metronidazole (anaerobes may be responsible). Once the breast abscess is larger than 1 cm needle aspiration or incision drainage are usually required. Needle aspiration may need to be repeated.

## Other benign breast lumps

- *Lipoma*: soft, rounded, quite difficult to feel, may have a distinct edge.
- *Hamartoma*: fairly soft, discrete, no malignant potential.
- *Phylloides tumour*: mimics a fibroadenoma and may be quite similar histologically. Phylloides tumours may grow to become very large. They may recur following excision if a small amount of the lesion is left behind and they should therefore be removed with a clear histological margin. There are malignant variants of phylloides tumours that develop into fibrosarcomas.

## Breast malignancy

## Epidemiology

### Rates

The incidence of breast cancer in the UK is still increasing. Currently there are 40 000 cases diagnosed each year (1999). The mortality from breast cancer has been falling since the late 1980s. This is thought to be due to the therapeutic effect of Tamoxifen and more recently due to the beneficial effects of the National Breast Screening Programme (Figs 18.1 and 18.2).

### Risk factors

**Genetic**
Mutations in either of the two recognized breast cancer genes (BRCA1 and BRCA2) result in a very high chance of developing breast or ovarian cancer. Other genetic abnormalities associated with a higher than average breast cancer risk are Cowden's syndrome and ataxia telangiectasia.

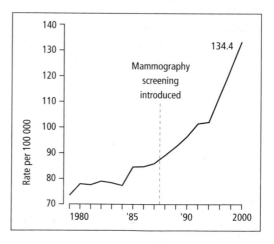

**Figure 18.1** Age standardized incidence of breast cancer in England and Wales.

## Hormonal

The following are associated with a higher than average risk of breast cancer: early menarche, late menopause, no full-term pregnancies, full term pregnancy occurring after the age of 40. Longer periods of breast feeding and multiple full-term pregnancies are associated with a lower incidence of breast cancer. The oral contraceptive pill has practically no effect on breast cancer risk. HRT is associated with a small increase in the risk of breast cancer which amounts to around 35% increase after 12 years of usage.

## Environmental

Radiation (such as that associated with the fall out from the atomic bombs in Japan) is associated with all sub-types of breast cancer. Alcohol increases the risk of breast cancer in a dose-dependent manner. Diet has a large effect on breast cancer risk. Diets rich in fresh fruit and vegetables are associated with a much lower risk of breast cancer (50% reduction). This risk reduction is probably partly related to vitamin C intake. Smoking is not related to breast cancer. The lowest incidence of breast cancer occurs in Japan, the highest risk in Western Europe and North America. Women migrating from one geographic region to another slowly develop the full breast cancer risk associated with their new environment.

## Presentation

Breast malignancy most commonly presents with a painless lump. Skin tethering is highly suggestive of malignancy. The characteristics of a malignant lump compared with a benign lump are compared in Table 18.1. For breast cancers around the nipple, inversion or distortion of the nipple together with nipple discharge may be presenting symptoms. Infrequently patients present with an enlarged axillary lymph node with no obvious palpable mass in the breast. Other less common symptoms and signs of breast cancer are peau d'orange, distortion of the shape of the breast, generalized enlargement of the breast, focal breast pain and skin changes (erythema or ulceration). Paget's disease of the nipple is always associated with an underlying malignancy. This may be invasive or *in situ* disease. Paget's disease may look similar to nipple eczema being dry and scaly or may be beefy red and weeping.

**Figure 18.2** Age standardized mortality rates from breast cancer in women aged 55–69 years in England and Wales.

**Table 18.1** Clinical features of some common breast lumps.

|  | **Fibrocystic** | **Cyst** | **Fibroadenoma** | **Cancer** |
|---|---|---|---|---|
| *Tender* | Yes | Yes | No | No |
| *Discrete* | No | Yes | Yes | Usually |
| *Surface* | No edge/surface | Smooth | Smooth | Irregular/smooth |
| *Consistency* | Normal to firm | Firm to hard | Firm | Firm to hard |
| *Shape* | Nodularity/ridge | Round | Round/elipse/lobulated | Rounded |
| *Overlying skin* | Normal | Normal | Normal | Tethering |
| *Multiple lesions* | Yes | Yes | Yes | No |

## Staging

- Stage 1: breast cancer confined to the breast.
- Stage 2: involvement of the breast and axillary lymph nodes.
- Stage 3: locally advanced disease involving the breast with muscle fixation or skin involvement.
- Stage 4: metastatic disease.

Breast cancer can be more accurately staged according to the TNM classification.

- **T** relates to the size of primary tumour:
  - T1 = 2 – 20 mm,
  - T2 = 21 – 50 mm,
  - T3 = 51 or more mm.
- **N** refers to the regional lymph node status:
  - N0 = node negative,
  - N1 = mobile ipsilateral nodes,
  - N2 = immobile, fixed or matted nodes,
  - N3 = internal mammary node involvement.
- The **M** classification whether there is metastatic disease that:
  - M0 = no detected metastases,
  - M1 = metastatic disease.

Primary breast cancer is usually simply staged by performing:

- chest X-ray to look for pleural or pulmonary disease;
- liver function test or a liver ultrasound looks for hepatic metastases;
- large tumours (over 4 cm) or high-grade tumours (3) would additionally have staging involving a bone scan.

## Investigation and diagnosis

Investigation of any breast lump is based on the principle of triple diagnosis.

- Clinical assessment.
- Radiological imaging.
- Cytological or histological verification.

It is only if all these three types of assessment are entirely benign that a lump can be left without further investigation.

Invasive breast cancer shows up on a mammogram by producing either:

- a dense (white) mass,
- an area of distortion of the breast parenchyma or microcalcification.

On mammography, a malignant mass will appear spiculate with ill-defined edges. Breast distortion may occur without a mass, particularly in the case of a lobular carcinoma. Malignant microcalcification is focal, relatively fine and heterogeneous. The sensitivity of mammography for detecting a malignancy is around 85%.

An *ultrasound scan* will show a malignant mass as an echo-poor focal area that interrupts the normal transverse breast architecture. The lesion is ill-defined and is usually taller rather than wider. There may be a dense acoustic shadow. The sensitivity of breast ultrasound for the diagnosis of malignancy is between 75% and 80%.

*Needle cytology* is carried out without local anaesthetic. The specimen, which usually amounts to just a drop or two of blood-stained-tissue fluid, is spread onto glass microscope slides. These can be air dried. No immediate staining is required although this is carried out later in the laboratory. The breast cytopathologist requires five clusters of duct epithelial cells to be able to make a definitive diagnosis. An alternative to fine needle aspiration cytology (FNAC) is core-needle biopsy. This is now being carried out much more frequently as it gives additional information regarding the architecture of the lesion. It is performed under local anaesthetic with a core-needle-biopsy gun and needle varying between 14 and 11 gauge. It is possible to perform cytological examination of the cells on the surface of the core by simply rolling the tissue core between two microscope slides. This gives an accurate answer in less than an hour (touch imprint cytology). A core biopsy will require at least 48 hours for histological examination.

*Magnetic resonance imaging* (MRI) may be used to diagnose breast malignancy. It is particularly sensitive (95–100%) but the specificity is much lower (65–70%). Examination needs to be carried out with contrast during the first half of the menstrual period. Benign breast lesions such as fibroadenomas may enhance, but the enhancement characteristics are generally different in benign compared to malignant lesions.

## Treatment

### General strategy

Breast cancer, when confined to the breast or the axillary lymph nodes, is curable. Metastatic breast cancer is not. More than 90% of patients present with primary breast cancer (stage 1 or 2) with no evidence of metastatic disease. However, at this stage micro-metastases are probably present in some patients and these are often the patients who later relapse systemically. The treatment of primary breast cancer is therefore to eradicate the malignancy from the breast and axillary lymph nodes and to provide some type of systemic (adjuvant) treatment to try and eliminate any micro-metastases. The presence or absence of micro-metastases is not known in any one individual patient although the likelihood of micro-metastases can be estimated by taking into consideration the lymph node status and the size and grade of the tumour.

When considering the treatment of primary breast cancer think of three anatomical boxes, each of which will receive its own treatment. The treatment strategy for each box has either no or only marginal impact on the other two anatomical areas and each should therefore be formulated independently. The treatment of primary breast cancer should therefore involve adequate treatment of the:
- breast itself (breast primary);
- axillary lymph nodes;
- micro-metastases.

### The treatment of a breast primary

#### Surgical treatment
The most effective modality utilized in the treatment of breast cancer is the surgical treatment of the primary. The aim of surgical treatment is to achieve complete removal of the primary lesion together with any satellite lesions and any associated ductal carcinoma *in situ* (DCIS). Mastectomy is one effective way of removing a primary lesion although it is now well established that a lumpectomy, if carried out in conjunction with breast

radiotherapy (breast conserving therapy), is as effective as mastectomy both in terms of local control and overall survival. Lumpectomy is not appropriate for large tumours (generally over 4 cm), for multifocal tumours (unless the lesions are small and closely applied to one another) or lesions associated with very extensive ductal carcinoma *in situ*. For these cases and for patients who cannot, for one reason or another, undergo breast radiotherapy (serious heart or lung disease) mastectomy is the only safe option. In the case of large tumours primary chemotherapy (neo-adjuvant chemotherapy) can be employed at the outset to shrink the tumour to a size that is amenable to a lumpectomy and radiotherapy.

Opinion is still divided over the importance of clear surgical margins following breast lumpectomy. It is certain that widely involved margins are associated with a much higher rate of local recurrence. Focally involved margins or close margins (1 mm or less) are associated with a small increase in local recurrence rates compared with widely clear margins.

Mastectomy as performed by Halstead in the early part of the twentieth century involved removal of not only the breast but also the axillary nodes and pectoralis minor and pectoralis major. This was termed a radical mastectomy. It is now known that it is not necessary to remove either of the pectoral muscles since primary breast cancer only infrequently infiltrates the skeletal muscle. Removal of the breast and axillary lymph nodes is termed a modified radical mastectomy.

#### Breast radiotherapy
Radiotherapy to the breast following lumpectomy is a critical and irreplaceable part of breast-conserving therapy for primary breast cancer. If breast radiotherapy is not possible then mastectomy is the only safe alternative. The radiotherapy course takes 6 weeks and involves daily fractions (30 fractions). It is usually associated with a skin reaction that comprises erythema and sometimes peeling of the skin.

Breast radiotherapy can be given to the chest wall following a mastectomy. It is shown to be effective in reducing local recurrence rates in the patients with positive axillary nodes, high grade tumours and large tumours. There is some evidence that irradiation of the supraclavicular fossa and internal mammary nodes in addition to the chest wall may produce a small improvement in overall survival.

## Treatment of the axilla

All patients with primary breast cancer (stage 1 and 2) undergo surgery to the axilla. In most instances this involves axillary nodal clearance to level 2 or 3. At least 10 to 50 lymph nodes are removed. This surgical procedure achieves two main functions. First of all axillary node clearance is a very effective means of controlling potential axillary disease. The likelihood of axillary recurrence without any axillary treatment is around 30–35%, whereas following axillary node clearance the risks of recurrence are only around 1%.

Axillary node clearance is also very important in staging the axilla. The status of the axillary nodes is the best prognostic indicator that is available in patients with breast cancer, and other aspects of the treatment such as adjuvant systemic treatment and chest wall radiotherapy are decided based largely on the axillary node status. Not only the presence or absence of axillary disease but the number of axillary nodes that are involved is important. Axillary nodal clearance therefore provides invaluable information.

Axillary node clearance is associated with significant morbidity. The most serious problem associated with this type of surgery is arm lymphoedema. This occurs to a variable degree but is serious enough to impact on a patient's lifestyle in around 15% of cases. Arm lymphoedema is more common in older women and in women who are overweight. Other problems following axillary nodal clearance include an alteration in the sensation of the skin of the upper arm due to interruption of the intercostobrachial nerve, pain in the arm and an increased susceptibility to serious infections in the ipsilateral upper limb.

Less radical axillary node dissection may be undertaken (level 1) but it is not entirely clear whether this makes very much impact on the postoperative morbidity. A new alternative is sentinel node biopsy. In this technique blue dye or an isotope labelled colloid tracer are injected close to the breast primary and are used to identify one or two axillary lymph nodes that are termed sentinel nodes. In theory, if the sentinel nodes are clear of metastatic disease then all the other axillary nodes are also negative and full axillary clearance is not required. Sentinel node biopsy is associated with much lesser morbidity since only one or two lymph nodes are removed. Of course if the sentinel node is affected by metastatic disease a second operation is required to complete the axillary clearance. Sentinel node biopsy has the potential for avoiding axillary clearance in more than 50% of patients with breast cancer but the accuracy of the technique and the consequences of sentinel node biopsy on overall survival have still to be assessed.

## Adjuvant systemic treatment

Adjuvant systemic therapy aims to eliminate any micro-metastatic disease that may be present but undetectable at the time of primary diagnosis. Adjuvant systemic treatment is given following primary breast surgery and involves hormonal treatment, chemotherapy or both.

### Adjuvant chemotherapy

Adjuvant chemotherapy is usually given as soon after primary breast surgery as is safe (2–3 weeks). New combinations of chemotherapy drugs that are normally used are either CMF (Cyclophosphamide, Methotrexate or 5-Flourouracil) or FEC (5-Flourouracil, Epirubicin and Cyclophosphamide). Usually six cycles of this treatment are given. Depending on the regime employed there is a 3 or 4 week gap between each cycle meaning that chemotherapy continues for between 4.5 and 6 months. Common side effects include tiredness, nausea, hair loss, stomatitis and infection. Adjuvant chemotherapy is much more effective in younger (pre-menopausal) women and in women who are node positive. It is rarely used in women over the age of 70 as there is little evidence of its efficacy in this age group. In younger women these drug combinations may cause infertility and this side effect needs to be very carefully explained to patients.

### Adjuvant hormone therapy

Hormone therapy is effective in breast cancer because at least 75% of breast malignancies are composed of cells which depend primarily on oestrogen as a growth factor. These tumours are identifiable by immunohistochemical staining to reveal the oestrogen receptor. It is only breast cancers that express the oestrogen receptor that are amenable to adjuvant hormonal treatment.

The most common hormonal agent used in the adjuvant setting is Tamoxifen. Tamoxifen is a selective oestrogen receptor blocker which fortunately effectively blocks the oestrogen receptor in breast duct epithelial and breast cancer cells. Tamoxifen is used in the adjuvant setting for a period of 5 years following surgery. It has a generally benign side effect profile and has only one significant drug interaction (with Warfarin). Common side effects are menopausal symptoms such as hot flushes and night sweats. The two serious side effects associated with Tamoxifen use are slightly increased incidence of endometrial carcinoma and a low incidence of deep venous thrombosis and pulmonary embolism. Adjuvant Tamoxifen reduces the rate of breast cancer recurrence by around a third and also reduces the chance of developing a primary breast cancer in the opposite breast by 35–40%.

The aromatase inhibitor class of drugs are currently being advocated and trialled as adjuvant treatments in primary breast cancer. It appears that they are slightly more effective than Tamoxifen. The drugs include Anastrozole, Letrozole and Exemestane. They work by blocking the production of oestradiol from adrenal precursors in peripheral adipose tissue. The production of oestradiol in the ovaries is not dependent on aromatase and the aromatase inhibitors are therefore only effective in postmenopausal women. They have a better side effect profile than Tamoxifen and in particular do not increase the incidence of endometrial carcinoma.

Measures that effectively reduce circulating oestradiol in premenopausal women are also effective as adjuvant treatments. These include

bilateral oophorectomy or Zoladex. Zoladex is a GnRH agonist which suppresses oestrogen secretion in the ovary. It is given by Depo injection either every one or three months. For premenopausal women it can be given in addition to Tamoxifen with enhanced effect. Zoladex or oophorectomy drastically reduce the circulating oestradiol in young women and both are associated with significant bone loss.

## Ductal carcinoma *in situ*

*Pathology*

It is now established that ductal carcinoma *in situ* (DCIS) is the precursor lesion to invasive breast cancer. The individual cells are derived from the breast duct epithelium and are similar morphologically to those found in invasive breast cancer. The critical fact that differentiates DCIS from invasive breast cancer is the lack of invasion. The atypical cells that characterize DCIS remain within the breast ducts and as a consequence do not have the ability to spread to either the regional lymph nodes or to cause metastatic disease. As with invasive breast cancer DCIS is divided into three histological grades (low, intermediate and high grade). The higher grade of DCIS particularly can be associated with cell necrosis and subsequent secondary calcium deposition. This ductal microcalcification is detectable on mammography and is the most common way for DCIS to be diagnosed.

*Natural history*

The natural history of DCIS depends on the grade of the malignant change. High-grade DCIS is very likely to develop into invasive malignancy over a fairly short term. When it does so it develops into higher grade invasive carcinoma (usually grade III). Low-grade DCIS (various types) may never turn into invasive carcinoma, the progression towards invasive disease is much slower, and if invasive disease does occur it is usually of low grade (grade I).

*Presentation and diagnosis*

It is unusual for DCIS to form a palpable mass. Most patients who are diagnosed with DCIS have only a mammographic abnormality, usually consisting of microcalcification of the ductal type. This is typically focal, fine and heterogeneous with branching forms. Suspicious microcalcification is further investigated with stereotactic core needle biopsy or mammotome biopsy.

*Treatment*

Ductal carcinoma *in situ* is confined to the breast. No treatment to the axillary lymph nodes is required. There is no chance of metastatic disease as long as there is no invasive breast malignancy. For this reason the treatment of DCIS does not involve adjuvant systemic treatment such as chemotherapy.

The principle treatment modality for DCIS is surgery. Complete excision with clear margins is required. This may be achieved by mastectomy (for extensive areas of DCIS) or by local excision (for focal areas of DCIS measuring less than 4 cm). Following local excision, breast radiotherapy further reduces the chance of recurrence. For patients with low-grade DCIS the chance of recurrence is anyway very low and radiotherapy is not usually given. It is, however, normally part of the treatment for high grade DCIS. Patients with intermediate grade DCIS may or may not have breast radiotherapy depending on the size of the lesion and the margins. The recurrence rate for DCIS following mastectomy is 1%. The recurrence rate for high grade DCIS following wide excision is between 25% and 30%. If radiotherapy is used in addition to local surgery the recurrence rate is approximately halved. Recurrence of DCIS is in the form of *in situ*

disease in 50% of cases and in the form of invasive breast cancer in the other 50%.

## Breast cancer screening

Breast cancer screening using mammography is a good example of effective population screening. In the UK it has been offered to women between the age of 50 and 70. Screening involves mammograms without clinical examination performed at three yearly intervals. Breast screening using mammography has proven to be effective between the ages of 40 and 50 but more frequent mammography (annual) is required. This is not currently part of the NHS Screening Programme.

Breast cancer screening using mammography can be made more sensitive in a number of ways. The mammograms can be double reported (reviewed independently by two radiologists) and the X-rays can be carried out in two perpendicular views on each screening visit rather than as a single view. These changes are expensive but are gradually being introduced into the National Breast Screening programme. In the UK women over 70 can still elect to continue with mammographic screening but they have to request this by contacting the screening unit themselves.

## Web links

More information on benign and malignant breast conditions can be obtained at www.breast-cancer-information.com.

---

**Self-assessment**

**18.1** What are the four stages of Breast Cancer Screening?

**18.2** List the risk factors for breast cancer.

**18.3** Which of the following agents are used in adjuvant therapy?

    (a) Zoladex.

    (b) Anastrazole.

    (c) Cisplatin.

    (d) Provera.

    (e) Methotrexate.

**18.4** List the three main areas that should be treated in a case of primary breast cancer.

# Chapter 19

# Screening for gynaecological cancer

## Cervix

The best known screening service is for carcinoma of the cervix; this should be a preventable disease because:

• there is usually a phase of premalignancy, dysplasia or intraepithelial neoplasia;

• the cervix is a relatively accessible organ to examine;

• cells can easily be obtained in the premalignant phase.

The biggest problem is getting to women liable to develop a carcinoma of the cervix to take part in the screening.

## Current position

In the UK screening is aimed at all women at risk from within five years of starting sexual activity (usually 15–20 years) to the age of 65 years. After this the development of premalignant lesions is rare.

The screening service for cervical cancer aims to recall women aged 20–64 years every 3 years. It is possible that some carcinomas will grow very rapidly, but for the majority a cervical smear performed every three years will pick up the pathological warning signs. Three-yearly smears detect 91% of the premalignant conditions. Increasing the smear frequency to yearly only improves the pick-up rate to 93%; trebling the work load thus improves results by only 2% (see Box 19.1).

Smear tests are offered at most places where women attend for obstetric or gynaecological procedures. Thus they may be done at:

• GP surgeries;

• antenatal clinics;

• family planning clinics;

• genitourinary medicine clinics;

• gynaecology out-patient clinics;

• well-woman clinics.

Since the average age group of women with premalignant conditions is older than the reproductive age group, the most appropriate place for smear tests is the GP surgery, using a well-organized computer-generated record system with an age–sex register (call–recall system from Health Authority); those who do not accept their invitation must be reinvited. There must also be some system of ensuring that the results are returned to the woman promptly. This is now achieved through computer technology so that each woman receives a letter saying either (a) that her result is normal or (b) that she should contact her doctor. All smear results are sent to the woman's GP, irrespective of where the smear is taken.

This requires an enthusiastic GP service which is appropriately funded. In the UK, the National Health Service offers incentives to GPs to ensure that a high percentage (>85%) of those in the appropriate age groups have their smears at correct intervals.

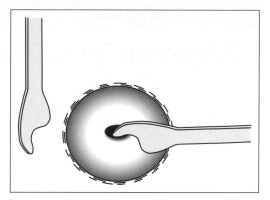

**Figure 19.1** Smear taken from a nulliparous cervix with the shaped end of an Aylesbury spatula.

## Taking a smear

The smear can be taken by anyone competent to perform a vaginal examination; thus it can be done by a gynaecologist, a GP, a community clinic doctor, a trained midwife or a nurse.

After discussion, the woman is positioned on the couch and a warmed speculum is passed to expose the cervix. A glass slide should be labelled prior to undertaking the examination. The slide is marked in pencil with the woman's name, date-of-birth, date-of-test and hospital number/NHS number if known. A spatula is then used to scrape the whole squamocolumnar junction (SCJ). If the external os is regular, the pointed end of a spatula can be passed into the canal and rotated by 360° (Fig. 19.1). If the cervical os is stenosed, the brush end of a cytobrush should be used (Fig. 19.2). This is common after surgery to the cervix for cervical abnormality or in postmenopausal women. The most commonly used spatula is the Aylesbury spatula with its elongated beak to go up the cervical canal.

The material removed on the tip of the spatula should be smeared onto the glass slide and fixed immediately to prevent the cells drying in air. The slide can go straight into the fixative medium or be sprayed with the fixative aerosol which dries rapidly, fixing the cells and nuclei. The slide can

**Figure 19.2** Smear taken from a stenosed cervix with the brush end of a cytobrush.

then go to the laboratory through the post or by messenger.

The cytopathologist will need certain basic information about the woman in order to interpret the findings carefully.
• The age of the woman.
• Menstrual cycle and date of last menstrual period.
• Any irregular vaginal bleeding.
• Is she pregnant?
• Any current hormone therapy (including oral contraception)?
• Presence of intrauterine device.
• Clinical state of the cervix.

## Examination of the smear

Do not take a smear during menstruation for red cells obscure the epithelial cells at microscopic examination. However, if the woman has irregular bleeding it is impossible to avoid this. A note should be made to the pathologist if this occurs.

At the laboratory the smear is stained and examined by cytotechnicians. If any abnormality is detected, the smear will be passed to a cytopathologist.

*False negative results*

These occur when a woman has premalignant changes in her cells but these are not reported. Incidence is unknown but from data on women who do develop carcinoma of the cervix, it is probably between 10 and 30%. Causes include:
- error in taking the smear:
  (a) non-representative sample of cells;
  (b) not from SCJ;
- a misinterpretation in the laboratory itself;
- incorrect typing of the report from the laboratory.

*False positive results*

This happens when the smear is reported as having a greater degree of malignant change than exists. This is caused by:
- misinterpretation by the cytologist;
- infection;
- pregnancy;
- incorrect typing of results on the report;
- incorrect interpretation of the report by the clinician.

## Grading the smears

Originally the grading of smears was according to the classification of Papanicolaou. This has changed so that cytological grading is different from histological grading (p. 261). Cytologists grade the smear according to the appearances of the cells they see. For a satisfactory smear they must receive a sample with cells from the SCJ—in other words cells that are undergoing metaplasia from columnar to squamous cells since these are the cells most likely to undergo neoplastic change. The features assessed are:
- Nuclear/cytoplasmic ratio (amount of cytoplasm should be twice that of the nucleus).
- Shape of the nucleus (poikilocytosis).
- Density of the nucleus (koilocytosis).
  Other features that may be present:
- Inflammation—the presence of leucocytes.
- Infection—presence of *Trichomonas*, *Candida*, diplococci.
- Evidence of mitosis.
  The cytologist will classify the smear accordingly:
- Insufficient for adequate assessment—no cells seen from the SCJ.
- Inflammatory—excessive numbers of leucocytes, *Candida* or *Trichomonas* seen.
- Borderline—some nuclear changes but indeterminate.
- Mild dyskaryosis—cells have irregular enlarged nuclei with a change in the chromatin pattern. The nuclear membranes may be slightly irregular.
- Moderate dyskaryosis—as mild, but the nucleus is enlarged to <50% of the cell size.
- Severe dyskaryosis—the nucleus is enlarged to >50% of the cell size. The nuclei vary in size and shape and the nuclear membranes are irregular.
- Possible invasive carcinoma—mitotic figures seen.

The relationship of the degree of dyskaryosis to the histological findings at biopsy or removal of the affected area is not absolute.

All women with a smear showing mild/moderate/severe dyskaryosis/invasion should be referred to a colposcopy clinic where the cervix can be examined under magnification. Inflammatory smears should be treated with antibiotics (metronidazole 400 mg t.d.s. for 7 days) or antifungal agents as appropriate and the smear repeated three to six months later. All women with a smear showing mild dyskaryosis or greater should be referred to colposcopy. Women with a borderline smear should have the smear repeated within 6 months. If the woman has two consecutive borderline or inadequate smears she should be referred to colposcopy. In addition, a woman who has had three abnormal smears in the preceding 5 years, that may not have been consecutive, should be referred for colposcopy if she has not already been seen in a clinic (Box 19.2). All women with moderate or severe dysplasia or evidence of invasive carcinoma should be seen in the colposcopy clinic within six weeks of diagnosis.

It is very important when telling women the result of their smear test to emphasize that they do not have cancer but if nothing was done they could develop cancer in time. Treatment now will cure the problem in 98% of cases.

## Colposcopy

A speculum is passed and the cervix visualized as for a smear. 4% Acetic acid is painted onto the surface of the cervix with a cotton wool swab. Abnormal cells at the SCJ will stain white with this liquid because of their increased glycogen content (Acetowhite). The speed and the density of the white colour are proportional to the degree of abnormality. The abnormal areas are noted and drawn in diagrammatic form in the notes. Additional features that can be looked for that have been associated with microinvasive disease are:
• mosaicism (tile like formation of the cells);
• punctation (small dots on the surface of the cervix);
• new vessel formation (using a green light filter);
• the upper limit of the abnormality inside the cervical canal must be seen.

Iodine solution is then painted onto the cervix. Normal squamous epithelium will stain dark brown with this solution while abnormal cells and

normal columnar epithelium will remain unstained. This delineates the area more accurately but does not give an idea of how severe the lesion may be so acetic acid should always be used first.

Once the lesion has been defined a biopsy is taken and the treatments, with a local anaesthetic cervical block, may be:
• *Cryotherapy.* The abnormal area is frozen with a liquid nitrous oxide probe.
• *Laser.* Suitable for small mild/moderate lesions where the limits are clearly visible on the surface of the cervix.
• *Loop excision of the transformation zone (LETZ).* The abnormal area is removed using a red-hot loop (diathermy). This goes to a depth of 1 cm down the cervical canal ensuring that the whole of the transformation zone is removed. A large loop excision (LLETZ) is sometimes employed if the area is more extensive.

Suitable for extensive, moderate or severe lesions with no evidence of invasion.
• *Formal cone biopsy.* This has to be undertaken under general anaesthetic. A specially shaped knife is used bent inwards so that a cone of the cervix is removed to a depth of 1.5–2 cm. This is useful in cases where microinvasion is suspected and is the most likely procedure to cause later problems in pregnancy: either cervical incompetence or cervical stenosis.

## Cervical intraepithelial neoplasia (CIN)

This is a purely histological diagnosis. Biopsies or samples from a LLETZ or cone biopsy are graded into:
• CIN 1—the outer third of the epidermis contains cells with a reduced cytoplasmic/nuclear ratio and increased nuclear density.
• CIN 2—the outer two-thirds of the epidermis contains abnormal cells.
• CIN 3—the entire depth of the epidermis contains abnormal cells but the basement membrane is intact.
• Microinvasion—the entire depth of the epidermis contains abnormal cells and there are small breaches in the basement membrane with abnormal cells invading to a depth of <3 mm.

---

**Box 19.2 Indications for referral to colposcopy**

Two consecutive borderline smears
Mild dyskaryosis
Moderate dyskaryosis
Severe dyskaryosis
Three abnormal smears in the preceding 5 years that may not have been consecutive if she has not already been seen in a clinic
Two consecutive smears inadequate for assessment (particularly in postmenopausal women)
(British Society for Cervical Cancer Prevention 2003)

Following treatment, all women should have a repeat smear at 6 months and, if normal, check smears every year for 5 years.

## Effectiveness of cervical screening

If cervical screening were totally effective, carcinoma of the cervix would be eliminated. Approximately 1300 women still die annually from this condition in the UK so the cervical screening programme has obviously not been so effective. Countries with a more effective cervical screening programme than the UK's report a diminution in deaths from carcinoma of the cervix (Fig. 19.3).

In practice, no screening programme, however, can have perfect success in controlling disease because:
• screening may not reach all the population at risk;
• there will be false negatives;
• the infrequency of screening may miss a rapidly progressive case;
• treatment as a result of screening may be incorrectly given;
• the treatment that follows screening may not be effective;
• recurrences may occur after even apparently successful courses of treatment.

In actuality, the majority of women in the UK who now die from clinical carcinoma have never had a cervical smear.

Rapidly progressive cases are rare, but women with a carcinoma of the cervix can have had a normal smear performed within a year or so, but this is unusual. The more aggressive cases tend to occur in younger women and are often glandular in origin giving rise to adenocarcinoma rather than the more common squamous carcinoma. Glandular abnormalities are more difficult to detect on routine screening.

## Benefits of cervical screening

A screening programme should aim to benefit the individual first (Box 19.1) and then society.

Society, however, can reap benefits or disadvantages from extending the cervical screening programme. If priority is given to cervical screening, monies have to be diverted from other resources and other services curtailed.

The cost/benefits of different aspects of cervical cancer screening can be assessed; an example is the frequency with which smears are taken. The financial benefits to society of a successful cervical screening programme would be the avoidance of expenditure in treating advanced cancer and the extra years of productivity of people who have survived.

## Conclusion

In the UK, the cervical screening programme has reduced the incidence of deaths from cervical cancer but it is by no means perfect. In order to achieve a three-yearly smear for the 20 million women at risk, a more organized system of screening is now provided, but will take a few years to come into full effect.

## Ovary

Cancer of the ovary is a significant cause of premature death in women (Fig. 19.4). It is often diagnosed late because of its lack of symptoms and it commonly spreads quickly and widely (Chapter

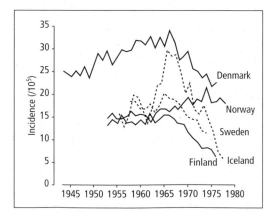

**Figure 19.3** Incidence of cervical cancer in the Nordic countries. Norway was the only country with no cervical cancer screening programme.

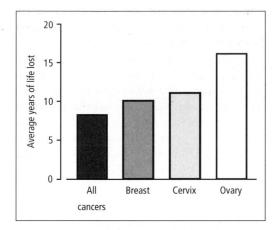

**Figure 19.4** Average years of life lost from different cancers.

20, p. 272). Hence, a screening test would be helpful. At present, two methods are possible.

• Serum marker CA125:

(a) 25% of those with ovarian carcinoma are positive five years before clinical diagnosis;

(b) 50% of those with ovarian carcinoma are positive one and a half years before clinical diagnosis.

(c) Additional serum markers for epithelial ovarian cancers include CA19.9 and CEA. Tumours of embryonic origin produce high levels of alphafetoprotein (AFP), lactase dehydrogenase (LDH) and/or human chorionic gonadotrophin (HCG).

• Ultrasound—high sensitivity for ovarian tumours, but:

(a) high false positive rate leading to unnecessary surgery;

(b) depends on experience and equipment which is not universally available;

(c) needs expert ultrasonographers who are not widely available.

Hence, serum CA125 is first screen and ultrasound the backup. A modest increase in earlier diagnosis could reduce death rates.

## Endometrium and vulva

Cancer of the endometrium and vulva tends to bleed early and so is detected on clinical grounds. There are no useful screening programmes.

## Breast

Screening for breast cancer—mammography—is considered in Chapter 18.

---

**Self-assessment**

**19.1** OSCE question: At the next station you are expected to take a cervical smear from the pelvic floor model provided. (Some universities may use gynaecologically trained assistants—women who have volunteered to assist in the training of medical students and doctors in performing vaginal examinations). Find a pelvic floor model and practise doing a vaginal examination and taking a cervical smear as if in an examination.

**19.2** Which of the following statements are true?

(a) Cervical screening should be offered to all women from age 20–64.

(b) Cervical screening gives an accurate diagnosis of the degree of cervical intraepithelial neoplasia.

(c) Women with an abnormal cervical smear graded moderate dyskaryosis should be referred for colposcopy.

(d) Women with an abnormal cervical smear graded moderate dyskaryosis should have a repeat smear performed 6 months later.

(e) Cervical smears taken during pregnancy are more likely to give a false negative result.

**19.3** A woman of 35 is referred to colposcopy with a smear result of severe dyskaryosis. Place the following description of the examination in the correct order.

(a) A biopsy is taken of an unstained area.

(b) A note is made of the areas that turn white and how rapidly they do so.

*Continued on p. 264.*

**Self-assessment** *Continued*

(c) The area is excised using loop diathermy under local anaesthetic.

(d) 4% acetic acid is painted onto the cervix.

(e) Iodine solution is painted onto the cervix and the unstained areas noted.

**19.4** List the six main reasons why the UK cervical screening programme is not 100% effective.

**19.5** List the five measures that have been put in place to try to improve the effectiveness of screening in the UK.

# Part 5

# The older woman

# Chapter 20

# Malignant gynaecological conditions

Cancer Registries collect data about every new case of malignant disease diagnosed in that catchment population. In the UK, data come from:

- hospital in-patient statistics;
- pathology registers;
- radiotherapy registers;
- oncological out-patient clinics;
- colposcopy clinics.

Registries also get death certificates of all cancer deaths in their population, so giving a measure of the total incidence of gynaecological cancer. Mortality rates of malignant disease come from death certificates and are published by the Office of Population Censuses and Surveys (OPCS). Thus, there are two distinct sources of epidemiological data about malignant disease:

- the living—prevalence and incidence rates;
- the dead—mortality rates.

In 2000, three gynaecological cancers featured amongst the 10 most frequent cancers among females. Some 5400 women were reported with new cases of carcinoma of the ovary, 2424 with invasive carcinoma of the cervix and 4730 with carcinoma of the body of the uterus. Thus, carcinoma of the ovary has overtaken that of the cervix in the last 20 years as the commonest gynaecological cancer. In 1973 registrations for cervix and ovary were respectively 4065 and 3819.

In 2001, the deaths reported of the same three cancers were 3807, 947 and 853. No precise mathematical ratios can be derived because the data are of different populations in time—however, this provides an indication of the poor prognosis of cancer of the ovary compared with that of the cervix/uterus; over the years the prognosis for ovarian cancer has remained unchanged. The five-year follow-up data are given in Table 20.1. These differences may represent:

- a real change in the prevalence of a condition;
- a more complete reporting system;
- better diagnostic facilities for making an early diagnosis.

There is a trend of increasing incidence of cervical cancer in younger women. There has been a 20-fold increase in the number of women aged under 35 presenting with cervical carcinoma. Many of these will have adenocarcinoma rather than squamous cell carcinoma which is harder to detect on routine screening and has a poorer prognosis. The numbers remain small and there is no evidence that the overall mortality for cervical cancer is increasing.

The geographical incidence of carcinoma of the cervix was highest in Central and Southern America, decreasing as it crossed Europe and Africa to Asia and the Far East. This apparent trend no longer exists. There are many local variations; for example, Portugal has a very high rate of carcinoma of the cervix while its close neighbour, Spain, has a very low one, yet their economic and social characteristics are very similar.

**Table 20.1** Approximate five-year survival rates for gynaecological cancer in Europe in 2000.

| Condition | Five-year survival rates (%) by stage | | | |
| --- | --- | --- | --- | --- |
| | I | II | III | IV |
| Carcinoma of the ovary | 95 | 70 | 40 | 31 |
| Carcinoma of the endometrium | 96 | 65 | 50 | 26 |
| Carcinoma of the cervix | 92 | 70 | 51 | 16 |

## Gynaecological cancer mortality rates

The standardized registration rates of women dying in 2000 of three major gynaecological malignancies show an increase in ovarian cancer cases in a decade, a reduction of endometrial cases, while cervical cancer cases stay the same. Such rates cannot be compared directly with incidence rates for the latter takes place many years before the former. Five-year survival rates after treatment may be a slightly more precise measure. Since cervical carcinoma may recur up to 10 years, a longer time interval than five years may be required. The 15-year survival rate is currently about 40%. There are few recurrences of carcinoma of the endometrium after five years and so that index is a reasonable one; one can say that about two-thirds of women with endometrial cancer are cured.

The survival rate of carcinoma of the ovary is poor and probably reflects the fact that only about a fifth of diagnosed patients are cured. It may be in the future that, with more drastic surgery and chemotherapy, this might be improved, but it is still mostly due to late diagnosis of the disease.

Subdividing these coarse five-year survival rates into stages gives a better idea of the problem. For example, in the UK most carcinoma of the cervix is either Stage I or Stage II when diagnosed compared with developing countries when it is either Stage III or even IV.

## Cancer of the cervix

Cancer of the cervix arises most frequently from the squamous epithelium at its junction with the columnar epithelium; it is predominantly a squamous carcinoma. A columnar cell type arises from the cervical glands inside the cervical canal, an adenocarcinoma. Malignant change may also arise in a cervical mucous polyp.

*Aetiology*
- Mainly in the age group 45 to 55.
- Rare in virgins.
- Coitus increases the risk:
  (a) very early coitus;
  (b) multiple sexual partners.
- Infection with the wart virus Types 16 and 18 and certain herpes.
- Rare in nuns, Jewesses and Arab women.
- More frequent in the lower social class groups; possibly hygienic factors may play a part.
- Cigarette smoking shows an associated higher risk.

*Pathology*
95% of the growths are squamous cell carcinomata from the squamocolumnar junction. About 5% are adenocarcinomata from the columnar cells inside the cervical canal.

Invasive cancers present as an ulceration of the cervix. In advanced cases, the cervix is replaced by an ulcerated, fungated mass of growth which is fixed to the surrounding structures. Spread may be:
- The vaginal fornices.
- The bladder.
- The body of the uterus.
- The broad ligaments which may cause obstruction of the lower ends of the ureters. A large blood vessel may be eroded causing severe haemorrhage.
- Lymphatic spread to the iliac, obturator, sacral, inguinal and para-aortic nodes.
- Bloodstream spread occurs comparatively late but may lead to metastases in the lungs, bones or elsewhere.

*Symptoms*
The symptoms of cancer of the cervix only begin when the surface of the growth becomes ulcerated. Hence, they appear later with endocervical growths. The chief symptom is a watery *discharge* (often offensive) and blood-stained discharge or bleeding, particularly after coitus. Later

frank, sometimes severe and continuous *bleeding* occurs, with the patient rapidly becoming anaemic.

### Physical signs

Early, the cervix feels hard and bleeds on touch. Later the cervix is ulcerated and friable. In advanced cases the vaginal vault is filled with an ulcerated mass and pieces of growth are detached by the examining finger; examination may provoke severe bleeding. In endocervical growths the cervix feels barrel-shaped.

The cervical smear may contain frankly malignant cells, but not always because the surface cells are often dead and atypical.

### Diagnosis

This depends on biopsy of the cervix. If the site and size of the lesion allow, a cone biopsy should be taken to include all the squamocolumnar junction and most of the cervical canal.

### Staging investigations

Staging for cervical carcinoma includes:
- Examination under anaesthetic, including rectovaginal examination to assess the size of the tumour, parametrial spread, extension into the rectovagina; septum.
- Cystoscopy and sigmoidoscopy to assess bladder and bowel involvement.
- Biopsy of the suspicious area.
- Chest X-ray.
- Intravenous urography (IVU).

Computerized tomography (CT) or magnetic resonance imaging (MRI) may be offered if available to give further information on tumour size and nodal involvement, but does not alter the FIGO staging which is determined by the above investigations.

### Differential diagnosis

Mainly from:
- cervical ectropion;
- tuberculosis may present in a proliferative form;
- other chronic granulomatous infections.

### Staging

Box 20.1 shows the clinical staging of cancer of the cervix.

---

| Box 20.1 | Staging of cancer of the cervix |
|---|---|
| Stage 0 | Intraepithelial carcinoma (carcinoma *in situ*). The growth remains within the epithelial layer of the cervix |
| Stage 1 | Cancer clinically confined to the cervix |
| Stage 2 | Growth has spread to the upper two-thirds of the vagina or into the parametrium but not as far as the pelvic wall |
| Stage 3 | The growth has spread to the lower one-third of the vagina or into the parametrium as far as the lateral pelvic wall |
| Stage 4 | Metastases have formed beyond the pelvis or growth has involved the bladder or the rectum |

---

This is a clinical classification; in fact 20% of Stage 1 cases are found at subsequent operation to have metastases in the lymph glands (i.e. would be Stage 3).

## Treatment of invasive carcinoma

The choice of treatment depends on many factors.
- The age and general condition of the patient.
- The extent and type of the lesion.
- Ideally all patients with cancer of the cervix should be seen by a gynaecological oncologist and a radiotherapist for consideration of all the factors of the individual case.
- The experience, resources and personal preference of the oncology team.

Renal function should be assessed by blood urea and intravenous urography. Urinary infection is often present and should be treated. Anaemia may also need treatment.

Ultrasound and CT scan may help identify spread in the pelvis or to lymph nodes.

Examination under anaesthesia is essential.
- The clinical extent of the growth is assessed.
- Hysteroscopy and curettage is performed and a biopsy taken in all cases, even those which seem the most obvious clinically.
- A rectal examination is important to exclude invasion of the rectum itself. The clinical extent of growth in the parametrium is also more easily felt rectally.

• Cystoscopy excludes involvement of the bladder.

## Radiotherapy

This is the first line of attack in advanced stages or in poor-risk patients. It cannot be used if the bladder is invaded owing to the risk of fistula formation.

Caesium is applied by various techniques; the most common is the Stockholm technique or one of its modifications. A tube containing 50 mg of caesium is put into the uterus and two ovoids or flat boxes containing a further 60 mg are packed into the vagina. Care is taken to give a minimal dose of radiation to the rectum. The caesium is left for 22 hours and three applications are usually given, the second a week after the first and the third two weeks after the second.

This older regimen has been replaced by the use of the cathetron; an empty container is inserted into the uterus and vaginal fornices and clamped into position. Its position is checked and several high-intensity cobalt sources are after-loaded and deliver the irradiation. The apparatus is contained in a sealed unit and radiation delivered by remote control, thus eliminating danger to staff.

Caesium may be used as a preliminary to surgery or combined with external radiotherapy to the lateral pelvic walls. Advanced techniques of irradiation such as cobalt or the linear accelerator may be used in advanced disease to give total pelvic irradiation.

## Surgery

Surgical excision is suitable for all Stage 1 and some Stage 2 cases. A Wertheim's radical abdominal hysterectomy is the treatment of choice removing the uterus, tubes, ovaries, broad ligaments and parametrium, the upper half or two-thirds of the vagina and the regional lymph glands (Fig. 20.1).

## Chemotherapy

Increasingly multiagent chemotherapy with cis-

**Figure 20.1** The extent of pelvic tissue removed at a Wertheim's radical abdominal hysterectomy.

platinum, vinblastin and bleomycin is used in combination with radiotherapy.

## Pelvic exenteration

In some advanced cases where carcinoma of the cervix has spread, extensive surgery must be undertaken as the only hope of cure for the patient. It is reserved mainly for patients in good general health with extensive disease involving the bladder or rectum.

*Anterior exenteration* consists of removing the uterus and adnexae, the vagina, the bladder and the urethra. The ureters are implanted into the colon or into an ileal loop opening on to the abdominal wall.

*Posterior exenteration* removes the uterus and adnexae, the vagina, descending colon and rectum, leaving a colostomy. This is suitable for posterior growths involving the colon or rectum.

In *total exenteration* the two operations are combined and the patient left with an ileal loop and a colostomy.

## Results of treatment

These are best assessed by a 5-year follow-up which shows in most centres a cure rate of up to 80% with Stage 1 and about 10% with Stage 4.

This range of cure emphasizes the value of early diagnosis and treatment; the tragedy is that so many women do not receive treatment until the disease is advanced.

## Complications of treatment

Complications may follow treatment with irradiation or surgery. Radiotherapy treatment can flare up infection in the renal tract, or exacerbate pelvic abscess. Caesium proctitis may prove troublesome.

The mortality risk at the operation of Wertheim's hysterectomy is now only 1% in experienced hands. In addition to any complications of a severe abdominal operation, there is a risk of ureteric fistula which has been reported as high as 8% of patients submitted to Wertheim's hysterectomy after irradiation.

## Palliation

When nothing can be done to cure the patient of cancer, everyone concentrates on making her last weeks or months as comfortable as possible. Death may occur mercifully from uraemia or haemorrhage, but many women suffer severe and intractable pain in the final stages of the disease.

Analgesics must be used liberally in sufficient amounts to relieve pain. Epidural anaethesia and/or nerve blocks may be helpful. Chordotomy is sometimes used in intractable pain. If there is severe rectal pain, colostomy may be necessary. Morphia and heroin are of great help here and must be retained in the profession's therapeutic armamentarium, prescribing and dispensing being under strict control. Addiction is not a concern in those with advanced pelvic cancer and dosage should be liberal once started.

## Malignant tumours of the uterus

### Choriocarcinoma

A malignant tumour arising from chorionic tissue following a hydatidiform mole, abortion or pregnancy and is considered in Chapter 7.

### Endometrial carcinoma

*Aetiology*
• Mean age of presentation is 56 years. Four-fifths of the women are menopausal and it is rare under the age of 40.
• Associated with hyperoestrogenic states:
 (a) obesity;
 (b) diabetes;
 (c) late menopause;
 (d) prolonged use of unopposed oestrogens;
 (e) oestrogen secreting tumours;
 (f) long-term tamoxifen usage.
• May be associated with:
 (a) previous pelvic irradiation;
 (b) lower parity.

*Pathology*
• Usually an adenocarcinoma.
• More often well differentiated than anaplastic.
• May be associated with squamous metaplasia where, if excessive, becomes an adenocanthoma.
• May be associated with pyometra or haematometra, secondary to cervical stenosis.
• Spreads by invasion through the myometrium and by filling the uterine cavity.
• Spreads via cervical lymphatic drainage involving the iliac and para-aortic nodes.
• Tumours of upper uterus may spread along the lymphatics in the round ligaments to the deep inguinal nodes.
• In advanced cases, the bloodstream spread may carry to the lungs, liver and to the bones.

*Symptoms*
• Postmenopausal bleeding: this symptom should be assumed to be caused by carcinoma of the endometrium until proved otherwise.
• Bloodstained discharge.
• Irregular bleeding.

*Signs*
• Less commonly, uterine enlargement.
• Bleeding through the cervix.

*Investigations*
• Ultrasound to assess dimensions of any tumour and to show endometrial thickness.

*Staging*

Box 20.2 shows the clinical staging of endometrial cancer.

*Treatment*

The treatment of uterine carcinoma is usually surgical.

• The surgical management of well differentiated carcinoma involves a total abdominal hysterectomy and bilateral salpingo-oophorectomy (TAH/BSO). The role of pelvic lymphaedectomy is being assessed in the MRC ASTEC trial.

• In women with high grade disease (grade 3 or grade 2 with >2 cm invasion), or in women with >50% myometrial invasion or cervical involvement, or in women with adverse pathological subtypes (adenosquamous, clear cell or papillary serous carcinoma), a full staging laparotomy involving omental biopsy, lymph node sampling and inspection of the upper abdomen is required in addition to the TAH/BSO.

• Radical hysterectomy is indicated if there is cervical involvement.

Radiotherapy is rarely employed alone unless the patient is unable to withstand a surgical procedure. It may be used as adjuvant treatment if adverse factors are identified in the pathology review:

• >50% myometrial invasion;

• poorly differentiated high grade disease;

• adenosquamous, clear cell or papillary serous carcinoma;

• positive pelvic lymph nodes.

The pelvic lymph node status determines whether radiotherapy is given to the vault alone or to the vault and the pelvic side wall.

Hormone therapy—progestogens inhibit the rate of growth and spread of endometrial carcinoma.

## Rarer tumours

## Sarcoma

Occurs in:

• childhood as sarcoma botryoides;

• postmenopausal women with a fibroid.

It is highly malignant, radioresistant, spreads by the bloodstream and is diagnosed late. Treatment is a total abdominal hysterectomy and bilateral salpingo-oophorectomy. Recurrences are treated with multiagent chemotherapy.

## Mixed mesodermal tumours

These arise from mesodermal cells of the ovarian ducts and may contain primitive muscle cells, myxomatous tissue, cartilage and glands. They present with abnormal bleeding and treatment is by hysterectomy or occasionally by exenteration. Vascular spread is common, prognosis poor.

## Carcinoma of the ovary

Primary carcinoma of the ovary is now the commonest malignant tumour found in gynaecology in the UK and an important cause of death in women, accounting for some 4000 deaths annually in England and Wales. It is a disease of middle and old age with 90% of cases in women above 45 years. It is often diagnosed late because of its lack of symptoms and it commonly metastasizes quickly and widely. Hence, a screening test would be helpful (Chapter 19).

Risk factors relate to ovulatory history and the past activity of the germinal epithelium:

• increased risk—no pregnancy;

• decreased risk—many pregnancies—use of oral contraceptives.

| Box 20.2 | Staging of endometrial cancer |
|---|---|
| Stage 1 | Carcinoma confined to the body of the uterus |
| Stage 2 | Extension to the cervix |
| Stage 3 | Extension outside the uterus but within the true pelvis |
| Stage 4 | Involvement of the:<br>(a) bladder<br>(b) rectum<br>(c) extension outside the true pelvis |

Ovarian carcinoma may be cystic, arising usually from a benign cyst, or solid. Solid epithelial carcinoma may be papillary or an adenocarcinoma, an undifferentiated carcinoma. It may arise in one of the special ovarian tumours such as granulosa cell tumour or dysgerminoma. Although accounting for only 1–2% of tumours, the latter are treatable using modern chemotherapy.

## Spread of ovarian carcinoma

The main route of spread of carcinoma of the ovary is transcoelomically via the general peritoneal cavity, to the greater omentum and the peritoneum of the pouch of Douglas in particular. Ascites is frequent. Malignant tumours are often bilateral. Spread by lymphatics leads to involvement of the para-aortic glands; further spread may involve the supraclavicular glands. Bloodstream spread is unusual, death generally occurs from complications resulting from massive transcoelomic peritoneal secondaries. Staging is shown in Box 20.3.

## Metastatic ovarian tumours

The ovary is a frequent site for secondary malignancy because of its rich blood supply. Adenocarcinoma is the commonest and the primary site may be the uterus, the other ovary, breast, stomach or large bowel. Secondary tumours in the ovary generally reproduce the cell structure of the primary growth.

The *Krukenberg tumour* is an uncommon form of secondary carcinoma of the stomach or large bowel. The ovaries are enlarged by solid tumours, usually bilateral, which may reach 20 cm. Histologically they are characterized by the presence of signet ring cells which have undergone mucoid degeneration so that the nucleus is pushed to one side by a droplet of mucin.

Possibly a small number of Krukenberg tumours are primary in the ovary; patients have been known to survive for many years after removal of Krukenberg tumours with no primary tumour found despite extensive investigation. This is not inconsistent with a microscopic slow-growing primary growth somewhere in the gastrointestinal tract which cures itself.

---

**Box 20.3  Staging classification of ovarian carcinoma**

| | |
|---|---|
| Stage I | Tumour limited to the ovaries |
| IA | Tumour limited to one ovary |
| IB | Tumour limited to both ovaries |
| IC | IA or IB with capsule ruptured<br>or<br>surface involvement<br>or<br>malignant cells in ascites/peritoneal washings |
| Stage II | Tumour involves one or both ovaries with pelvic spread |
| IIA | To tubes or uterus |
| IIB | To other pelvic tissues |
| IIC | IIA or IIB with malignant cells in ascites/peritoneal washings |
| Stage III | Tumour involvement of abdominal cavity |
| IIIA | Microscopic peritoneal metastasis beyond pelvis |
| IIIB | Macroscopic peritoneal metastasis >2 cm diameter<br>or<br>involvement of retroperitoneal or inguinal nodes |
| IIIC | Tumour in pelvis with involvement of small bowel<br>or<br>omentum |
| Stage IV | Distant metastases<br>Liver<br>Bowel<br>Pleural fluid with malignant cells |

---

## Investigation of ovarian tumours

*Imaging*
• Ultrasound scan—can reveal the size of the ovarian cyst as well as suspicious features of malignancy which include solid as well as cystic areas, spread through the capsule of the cyst/ovary, papillary growths within the cyst.

• CT/MRI scan of the abdomen and pelvis—more accurately delineates the spread of disease showing peritoneal deposits, omental deposits, para-aortic node involvement and/or liver metastases, ureteric obstruction (rare in ovarian cancer).
• Chest X-ray—shows pleural effusions and/or hilar lymphadenopathy.

*Blood tests*
• Tumour markers—CA125, CA199, CEA. If any of these are raised they are used postoperatively to track the success of treatment and the onset of recurrence.
• Liver function tests to detect spread to the liver.
• Urea and electrolytes.
• Full blood count.
The latter two do not help in staging the disease but are important for preoperative assessment.

## Treatment of ovarian tumours

The treatment of malignant ovarian tumours is surgical removal as soon as the tumour is diagnosed. If the tumour is apparently malignant and where ascites is present, laparotomy should always be undertaken. Ascites may be associated with a benign tumour such as a fibroma, and even if there are metastases the prognosis is not hopeless. It may be possible to remove secondary masses in the omentum and, if the primary tumour is removed, secondaries sometimes regress. An ovarian tumour, even if very large, is best removed intact. Tapping the fluid carries a risk of spilling the contents and contaminating the peritoneal cavity.

*Carcinoma of the ovary* should be treated initially by surgery which should involve total hysterectomy, bilateral salpingo-oophorectomy and omentectomy, though in young women a normal, uninvolved ovary might be left. In advanced cases, as much tumour as possible should be removed at a debulking operation and the greater omentum should be excised. A search should be made for peritoneal metastases, including those on the upper and under surface of the liver. A CT or MRI scan to check that the peritoneal cavity is free from secondary deposits may be carried out three to six months after the original operation.

Even in apparently advanced disease the ultimate prognosis appears to be improved by operative removal of the main tumour masses. The first operation offers the best chance of cure. It should be done by an experienced gynaecological oncologist, preferably working in a specialist centre of gynaecologic oncology, who will do the widest excision with the least damage to ureters, bladder or intestines.

Radiotherapy is not much used in the management of ovarian cancer; the tumours are rarely radiosensitive and radiation would have a deleterious effect on the bone marrow in the lumbar vertebrae.

Chemotherapy with cytotoxic agents gives more hopeful results. Cisplatin, one of the platinum compounds, given in intravenous infusion and repeated every four weeks, shows good results. Carboplatin is equally useful and has fewer side-effects. In combination with other agents such as Taxol, the platinum compounds give a significant improvement in results (see Box 20.4).

## Prognosis

The general prognosis for ovarian carcinoma is poor, less than 20% surviving for five years. Factors which worsen prognosis are:
• advanced stage of disease;
• poorly differentiated tumour;
• how much tumour remains after surgery.

---

**Box 20.4 Chemotherapy with cytotoxic agents**

*Single platinum agents*
• Cisplatin
• Carboplatin

*Combinations*
• Platinum agents plus cyclophosphamide
• Platinum agents plus cyclophosphamide plus doxorubicin
• Platinum agents plus Taxol

---

# Carcinoma of the fallopian tube

*Primary*
- A rare malignancy occurring in older women.
- Papillary carcinoma may be solid or alveolar.
- Sometimes there is a vaginal discharge of an orange–yellow colour.

Treatment is as for ovarian carcinoma.

*Secondary*
- Metastases in the tube most commonly come from cancer of the ovary or uterus.

# Malignant disease of the vulva

## Squamous carcinoma

Vulval carcinoma is less common than other gynaecological cancers. The squamous form is the commonest malignant tumour of the vulva. It occurs mainly in the older age group, with a peak incidence at about 60 years of age. The condition is associated with vulval dystrophy (Chapter 6).

*Pathology*
The primary growth is an ulcer with a raised, everted edge and indurated base. Multiple primaries may be found, sometimes the inner sides of both labia minora are involved. The growth may also arise on the clitoris.

*Methods of spread*
- The growth may spread by direct extension and contact to other parts of the vulva, vagina or anus.

Secondary spread is mainly by lymphatics. Owing to the rich lymphatic drainage of the vulva, the glands which tend to be involved are:
- superficial inguinal group of both sides;
- inguinal;
- femoral;
- iliac;
- aortic.

In untreated cases, the glands in the groin may break down to form a fungating ulcerated mass of growth.

*Clinical features*
Carcinoma of the vulva commonly begins as a small nodule, often unnoticed by the patient at first. It grows in size and becomes ulcerated with discharge and bleeding. It tends to grow on the inner surface of the labia minora in elderly women and may remain unnoticed except for slight discomfort and soreness from the discharge until an advanced stage.

*Differential diagnosis*
To differentiate malignancy from other causes of a lump in the vulva or of ulceration is the main problem. All lumps or ulcers of the vulva must be fully investigated including a biopsy.

*Treatment*
Treatment of carcinoma of the vulva is vulvectomy and dissection of all the superficial and deep inguinal glands and occasionally the iliac glands. The vulva itself is widely excised with the glands through separate incisions over each groin. Wide excision in advanced growths may have to include removal of the lower part of the urethra, vagina or anal canal depending on site.

In operable cases, a 5-year cure rate of about 70% is achieved. The prognosis depends mainly on involvement of the lymphatic glands.

RADIOTHERAPY
Carcinoma of the vulva is relatively radioresistant while the surrounding normal tissues are radiosensitive. Hence, it is not employed usually, but high-voltage treatment may be used for recurrences.

CHEMOTHERAPY
This is not a primary treatment for squamous epithelioma or cancer of the vulva, but as with carcinomas of the anus it is being used more often for recurrence.

## Intraepithelial neoplasia

In vulval intraepithelial neoplasia (VIN), the malignant cells are limited to the outer layers of the epidermis and there is no spread to the underlying tissues and no metastases. The whole layer is infiltrated with malignant cells.

*Clinical features*

The patient has irritation or soreness of the vulva. The appearance may be that of vulval dystrophy or there may be a red area with a serpiginous outline. VIN may remain dormant for years or may assume the characteristic of invasive carcinoma.

Diagnosis depends on biopsy.

Treatment is by a wide excision with a margin of healthy skin and epithelium.

## Basal cell carcinoma

This uncommon tumour presents as an indolent ulcer without invasion of the underlying tissues. Diagnosis is made by biopsy.

The treatment consists of local excision with a margin of normal skin.

## Malignant melanoma

Fortunately this highly malignant tumour is rare. It may present as a melanotic nodule or as a pedunculated tumour. The best treatment is to perform a vulvectomy and if nodes are involved, an *en bloc* dissection. Cases with diffuse spread of melanoma may be treated by radiotherapy.

---

**Self-assessment**

**20.1** Which of the following statements are true?
  (a) Carcinoma of the cervix is the most common gynaecological malignancy.
  (b) More women die of ovarian cancer than any other gynaecological malignancy.
  (c) Cervical cancer most commonly presents with postmenopausal bleeding.
  (d) Endometrial cancer most commonly presents with postmenopausal bleeding.
  (e) Ovarian cancer most commonly presents with postcoital bleeding.

**20.2** A woman of 48 presents with postcoital bleeding, her last smear was 8 years ago and was normal. She is otherwise well. On examination she has an ulcerated lesion on her cervix which bleeds on contact. The vulva, vagina and uterus all feel normal. Which of the following should be undertaken to investigate the cause of her postcoital bleeding?
  (a) CT scan of abdomen and pelvis.
  (b) Liver function tests.
  (c) Biopsy of her cervix.
  (d) Chest X-ray.
  (e) Hysteroscopy and curettage.

**20.3** A woman of 63 presents with a hard fixed abdominal mass noticed by her GP when she complained that her clothes were becoming tighter. Her menopause was 12 years ago and she has had no vaginal bleeding. She has no other abnormalities on examination. What is the most likely provisional diagnosis?
  (a) Stage 3 carcinoma of the ovary.
  (b) Stage 3 carcinoma of the cervix.
  (c) Stage 1 carcinoma of the ovary.
  (d) Stage 3 carcinoma of the uterus.
  (e) Stage 4 carcinoma of the ovary.

**20.4** Which of the following are useful preoperative staging investigations for the woman in Question 20.3?
  (a) Hysteroscopy and curettage.
  (b) CT scan of abdomen and pelvis.
  (c) Serum tumour markers.
  (d) Chest X-ray.
  (e) Urea and electrolytes.

**Self-assessment** *Continued*

**20.5** A woman of 63 presents with an offensive discharge from her vagina. She admits that her vulva has been very itchy and sore for several years. Over the last few months she has noticed occasional blood stains on her pants and a lump on her left labia. Her GP has treated her with antibiotics to no effect. Which of the following are the most appropriate investigations for this woman?
  (a) Examination and biopsy of her vulva.
  (b) High vaginal swab.
  (c) Abdominal palpation particularly in both groins.
  (d) Cervical smear.
  (e) Hysteroscopy and curettage.

# Chapter 21

# The menopause

The menopause is the cessation of normal menstruation. The climacteric is a longer period during which time the reproductive organs involute. These time zones overlap each other in time just as they do in youth with the two processes of menarche and puberty.

The mean age of menopause in the UK is 51 with a normal range from 45 to 56. Conventionally a woman has to stop menstruating for 12 months before she is considered to be postmenopausal.

## Physiology

At the end of reproductive life, the ovaries become less able to produce oocytes due to:
- a lack of primordial follicles, because all have been used;
- more refractory receptor function in the granulosa and thecal cells.

The falling oestrogen levels result in a large increase in follicular stimulating hormone (FSH). The endometrium does not proliferate.

The ovarian stroma produces androstenedione which converts in peripheral fat to oestrone, a weaker oestrogen than oestradiol, the steroid on which the woman has depended for much of her reproductive life. Menstruation stops due to a lack of cyclical oestrogen and progesterone.

## Symptoms

At the menopause 60% of women are relatively asymptomatic, 25% of women have mild symptoms and 15% have moderate to severe symptoms. The two commonest symptoms are:
- hot flushes;
- dryness of the vagina.

There is often a loss of libido, part of which is hormonal.

Mood swings, nervousness, anxiety, irritability and depression are all measured in this group of women. The decrease of oestrogens may reduce their modulatory role on brain monoamine synthesis.

Symptoms are found more commonly in those who had premenstrual tension or dysmenorrhoea. The symptoms are less frequent in Asian and Negro women, possibly associated with better maintenance of oestrogen levels by peripheral conversion in these groups.

Loss of collagen leads to uterovaginal prolapse and wrinkling of the skin.

## Hot flushes

These are the feeling of heat over the face and upper part of the body usually lasting for half to one minute. They are followed by perspiration of this area, which may render the woman wringing wet. These flushes usually last for a year or so and in up to a quarter of women at least four years. This is probably due to an increase in the sympathetic nervous system drive mediated through the central neurotransmitters. They come on more at night when in bed and can wake a woman up.

## Dry vagina

The cervix and vagina are oestrogen dependent. Secretions from the cervix and the surface glands are diminished and the vaginal epithelium becomes thinner, less elastic with a reduced blood supply; atrophic vaginitis follows. Dryness and, therefore, dyspareunia are common. Extra lubrication may be required or oestrogen cream.

## Other genital changes

The breasts become atrophic and the nipples flatten. The uterus becomes smaller. There is less support from the cardinal ligament, uterosacral and uteropubic ligaments so prolapse may occur (Chapter 22).

## Other symptoms

The lower oestrogen levels lead to atrophy of the urethra causing frequency of micturition, dysuria and urgency (urethral syndrome). This is commonly confused with symptoms of urinary tract infection but does not improve with antibiotics. The weakness of the supporting muscles and the cardinal ligaments allows stress incontinence to start at this age.

The pulling back of the posterior wall of the urethra often exposes the sensitive anterior wall which becomes inflamed. A small polyp or caruncle may occur on the posterior wall.

The reduction of oestrogens leads to an increase in the levels of low density lipoproteins, cholesterol and triglycerides. This is accompanied by a catch-up rate for women of coronary heart disease.

## Long-term symptoms

Most of the above symptoms disappear within a year or two but those on the skeleton stay for ever.

The calcium part of the skeleton is reabsorbed, whilst the collagen framework stays the same. This leads to osteoporosis (Fig. 21.1).

Women lose calcium at different rates and so the need for replacement oestrogens differs from one woman to another. Those with established osteoporosis should be treated with biphosphonates. In reproductive life, while oestrogen synthesis is high, women are protected from heart disease and coronary occlusion. After the menopause, this does not occur and ten years later, the rate of coronary thrombosis is as high in women as men. There has been some evidence that hormone replacement therapy (HRT) may decrease the incidence of ischaemic heart disease (IHD), but a more recent study amongst women at high risk of IHD has not

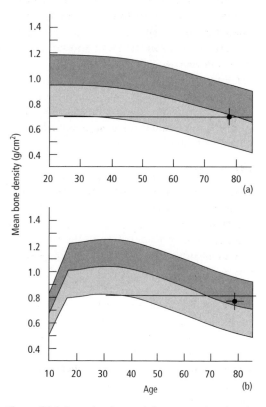

**Figure 21.1** Bone density graph for women showing the normal range for hip (a) and lumbar spine (b) against increasing age. The thickened line represents the threshold for increased risk of bone fracture. The filled circle is the result for a 77-year-old woman who is becoming osteoporotic.

demonstrated a protective effect. HRT does alter the lipid profile with a higher level of high density lipoproteins and lower cholesterol, but there is no definitive evidence that HRT reduces the risk of IHD in low-risk women.

## Postmenopausal therapy

The treatment for postmenopausal symptoms is:
1 acute oestrogen replacement for women who have symptoms, principally hot flushes and dry vagina;
2 more chronic replacement therapy for women who are losing oestrogen in order to prevent osteoporosis. Oestrogen is a potent factor in the maintenance of bone mineralization. Low oestrogen levels lead to a thinning of trabecular bone and eventually osteoporosis. This leads to an increased risk of fractures of the hip and wrist and compression fractures of the vertebrae resulting in a dowager hump.

The giving of symptomatic oestrogen replacement is the more straightforward therapy.

The aim should be to use the lowest effective dose of oestrogen for the shortest period of time. It is usual to give it in a cyclical fashion of 28 days. This causes remission of symptoms in most women, once the correct dose is achieved.

Progestogens are added in the second half of the cycle in all women who have a uterus to prevent a build up of endometrium with possible hyperplasia, or atypical hyperplasia and then malignancy.

Owing to the cyclical nature of the treatment, the endometrium which develops during the oestrogen phase is shed after withdrawal and so there appears to be a continuation of menstrual periods (usually light).

## Types of HRT

The hormone may be given in a number of ways, as described below.

### Orally

This is the commonest and the most convenient. Compliance may be patchy and patients may forget, rendering the therapy ineffective.

### Transdermal patches and gels

Oestrogen and progestogens are readily absorbed through the skin. There is the advantage of the oestrogen not having to pass through the portal system after absorption, where much would be destroyed. Hence, higher tissue levels of the oestrogens are achieved. The patches only need to be changed every third/seventh day and so compliance is higher. More recently, sprays have been developed.

### Implants

Oestrogens can be given in a retard preparation by implantation under local anaesthesia. The pellets can be inserted into the abdominal wall or the thigh under the fascia lata. They last up to six months and are easily replaced so compliance is not relevant. Occasionally the oestrogens are given with testosterone to provide some stimulus to the libido but this reduces the cardioprotective effect of oestrogen.

Repeated use of oestrogen implants can lead to very high levels of oestrogen. As the implant wears off the woman may experience menopausal symptoms even though the serum oestradiol levels are still within or above physiological levels. This may lead to women requesting their implants more and more often leading to dangerous levels of oestradiol with an increased risk of thrombosis. Early replacement of implants should therefore be avoided.

Progesterones should be taken by mouth during the second half of each cycle in order to get a withdrawal bleed and prevent build-up of the endometrium in women with a uterus.

This method is most commonly used by women who have had a hysterectomy.

### Vaginally

Steroids are absorbed through the vaginal epithelium, but a large dose is needed in the vagina to get a reasonable dose inside the body. However, if vaginal dryness is the main symptom, this is a good route.

### Preparations

1 Orally—Progynova, oestradiol or Premarin

(oestrone). Progestogen—norethisterone 1 mg a day for last 10 days.

**2** Subcutaneous implant—50–100 mg oestradiol (with 100 mg testosterone).

**3** Patches of oestradiol 25 or 50 µg with norethisterone acetate 1 mg (12 days).

**4** Vaginal application—oestriol or oestradiol as a cream or pessary high in the vagina twice a week.

**5** Non-bleed preparations. These can be either oestrogen with continuous progestogen or non-oestrogenic compounds (Tibolone) that mimic oestrogen's effect on menopausal symptoms and bone.

All treatments should be given for two years or to the age of 55. If the uterus has been removed previously, the supplementary progestogen is not required. Unless treatment is stopped for an interval, the doctor and the patient will never know if the treatment is still required.

## Side effects of HRT

Hormone replacement therapy has minimal side effects. A few women may experience abdominal bloating and breast tenderness which usually resolves after 2 or 3 months.

## Complications of HRT

### Malignancy

There is no evidence of any increase in malignancy of the *cervix* or *ovary*.

Neoplasia of the *endometrium* may follow unopposed oestrogen; the risk increases with the duration of use:

- 3–6-fold after five years of use.
- 10-fold after ten years.

Adding cyclical progestogens virtually eliminates this risk.

Breast cancer is stimulated by higher oestrogen levels. Meta-analysis indicates that the relative risk of *breast cancers* is about ×1.3 up to ten years and exceeds this with longer-term therapy. Continuous combined preparations have been shown to increase the risk of breast cancer two-fold after 5

years and three-fold after 10 years of use. The increased risk declines back to baseline within 5 years of stopping treatment. Obviously, a woman with a family history of breast cancer should be counselled before starting HRT.

### Continued periods

The risk rates of cancer of the ovary and cervix are unaffected. Regular monthly bleeding going on into the 60s is a nuisance. It often reduces in amount but still occurs. In an attempt to prevent this, progestogens may be given in a wider spread but lower dose throughout the cycle.

Tibolone (2.5 mg daily), a gonadomimetic, possesses weak oestrogenic, progestational and androgenic properties. It can be used to treat flushes, psychological and libido problems and is not accompanied by regular withdrawal bleeding symptoms though it is not absolute especially if used on women early in the menopause.

Some women have a weight gain due to water retention when they start the oestrogens but this settles after a few months. Some women get a depression like premenstrual tension during the progestogen phase. Changing the dose of added progestogens will help this.

### Uterine enlargement

Hyperplasia of the uterus may lead to an increase of bleeding. Any pre-existing fibroids may rarely continue their growth, whereas normally after the menopause their growth stops.

## Postmenopausal bleeding

Postmenopausal bleeding is bleeding from the genital tract occurring six months or more after the menopause. It is a serious symptom which may indicate the presence of malignant disease in the genital tract. Every woman with postmenopausal bleeding should be assumed to have a carcinoma until a full investigation has proved to the contrary.

The chief causes are:

*The vulva*
- Carcinoma.
- Urethral caruncle.

Rectal bleeding and haematuria must be excluded.

*The vagina*
- Carcinoma.
- Vaginitis, especially atrophic vaginitis.
- Foreign bodies, especially pessaries.

*The cervix*
- Carcinoma of the ectocervix.
- Carcinoma of a cervical canal polyp.
- Benign cervical polyp.

*The endometrium*
- Carcinoma.
- Sarcoma.
- Mixed mesodermal tumours.
- Polyp.
- Atrophic endometritis.

*The fallopian tube*
- Carcinoma.

*The ovary*
- Feminizing tumours.
- Granulosa cell tumour.
- Theca cell tumour.

## Investigation of postmenopausal bleeding

- Inspection of vulva and urethra.
- Cervical smear.
- Bimanual vaginal examination.
- Transvaginal ultrasound scan.
- Hysteroscopy and endometrial biopsy.

## Hormone treatment

Withdrawal bleeding may follow administration of oestrogens for menopausal symptoms. This should not be assumed to be the cause of any post-menopausal bleeding until a full investigation including cytology and curettage has excluded more sinister causes.

---

**Self-assessment**

**21.1** OSCE question.

**Candidate's instructions:** You are the junior doctor seeing a Mrs Hilda Black, a 48 year-old for her preoperative assessment. She is about to be admitted for a total abdominal hysterectomy and bilateral oophorectomy for menorrhagia which has not responded to medical therapy. She wishes to discuss her options for hormone replacement therapy (HRT). You are expected to answer her questions.

**Role-player's instructions:** You are Mrs Hilda Black, a 48-year-old housewife. You have had very heavy, painful periods for the last 5 years. You have tried all forms of medical therapy with minimal improvement and have finally decided to have a hysterectomy. The consultant has discussed removal of your ovaries and as your grandmother died of ovarian cancer you have decided to have them removed as well. The consultant gave you some leaflets on hormone replacement therapy but they have left you rather confused. You have come to the hospital for your preoperative check up and have a list of questions you wish to ask the doctor about your options for HRT.
1 What sort of HRT will I need to take?
2 How long should I take it for?
3 What are the side effects?
4 How will I take it?
5 What are the benefits of taking HRT?
6 What are the possible long term risks of HRT?
Try not to allow the candidate to take a history from you and move on to the questions.

**Self-assessment** *Continued*

**21.2** A woman of 53 presents with vaginal bleeding. Her menopause was four years ago and she has been on oral cyclical HRT since then. She is very happy with her HRT but has noticed that she has been bleeding between her packets. The bleeding lasts for a few days and can be quite heavy. Which of the following diagnoses are possible causes of her bleeding?

(a) Endometrial polyp.
(b) Subserosal fibroid.
(c) Atrophic vaginitis.
(d) Ovarian cancer.
(e) Cervical cancer.

**21.3** List the investigations which should be undertaken in this woman with reasons.

# Chapter 22

# Pelvic floor disorders

In the majority of adult women, when standing, the uterus is anteverted, the fundus directed forwards, and anteflexed, the body of the uterus bent forward on the cervix.

However, vaginal examinations always take place with the woman lying down. Then the body of the uterus often angles back to become axial, i.e. in line with the long axis of the vagina. Hence, while it is true that in the anatomical position four-fifths of uteruses are anteverted and one-fifth retroverted, at vaginal examination, about 40% are anteverted, 40% axial and 20% retroverted.

The structures which maintain the position of the uterus are:
- the cardinal or transverse ligaments;
- the uterosacral ligaments.

These are attached to the sides of the supravaginal cervix and lower uterus, leaving the body of the uterus mobile in all directions and capable of growth during pregnancy. The normal uterus is mobile, altering its position when the bladder or rectum becomes distended.

The secondary support of the uterus is the muscular pelvic floor (see Chapter 1).

## Prolapse

Prolapse is a downward descent of the female pelvic organs due to weakness of the structures which normally retain them in position. Both descent and prolapse are relative terms and perceived differently, but are more frequently encountered in women who have borne children and rarely in nulliparous women. Prolapse does not usually become apparent until after the menopause when there is general shrinking and weakening of the supports of the pelvic organs. It is less common in people of African descent.

A prolapse resembles a hernia for there is protrusion of part of the abdominal contents through an aperture in the supporting structures. Protrusion takes place between the two levatores ani and, in more severe cases, through the orifice of the vagina.

## Classification

Six components of a genital prolapse (Fig. 22.1) are recognized.

**1** *Dislocation of the urethra*—the urethra is displaced downwards and backwards off the pubis. It may be also dilated becoming an urethrocoele. This arises from damage to or weakness of the triangular ligament.

**2** *Cystocoele*—hernia of the bladder trigone following weakness of the vaginal and pubocervical fascia. The bladder base descends and later a bladder pouch is formed which may contain residual urine increasing the risk of a urinary tract infection.

**3** *Uterine prolapse*—descent of the uterus and cervix.

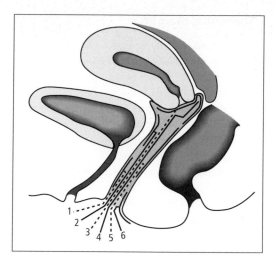

**Figure 22.1** Analysis of the areas involved in a prolapse. 1. Dislocation of the urethra. 2. Cystocoele. 3. Descent of cervix and uterus. 4. Enterocoele. 5. Rectocoele. 6. Deficient perineum.

(a) *First degree* with a descent of the uterus, but the cervix remains within the upper vagina.

(b) *Second degree* uterine descent when the cervix reaches down to the vulva on straining, but does not pass through it.

(c) *Third degree* or *procidentia* when the cervix and some or all of the uterus is prolapsed outside the vaginal orifice. In practice the fundus of the uterus usually remains within the vagina, but there is an associated inversion of the vagina.

**4** *Enterocoele* or pouch of Douglas hernia—a prolapse of the upper part of the posterior vaginal wall. The hernia contains the peritoneum of the pouch of Douglas often with a loop of bowel. Enterocoele may occur concurrently with other types of genital prolapse, especially procidentia. It is also seen in prolapse following a hysterectomy.

**5** *Rectocoele*—a prolapse of the lower part of the posterior vaginal wall due to weakness or divarication of the levatores ani; the rectum bulges into the vagina.

**6** *The perineal body* —this may be deficient and part of the anal canal may bulge into the vagina. It follows inadequately sutured tears after childbirth or by failure of healing in such tears.

## Symptoms

Symptoms of genital prolapse are variable and do not bear much relation to the physical signs found on examination but more to the degree of traction on the pelvic ligaments. The symptoms tend to worsen with the day's activities and can be relieved by lying down. The commonest complaints are:

- A feeling of fullness of the vagina.
- A lump coming down.
- A dragging sensation or bearing down in the back or lower abdomen.
- Vaginal discharge due to congestion of the cervix, an ulcer of the ectocervix or cervical ectropion. A bloodstained discharge may occur if there is ulceration.
- Difficulty with coitus may be experienced if the cervix protrudes or is greatly elongated.
- Urinary symptoms include:

  (a) *frequency* of micturition is common and is often daytime only;

  (b) *nocturnal frequency* may be present if there is added cystitis;

  (c) *urgency* of micturition due to weakness of the bladder sphincter mechanism and urge incontinence may occur in some cases;

  (d) there may be *difficulty in emptying* the bladder completely and the woman may find she has to push the prolapse up with a finger to complete the act of micturition;

  (e) complete *retention of urine* follows urethral overstretch;

  (f) *stress incontinence* when mild is common in women even without prolapse. This is considered later in this chapter.

- Rectal symptoms: many women with prolapse complain of constipation and this may be due to difficulty in emptying the rectum completely because it bulges into the vagina. Others notice discomfort on sitting on a firm surface; the vaginal wall over the rectocoele can bulge down between the labia. With age, the labia become atrophic and less protective and the prolapsed vagina is exposed to trauma when sitting on hard surfaces.

## Physical signs

The woman should first be examined in the dorsal position when she is asked to strain and cough. While she does, the anus may be supported to spare her the embarrassment of an involuntary escape of flatus or faeces. In case of doubt, she may be asked to stand up or walk about for a short time before testing for prolapse again on the bed.

The degree of descent of the cervix is tested with a finger in the vagina. The woman is then asked to adopt the Sim's position (Fig. 22.2). She lies on her left side with her left leg straight and her right leg bent up against her abdomen. Her right arm and shoulder should be turned away from you and her buttocks towards the edge of the couch nearest to the examiner. The Sim's speculum is then gently introduced along the posterior wall of the vagina. A cystourethrocoele is usually obvious and the distance from the introitus to the bulge can be measured using a special ruler. The woman is asked to cough and any leakage of urine and/or descent of the cervix is noted. As the speculum is withdrawn any posterior vaginal wall prolapse can be noted.

Where there is a complaint of stress incontinence, examination is best made with some urine in the bladder; the urethra and bladder neck may then be supported with two fingers to demonstrate that this manoeuvre controls the incontinence.

## Differential diagnosis

The diagnosis of prolapse is not difficult but it can be hard to decide if it is the cause of the patient's main symptoms. It must be distinguished from:
- vaginal or periurethral cysts;
- tumours of the vagina;
- a diverticulum of the urethra;
- urethral caruncle;
- urethral mucosal prolapse.

Symptoms similar to those of prolapse may be caused by:
- varicose veins of the vulva;
- haemorrhoids;
- rectal prolapse;
- cystitis;
- vaginitis with congestion of the vagina;
- pressure from a large abdominal tumour.

Stress incontinence must be distinguished from other causes of incontinence of urine such as urge incontinence and incontinence due to neurological disease.

## Prevention

Careful management of labour is important. The woman must be discouraged from bearing down before full dilatation for this may overstretch the uterine supports. The second stage of labour should not be prolonged unduly; episiotomy and

Inserted Sim's speculum

**Figure 22.2** The left lateral position or Sim's position.

low forceps extraction may reduce the risk of later prolapse. Episiotomies and tears must be carefully sutured in layers. Postnatal exercises should be encouraged after every labour. All women should see a physiotherapist to help with this.

Prevention of vault prolapse after hysterectomy is helped by suture of the cardinal and uterosacral ligaments to the vaginal vault. Subtotal hysterectomy is more likely to lead to vault prolapse than total hysterectomy, even though many women ask for the former.

## Treatment

Treatment of prolapse may be palliative or surgical.

## Physiotherapy

This can be successful, chiefly in young women after recent childbirth where the vaginal walls and pelvic floor are mainly affected. It is less effective in vault prolapse. Exercises to strengthen the pelvic floor muscles are carried out under the supervision of a physiotherapist including the voluntary retention of weighted cones in the vagina to strengthen the pelvic muscles. This may be combined with electrotherapy to the pelvic floor muscles.

## Palliative treatment

Many types of pessary and support have been devised for prolapse. Their use is only temporary, the better cure being a repair operation. With modern techniques of surgery and anaesthesia, operation can safely be undertaken in the majority of cases of prolapse.

The indications for pessaries are:
- prolapse during pregnancy;
- prolapse immediately after delivery;
- when another pregnancy is desired within a short time;
- in patients unfit for operation on medical grounds;
- in patients who decline an operation.

## Pessary treatment

A plastic ring pessary which fits well surrounds the cervix, pointing slightly forward, and resting between the posterior fornix and the anterior vaginal wall. It supports a vault prolapse by stretching the vaginal wall while a cystocoele is directly supported by it. It is less successful in controlling a rectocoele; if the perineum is deficient, the pessary will tend to slip or even fall out.

Pessaries are made in 5 mm sizes from 50 to 120 mm.

There are a few cases where a ring pessary fails to control prolapse and operation cannot be performed. In these cases there are other appliances. The cup and stem pessary consists of a sheet of vulcanite or plastic with a stem to which are attached tapes which are tied to a belt. It is removed at night for cleaning and is thus less likely to cause ulceration. It is a useful long-term pelvic floor support, but rarely used.

*Disadvantages*
- Ulceration of the vagina and cervix.
- A neglected pessary may become embedded in the vaginal wall and may only be removed with great difficulty.
- A carcinoma of the vagina may develop.

## Surgery

The best results from operations for repair depend on the degree of descent of the various components of the genital tract together with the judgement and expertise of the surgeon.

Many surgeons perform *vaginal hysterectomy* when operating for prolapse, an operation of choice when prolapse is combined with menorrhagia or where there are small uterine fibroids. Vaginal hysterectomy is preferred in cases of uterine procidentia.

*Anterior colporrhaphy and posterior colpoperineorrhaphy*
These operations are designed to restore the support to the vagina from the levator ani and muscles of the perineum. Women with urinary symptoms

and vaginal prolapse should all undergo urodynamic investigation prior to deciding on surgical treatment (see p. 291). The reasons for doing urodynamics include:

**1** If genuine stress incontinence is demonstrated vaginal surgery is not the treatment of choice.

**2** If the patient has detrusor instability vaginal surgery may make it worse and there is an increased risk of postoperative urinary retention and/or infection.

**3** The first operation for urinary problems gives the best chance of success and it is therefore essential to opt for the operation with the highest cure rate.

New surgical techniques for uterovaginal prolapse have been introduced. These include sacrospinous fixation where the uterosacral ligaments are fixed to the sacrospinous ligament via the vaginal or abdominal route.

*Anterior colporrhaphy* and *posterior colpoperineorrhaphy* may be combined with *amputation of the cervix* and shortening and suture of the cardinal ligaments; this is the Fothergill or Manchester operation.

The reasons for amputating the cervix are:
• the supravaginal cervix may be elongated;
• after suture of the cervix, repair of the vaginal vault is more satisfactory;
• the cervix is often unhealthy and infected;
• a possible site for future carcinoma has been removed.

The cervix should not be amputated in young women who may wish to bear children and in cases where there is no vaginal vault prolapse.

Abdominal operations may be combined with prolapse repair. Abdominal hysterectomy may be required for large fibroids and the prolapse may be repaired under the same anaesthetic or later. Removal of a large tumour may itself lead to cure or improvement of prolapse.

Stress incontinence presents surgical challenges. It can occur with or without prolapse.

## Preoperative care

Preparation for operation is most important. The general condition of the patient is assessed and treatment given for conditions such as obesity and chronic cough. Cardiovascular disease and mild diabetes are common in middle-aged women and may need preoperative treatment.

Ulceration of the vagina can follow exposure of the vaginal tissues outside the body in a procidentia or from long-wearing of a ring pessary. The risk of ulceration and infection are reduced by regular changing of the pessary (6-monthly) and using regular topical oestrogen cream. Elderly women find the changing of the pessary uncomfortable because the introitus is commonly less elastic and partially stenosed. It is important that the change is performed by a well trained professional. The pessary can be made more flexible by pre-soaking it in warm water. Regular changes over a long period of time may be unacceptable to some women and it is common for women to ask for surgical intervention after a few years of using a pessary.

Urinary tract infection is common and must be treated. Urge incontinence and detrusor muscle instability should be treated with antispasmodics and surgery postponed until this urogynaecology aspect is fully investigated and treated.

## Postoperative care

Early movements and deep breathing are encouraged and the patient should get out of bed as soon as possible. The use of a lavatory or commode in private helps to overcome difficulties with micturition and defaecation. Laxatives are given as required.

Postoperative complications in the first two weeks are:
• *Chest complications* associated with general anaesthesia.
• *Retention of urine* and urinary tract infection. Retention usually requires catheterization. If extensive dissection, especially of the perineal tissues, is carried out during the operation, an indwelling Foley catheter should be inserted at the operation. The bladder should be drained continuously for three to five days and the catheter then clamped intermittently for a day to reintroduce the sensation of bladder filling. An antibiotic agent should

be given during continuous catheterization to prevent urinary infection.

• *Local sepsis* is unusual with the use of antibiotic prophylaxis.

• *Haemorrhage* may be primary, reactionary or secondary. Blood transfusion may be required and in secondary or reactionary haemorrhage, resuturing of the vagina or cervix to arrest bleeding and packing of the vagina may be needed under anaesthesia in the operating theatre.

• *Pelvic vein thrombosis* and *pulmonary embolism* may occur.

There are remote complications.

• *Vaginal discharge* may persist for some weeks. In some cases it is due to granulation tissue in the scars which are best treated with silver nitrate sticks. Sutures used in the repair may not be absorbed. They can be nicked and any excess suture material removed at two weeks.

• *Urinary complications* include frequency due to irritable bladder or chronic infection. Rarely a vesicovaginal or urethrovaginal fistula develops.

• *Dyspareunia* is common and may be caused by leaving the vagina too small; care must be taken not to reduce the vaginal circumference, especially if a posterior repair follows an anterior wall operation. Dyspareunia may also result from disuse of the vagina due to fear. Senile atrophy may also be seen in the age group of those having repair operations.

## Future pregnancies after repair

Successful pregnancy can be achieved after prolapse repair though if the cervix has been amputated there may be an increased tendency to miscarry. Caesarean section is advisable in most cases especially if there is fibrosis of the remaining cervix, if there has been an extensive vault repair or where operation has been done for severe stress incontinence.

Vaginal delivery may rarely be allowed.

## Urogynaecology

## Physiology

The bladder has two main functions in the human.

• To act as a reservoir for the storage of urine.

• To empty this reservoir away from the skin of the body at an appropriate time and appropriate place.

Acting as a reservoir, the normal bladder:

• is lined with waterproof transitional epithelium which does not allow diffusion of the urinary electrolytes across its wall;

• has a high compliance, accommodating a large volume of urine (300–500 ml) with a rise of intravesical pressure to only 15 cmH$_2$O;

• is able to expand suprapubically and extraperitoneally without hindrance or constraint by bone or pelvic viscera;

• maintains the pressure in its outflow tract along the urethra at a higher level than intravesical pressure thus preventing leakage of urine.

The bladder is an efficient expulsive organ:

• The smooth detrusor muscle is richly innervated by the parasympathetic nervous system outflow of sacral roots 2, 3 and 4.

• At the onset of micturition, the pelvic floor striated muscle is voluntarily relaxed, reducing the intraurethral pressure. The background inhibition of the sacral reflex arc is suppressed. Efferent impulses pass to the detrusor muscle causing a rise in intravesical pressure. This then exceeds the intraurethral pressure and leads to the passage of urine down the urethra.

## Urinary incontinence

The involuntary loss of urine may be due to:

• true incontinence from a urinary fistula;

• genuine stress incontinence;

• detrusor instability (urge incontinence);

• overflow incontinence;

• reflex incontinence.

### Urinary fistula

A pathological tract may open between a part of the urinary system and the epithelial surface of the

vagina or occasionally the skin. These tracts bypass the normal controlling mechanisms causing development of continuous (true) incontinence. They can be congenital or follow major surgery, operative delivery or disease such as cancer of the cervix.
• Congenital (rare); the ureter draining the upper pole of one kidney opens on the anterior wall of the vagina. It presents in children with continuous urinary loss. This may result in poorly functioning renal polar hydronephrosis or an ectopic hydroureter.
• Caused by surgery—avascular necrosis leads to weakening of the wall of the ureter or bladder and the development of a ureteric or vesicovaginal fistula.

    (a) Gynaecological surgery, particularly if there has been anatomical distortion by infection, endometriosis, carcinoma or by preceding small blood vessel damage (endarteritis) caused by irradiation.

    (b) Obstetric trauma, in association with obstructed labour where the presenting part causes avascular necrosis of the bladder base or sometimes the rectum, causing the development of a vesicovaginal or rectovaginal fistula respectively.

## Genuine stress incontinence

An involuntary loss of urine occurs from the urethra, when the transmitted intra-abdominal pressure causes a rise of the intravesical pressure which exceeds the intraurethral pressure in the absence of a detrusor contraction. Approximately 25% of older women have mild problems and 5–10% severe.

*Symptoms*
Involuntary urine loss associated with a sudden, usually unexpected, rise of abdominal pressure such as coughing, sneezing, laughing or lifting.

*Physical signs*
The coincidental downswing of the bladder neck leads to urinary leakage from the urethra; often only a few ml are passed.

About 50% are associated with prolapse of the vagina.

## Detrusor instability

Incidence—8–10% increasing with age.

*Aetiology*
Incompletely understood but may be due to:
• an abnormality in the central nervous system when anxiety and stress result in the loss of ability to inhibit the detrusor reflex and, therefore, the development of detrusor contraction;
• a recognized neurological defect, such as spinal trauma, demyelinating disorders or epilepsy;
• intense bladder inflammation, particularly in the elderly.

*Symptoms*
• Urgency of micturition leading to urge incontinence—an inability to hold on.
• Frequency of micturition both by day and night.
• Often associated with stress incontinence.

*Diagnosis*
The demonstration of detrusor contraction (more than $15\,cmH_2O$) on cystometry, provoked by bladder filling or straining and the movement or sound of running water.

## Overflow incontinence

Loss of urine when the bladder has become filled, usually associated with either:
• obstructive surgery to the bladder neck;
• denervation of the detrusor muscle (usually by extensive pelvic surgery, neurological defects, diabetes).

*Symptoms*
• The frequent passage of small volumes of urine.
• Hesitation of micturition.
• A slow stream.
• A sensation of incomplete emptying.
• Involuntary leakage when bending or getting out of a chair.

*Physical signs*
• A palpable bladder.
• Leakage on elevation of bladder base.

- On cystometry, slow urine flow rate.
- High residual urine.
- Risk of back pressure to upper urinary tract if chronic.

## Reflex incontinence

Reflex involuntary voiding is associated with sensory stimulation of the sacral 2, 3 and 4 segments. This develops when the higher centres are cut off from the sacral reflex arc and thus micturition ceases to be centrally suppressed. It is triggered when there is a significant increase of the afferent impulses to the sacral segments 2, 3 and 4 either from the bladder or the somatic nerves.

Detrusor contractions are often associated with a simultaneous contraction of the pelvic floor (detrusor dyssynergia) causing partial obstruction of urine flow, unlike the relaxation in centrally organized normal micturition.

## Urodynamic investigation of incontinence

- Bladder behaviour can be assessed by keeping fluid output charts to measure the frequency of the volumes of urine passed during the day, with a diary of fluid intake.
- Cystometry (with subtracted abdominal pressure) determines the presence or absence of involuntary detrusor contractions thereby differentiating the stable from the unstable bladder and these pressure measurements may be coupled with video radiological screening (Figs 22.3 and 22.4).
- The residual urine can be measured by catheter or pelvic ultrasound.

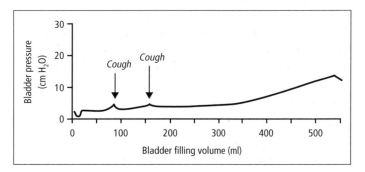

**Figure 22.3** Cystometry of a normal bladder filling with rise in intravesical pressure.

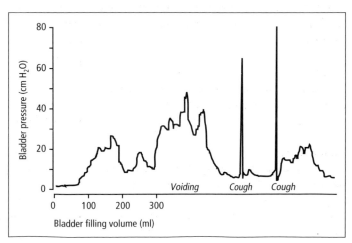

**Figure 22.4** Cystometry of filling of an unstable bladder.

• Measurement of urinary flow rate with pressure measurements differentiates the obstructed urethra from the poorly functioning detrusor.
• Ultrasound urograms outline defects of the bladder and upper urinary tract and retrograde urography to demonstrate ureteric and vesicovaginal fistulae.

## Treatment

### Stress incontinence

*Conservative*
• Mild urinary leakage (particularly postnatally)—with a good physiotherapist and patient motivation, pelvic floor exercises usually result in improvement.
• Reduction of weight, excessive physical exertion and the treatment of coughing also help.

*Surgical*
• Vaginal approach—anterior colporrhaphy with bladder neck buttress is a simple operation and permits repair of other prolapses at the same time. Long-term success rate in curing incontinence is approximately 40%.
• Sling operation—multiple varieties—using synthetic substances (nylon, prolene, Teflon, mersilene mesh, tension-free vaginal tapes) or natural tissues (e.g. round ligament or external oblique aponeurosis). Insertion is by open surgery or blind by directed needles through the retropubic space (e.g. Stamey procedure).
• Retropubic bladder neck suspension operations—suturing the vaginal wall to the pectineal ligament (Burch) or periosteum over the back of the pubic bone (Marshall–Marchetti–Krantz). These procedures are associated with an 85–90% cure rate of the incontinence but do not remedy much prolapse apart from that of the anterior vaginal wall.
• Paraurethral injection of collagens to stimulate fibrin formation.

### The unstable bladder

There is often a psychosomatic element (Fig. 22.5). The symptoms are improved by several means.
• Enthusiastic encouragement, with the help of urinary output volume chart, particularly by incontinence advisers, district nurses and doctors. If necessary, admission to hospital for intensive bladder training under close supervision.
• The use of anticholinergic drugs, e.g. oxybutynin, Pro-Banthine, imipramine.
• The use of vaginal oestrogen cream to reduce bladder irritability and the tendency of recurrent urinary infection.

### Overflow incontinence

• If obstructed, urethral dilatation or urethrotomy results in improvement.
• If due to weakened detrusor muscle—continuous drainage with a suprapubic catheter for two to three weeks to improve the tone of the detrusor often helps with subsequent bladder training. Occasionally intermittent self-catheterization can be of assistance although infection is common.
• α-agonists—bethanocol.

### Urinary tract infection

Almost all urinary tract infections develop from the upward spread of the bacteria along the 5 cm of urethra. Infections are associated with:

**Figure 22.5** Cystometry with detrusor muscle contraction and voiding.

• the upward passage of organisms during intercourse;
• catheterization;
• the incomplete emptying of the bladder leading to stagnant urine;
• atrophic urethritis from a lack of oestrogens;
• poor hygiene following defaecation or intercourse.

*Symptoms*
• Burning dysuria.
• Severe urinary frequency.
• Urgency of micturition.
• Suprapubic discomfort.
• Urine odour.
If the infection has spread beyond the bladder to the upper part of the urinary tract then:
• loin pain;
• vomiting;
• rigors.

*Investigations*
• Dipstick impregnated with nitrite sensitive amine to screen for bacteria.
• Mid-stream urine culture.

*Treatment*
• Encouragement of high fluid intake.
• Rest in bed if temperature is raised.
• Rapid use of appropriate antibiotics.
• Topical oestrogens in postmenopausal women.
• Educational hygiene encouraging postcoital micturition and correct wiping after defaecation.
• Bladder training with suprapubic catheter if the residual urine volumes are high.

## Urinary frequency

Is associated with:
• bladder irritants, e.g. coffee, cola and fortified wines;

• the presence of calculi;
• high fluid intake resulting in an increased urinary output;
• diabetes mellitus may present with polydypsia and polyuria;
• the use of diuretics;
• anxiety, tension and stress, e.g. outside the examination hall;
• development of habits and rituals associated with particular voiding patterns;
• insomnia leading to nocturia;
• the reduction of any peripheral oedema overnight resulting in increased kidney excretion, bladder filling and nocturia.

## Nocturnal enuresis

The involuntary voiding of urine into the bed-clothes whilst asleep.

*Aetiology*
Not fully known, but the following associations have been noted:
• deep sleep leading to the loss of suppression of the voiding reflex;
• impairment of the kidneys to concentrate urine whilst asleep, for example by the persistence of daytime renal excretion pattern;
• psychological disturbances such as great unhappiness;
• bladder instability in later life.

*Treatment*
• Frequent waking overnight to ensure regular voiding.
• The use of desmopressin and nasal sprays to suppress urine formation whilst asleep.
• Mattress alarms.
• Imipramine.

**Self-assessment**

**22.1** A woman of 52 is referred to the gynaecology outpatients by her GP. She is complaining of urinary incontinence. You are expected to take a history from her.

**Role-player's instructions:** You are Mrs Sarah Ball, a 52-year-old primary school teacher. Over the last five years you have been increasingly troubled by suddenly leaking small amounts of urine when you cough, run or do any form of exercise. You used to go to aerobic classes but have given them up. You are also finding it difficult at school—several of the children have commented on a smell of urine in the classroom and you feel very embarrassed. You empty your bladder between each class but still notice some leaking as you move round the classroom. You wear a panty-liner all the time which you find irritating. you have to get up to the toilet twice every night. The amount you pass is normal; occasionally you have to go again 5–10 minutes after emptying your bladder. You have noticed some backache and a feeling of something coming down. You have had three children all born vaginally—the first baby was delivered by forceps and you had a lot of stitches. Your last period was three years ago. Your last smear was two years ago and they have always been normal. You are not taking HRT because your mother died of breast cancer. You smoked 20 cigarettes a day until four years ago. Your weight has gradually increased since you stopped smoking. You are otherwise fit and well.

**22.2** Describe how you would examine and manage this patient.

**22.3** List five principal complications of vaginal repair operations (colporrhaphies).

**22.4** Define genuine stress incontinence.

**22.5** Which of the following are common symptoms of detrusor instability?

(a) Urgency.

(b) Slow urinary stream.

(c) Incomplete emptying.

(d) Nocturia.

(e) Frequency.

# Part 6

# Audit of obstetrics and gynaecology

# Chapter 23

# Statistics of reproductive medicine

The population of the world is increasing, although indications are that the boom of the earlier part of the last century is flattening off. In the UK the levels have been fairly steady since the Second World War.

Birth rates are measured in all countries that collect sufficient data. This means that developing countries with poor data sources are not very reliable in measuring birth rates.

The total birth rate is simplest:

$$\text{Total birth rate} = \frac{\text{Births per year} \times 1000}{\text{Midyear population}}$$

This requires a knowledge of not just all the births but a proper census of the population to derive the denominator (Fig. 23.1). However, it does not relate to the process of birth; no men have babies and few young women or those over 45 do; hence a more sophisticated measure is the general fertility rate:

$$\text{General fertility rate} = \frac{\text{Births per year} \times 1000}{\text{Women aged 15–45 years}}$$

This rate requires a more detailed data analysis of the censuses and is used in Western countries. The data for the last years in the UK are shown in Fig. 23.2.

A more readily understandable set of ratios is the completed family size but this can only be done retrospectively (Fig. 23.3).

In the UK the total birth rate is 14 per 1000 and the general fertility rate is 64 per 1000. The completed family size is 1.8, just below replacement level.

There are variations in the monthly birth rate which is highest from October to March. The rates by days of the week are highest on weekdays (see Fig. 23.4a).

As can be seen, the birth rate for babies under 2500 g provides a mirror image to the incidence of births and accounts for the higher perinatal mortality rates at the weekend (see Fig. 23.4b).

## Maternal mortality

### Definitions

Deaths of women while pregnant or within 42 days of delivery, miscarriage, termination of pregnancy, from any cause related to or aggravated by the pregnancy or its management but not from accidental or incidental causes. These deaths are further subdivided into direct and indirect causes; *direct* causes are those that result from obstetric complications, whilst *indirect* deaths are those resulting from pre-existing disease or disease that develops during pregnancy secondary to physiological changes of pregnancy.

### Major causes of maternal mortality

Maternal mortality has declined dramatically in the last 50 years in the UK (Fig. 23.5), but there are

**Figure 23.1** The total birth rate in England and Wales (1881–2001) showing numbers of births per thousand total population.

**Figure 23.3** Completed family size in England and Wales (1880–2000).

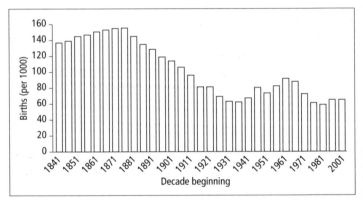

**Figure 23.2** The general fertility rate in England and Wales (1841–2001) showing numbers of births per thousand women aged 15–44.

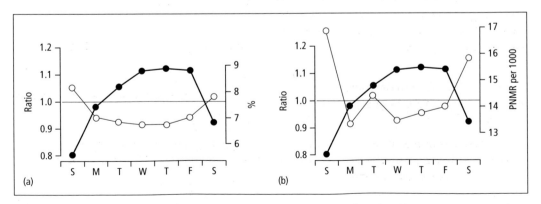

**Figure 23.4** Ratio of births by days of the week (for England and Wales) (•–•) against (a) percentage of babies born ≤2500 g (o–o) and (b) perinatal mortality rate per 1000 total births (o–o).

**Figure 23.5** Maternal mortality in England and Wales, 1900–1997.

still women who die as a consequence of pregnancy or labour. The major causes are secondary to hypertensive disease of pregnancy, thrombosis and haemorrhage which are discussed in more detail. Maternal mortality is expressed as deaths/1000 births or deaths/100000 maternities. In the three-year period 1997–1999 the maternal mortality rate (MMR) for direct and indirect deaths was 11.4/100000 maternities. In other words there was one death for each 9000 deliveries. The advances in medical care prior to pregnancy have led to more women with pre-existing medical conditions becoming pregnant. This has led to indirect maternal deaths making a larger contribution to the maternal mortality rate. In 1997–1999 the MMR for direct deaths was 5.0/100000 compared with 6.4/100000 for indirect deaths. In 1985–87 the rates were 6.1 and 3.8 respectively. However, the combined direct and indirect MMR has hardly changed over the past 15 years.

## Pregnancy-induced hypertension, pre-eclampsia and eclampsia (MMR: 0.7/100000)

Eclampsia is getting rarer. When it comes earlier in pregnancy (before 28 weeks) it has a worse effect. Death is from intracranial haemorrhage or renal failure.

To reduce deaths:
• Identify high-risk women.

• Check blood pressure frequently in pregnancy.
• Admit those with signs of pre-eclampsia.

This may be at home for lesser degrees rather than in hospital.

• Recognize biochemical and haematological aspects of HELLP syndrome (haemolysis, elevated liver enzymes, low platelets) (Chapter 10).

## Thromboembolism (MMR: 1.7/100000)

**1** A third are antenatal and two-thirds after delivery. A third of the latter follow Caesarean section.
**2** High-risk patients:
  • Over 35 years.
  • Obese.
  • Operative delivery.
  • Previous thrombosis.
**3** Half the deaths are with little warning of previous thrombotic episodes.

To reduce deaths:
• Prophylactic anticoagulation of high-risk patients.
• Avoid risk factors.
• Prompt effective treatment on suspicion.

## Abortion

**1** Usually after procured and illegal interferences.
**2** Patients die from haemorrhage, sepsis or renal failure.

To reduce deaths:
• Wider use of legal therapeutic abortion.
• Better contraception.

## Haemorrhage (MMR: 0.3/100000)

*Abruptio placentae*
Severe hypovolaemia leads to shock and later renal shutdown.

To reduce deaths:
• Central venous pressure monitoring.
• Adequate and quick blood replacement.

*Placenta praevia*
Repeated and increasing haemorrhage in last trimester of pregnancy. The severe degrees must be

treated by Caesarean section, which may be a technically difficult operation.

To reduce deaths:

• Pay more attention to warning bleeds in pregnancy.

• Have consultant in theatre for Caesarean section.

*Postpartum haemorrhage*
Usually from an atonic uterus but can follow cervical trauma.

To reduce deaths:

• Give oxytocic drug routinely at delivery.

• Deliver patients at risk in hospital where blood is available (see Chapter 13).

• Act promptly using a planned protocol.

*Ectopic pregnancy*
With reduction of deaths from other forms of haemorrhage this is becoming relatively more important.

To reduce deaths:

• Admit patients with suspicious symptoms.

• Act promptly on patients with actual symptoms.

• Be prepared to laparoscope on suspicion and do not rely on ultrasound and β hCG findings alone.

## Anaesthesia

Deaths associated with general anaesthesia are reducing greatly in the UK. Inhalation of acid stomach contents in labour under general anaesthetic leads to Mendelson's syndrome.

To reduce deaths:

• Wider use of regional anaesthetics (e.g. spinal epidural).

• If general anaesthetic essential, a senior anaesthetist involved and intubation with a cuffed tube.

## Other causes

All the other causes produce few deaths. Infection, once the killer of 1 : 5 women in childbirth, is much reduced (although still causing some deaths each year, mostly after Caesarean section in labour with prolonged ruptured membranes). Heart disease as a cause is diminishing, as rheumatic fever is better avoided or diagnosed and treated in childhood.

## Substandard care

In the UK every maternal death is reported to a central committee which publishes its confidential findings at three-yearly intervals. This is not a judicial enquiry and no blame is apportioned to any individual. It is a medical audit where the profession looks closely at its own work and tries to learn from mistakes. The committee tries to assess in each case if an avoidable factor was present: if there was 'some departure from the acceptable standards of satisfactory care'.

In a recent report, 50% of the deaths directly due to pregnancy and delivery were considered to have been avoidable by this definition. It was the patient who made the largest single contribution to this in the antenatal period by either not coming for care or else ignoring advice given. In labour, the hospital obstetricians and anaesthetists were associated with the highest incidence of substandard care incidents. This was mostly from not paying sufficient heed to warning signs and not having senior-enough doctors in the delivery suite. Shortage of staff and facilities is beginning to be reported in this category. Substandard care from general practitioners and midwives in these cases was rare.

The most important ways of reducing maternal deaths are:

**1** Improved access to antenatal care.

**2** Improved education in the population of the importance of antenatal care.

**3** More consultant obstetric and anaesthetic involvement on the delivery suite.

**4** Introduction of evidence-based guidelines for all areas of maternity care.

**5** Regular training of all staff including emergency drills for postpartum haemorrhage and shoulder dystocia.

## Near misses

Because maternal deaths are so few, even after national analysis, one cannot draw many statistical conclusions. However, an extended method can be used to increase the database. Here, one looks at women who have a firm diagnosis of a given, precisely diagnosed condition and examines the background even though they did not die. For example, one could look at those who have lost over two litres of blood at a primary postpartum haemorrhage. This would be a fairly well-defined group for the loss is so great and one would be able to compare the aetiology and management with that of women who died from postpartum haemorrhage. By so doing one would examine about six times as many cases. Similarly, one could look at the reasonably firm diagnosis of pulmonary embolism proven by a scan and, again, examine them as a larger group than those who died from the condition.

The idea of near misses as a method of examination is excellent for an individual hospital or group of hospitals that work as one, but is more difficult to apply regionally or nationally unless the definitions are firmly established.

## Risk management

Routine reporting of all incidents that affect the quality of care for the patient are reported to a risk management manager and lead clinician. These may appear minor (past notes unavailable in clinic) or major (delay in obtaining cross-matched blood in a case of major obstetric haemorrhage), however they can both have a major effect on the standard of patient care and the outcome for the mother and her child. All reports should be a purely factual account and not apportion blame to any individual. The manager and the lead clinician collect all the reports and investigate the problem. This process may highlight a problem in the system of care which needs to be rectified or a need for further staff education, either individually or as a group. Serious adverse incidents are usually investigated locally and then reported to the Strategic Health Authority together with recommendations for preventing such incidents reoccurring.

Patient complaints are investigated in a similar way and responses containing the facts of the case,

the findings of the investigation and the recommendations are sent to the patient. Patients have the right to request a formal meeting with the hospital after the investigation to express their views and make their own recommendations. Hospitals now employ patient advocates to help patients through this process. The direct communication to the patient reduces the number of cases that proceed to litigation.

Audit is used as a risk management tool. All maternity units in the UK are expected to follow evidence based multidisciplinary guidelines. These may be developed locally, by the Royal College of Obstetricians and Gynaecologists or the National Institute of Clinical Excellence (NICE). Each unit is expected to audit their care against these guidelines at regular intervals. Each audit should identify areas where the guidelines are not being followed or are inadequate. Recommendations are made to improve the standard of care and the audit repeated to ensure that the changes have improved care. This is called the audit cycle.

## Perinatal mortality

The perinatal mortality rate (PMR) is the total of stillbirths and first-week neonatal deaths occurring in every 1000 total births. In 1997 it was 7.9/1000 total births in England and Wales.

### Factors influencing PMR

**1** The mother's:
- Place of residence.
- Past nutrition and diseases.
- Education.
- Social class.

**2** The age and parity of the mother.

**3** An efficient health service.

**4** The definition of stillbirth and neonatal death. In the UK this was changed in 1991 to deaths after 24 completed weeks of gestation from a previous 28 weeks' limit. Hence, a small apparent increase for a short time appears.

Figure 23.6 shows the progressive reduction of PMR in 70 years.

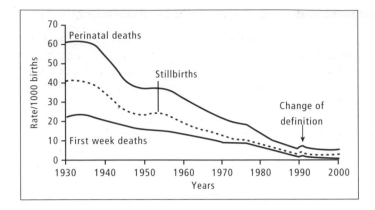

**Figure 23.6** Perinatal mortality, still-births and 1st-week neonatal deaths in England and Wales from 1930.

## Causes of perinatal mortality

Precise causes of perinatal death are often confused by a lack of autopsy information and an insistence on a single or primary cause of death on the certificate.

*Classification of causes of perinatal death*
**1** Macerated stillbirths without malformation.
**2** Congenital malformation in either stillbirths or neonatal deaths.
**3** Intrapartum perinatal deaths secondary to as-phyxia or trauma or both.
**4** Neonatal deaths as a result of immaturity.
**5** Other specific causes, e.g. Rh haemolytic disease.

*Small for gestational age (SGA)*
Two-thirds of neonatal deaths are associated with SGA. A high incidence of hyaline membrane disease and intraventricular haemorrhage is found.

*Congenital malformations*
A tenth of stillbirths and a quarter of neonatal deaths have a congenital anomaly. Malformations of the CNS and cardiovascular system are the most common.

*Asphyxia*
There is post-mortem evidence of asphyxia in a third of stillbirths and a tenth of neonatal deaths. This is due to:

BEFORE LABOUR
**1** Abruptio placentae.
**2** Placental failure:
• Pre-eclampsia.
• Hypertension.
• Postmaturity.
• Diabetes.

IN LABOUR
**1** Prolonged labour.
**2** Cord prolapse.

AT DELIVERY
• Impacted shoulder.
• Delayed onset of respiration.

*Birth injury*
Less than a tenth of neonatal deaths.

ASSOCIATED WITH
**1** Too fast a delivery:
• Precipitate delivery with immature fetus.
• Breech presentation with insufficient time for moulding of head.
**2** Too difficult a delivery:
• Disproportion.
• Badly performed operative delivery, particu-larly forceps.

*Infection*
**1** Intrauterine.
**2** Neonatal.

## Confidential enquiry into stillbirths and deaths in infancy (CESDI)

The Department of Health in conjunction with the Royal Colleges have set up a CESDI group in each of the old NHS regions. These assess, in a confidential way, all deaths from the 20th week of pregnancy through childbirth to the end of the first year of life. Although the groupings are disparate, one can derive a subset analysis of perinatal deaths leaving out the under-24-weekers (large numbers are terminations of pregnancy) and those after the first week of life when the perinatal period finishes among whom the major causes of death include sudden infant death syndrome.

Each CESDI group has research midwives who determine more details of each death reported by examining the hospital notes. The central committee then makes recommendations and finds if there is any degree of substandard care. In fact, in the most recent report of the Welsh CESDI group on intrapartum deaths in 1999 it was found that 52% had substandard care.

Recommendations follow from these groups and it is hoped that they can make as great an impact on perinatal deaths as the Confidential Enquiries in Maternal Deaths has made on mothers' care.

## Management of perinatal death

When pregnancy ends with the loss of a fetus or a neonate, particular care and support are needed for the couple involved. This is a difficult situation for the parents and relatives, and for the medical and nursing staff. Grief reactions commonly involve the following phases (Fig. 23.7):

**1** Initial denial of what has occurred.
**2** Attempt to apportion blame to themselves.
**3** Attempt to apportion blame to the doctors and midwives.
**4** Eventual acceptance of their loss which may take several months.

*Problems associated with intrauterine death*
• Intrauterine infection.
• Difficult induction of labour.
• Psychological and possibly psychiatric sequelae.
• Disseminated intravascular coagulopathy (DIC) if fetus retained for some weeks (rare).

*Management of labour*
**1** Confirm the diagnosis of intrauterine death by real-time ultrasound.
**2** Give the parents time to come to terms with their loss.

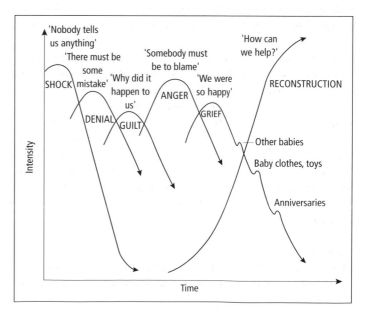

**Figure 23.7** Emotional response to bad news. (From Meadow R & Newell S. (2001) *Lecture Notes on Paediatrics*, Blackwell Publishing, Oxford.)

**3** Plan induction of labour at a time which is suitable for the parents but ensuring that they have a midwife to look after them throughout the period of induction and labour.
**4** Arrange facilities for the partner to stay throughout the procedure.

*Investigations*
**1** Hb (including $HbA_{1C}$).
**2** Cross-match and save serum.
**3** Kleihauer test.
**4** Clotting studies.
**5** Lupus anticoagulant and anticardiolipin antibodies (for SLE/APS).
**6** Fasting blood sugar and HbA (for diabetes).
**7** Liver function tests.

*Management*
**1** Induce labour with prostaglandin pessaries given every 3 hours.
**2** Do not rupture the membranes until the woman is in labour and the cervix is more than 4 cm dilated.
**3** Keep an accurate fluid balance chart.
**4** Give liberal analgesia. If the woman wishes an epidural ensure her blood clotting values are normal.
**5** Discuss whether the couple wish to see the baby after delivery. Parents should be encouraged but not pressed to view their babies.

• The babies should be photographed, clothed and looking as natural as possible. These photographs should be filed in case parents wish to see them much later—sometimes they ask a year or so later.

*Postnatal care*
The woman should be looked after by midwifery staff known to her in the antenatal period. The length of hospital stay is not determined by medical events but more by what the couple want. She may go home as soon as she wishes but should not have the feeling of being sent away. Her general practitioner and community midwife must be informed by one of the medical staff of the loss by telephone.
**1** Arrange for the mother to be seen by a specialist midwife who is skilled in counselling patients who have lost their babies.
**2** Ask if she wishes her baby to be baptized and buried; if so, arrange the procedure with the hospital chaplain or other religious leader according to the parent's request.
**3** Consent for post-mortem should be obtained from the parents.
**4** The following procedures should be undertaken:
(a) Heart blood should be sent for karyotyping and viral studies.
(b) Two polaroid photographs of the baby should be taken. One should be a general photograph and the other should be a close-up of the baby's face. In addition, foot and hand prints and a lock of hair are retained.
(c) X-ray the baby.
(d) If available, MRI of baby.
**5** The consultant should interview the parents before discharge from hospital and explain as far as possible the circumstances surrounding the death.
**6** The couple are met 4–6 weeks later with all the autopsy evidence to hand.
**7** The couple should be put in touch with a society, e.g. Stillbirth, Abortion and Neonatal Death Society (SANDS), or people who have experienced a similar problem.
**8** Lactation should be suppressed by means of a firm supporting brassiere. Bromocriptine or cabergoline should be offered.
**9** Women who had to have a hysterectomy or have one surviving twin may need professional psychotherapeutic help.

**Self-assessment**

**23.1** Give the definitions for the following.
  **1** Total birth rate.
  **2** General fertility rate.
  **3** Maternal mortality.
  **4** Maternal mortality rate.
  **5** Perinatal mortality rate.
**23.2** Give the three most common direct causes of maternal mortality.
**23.3** Give three measures that can be undertaken to improve standards of care.
**23.4** Give three maternal factors that affect the perinatal mortality rate.
**23.5** Following the death of a baby what investigations should be performed?

# Answers to self-assessment questions

## Chapter 1

### Answers

**1.1** (1) h, (2) g, (3) d, (4) b or j, (5) b or j

The uterine artery is a branch of the (1), (h) *Internal iliac* artery. The uterus is a hollow, muscle-walled organ in direct communication with the (2), (g) *fallopian tubes* and the vagina. Inferior to the uterine artery lies the (3), (d) *ureter*. The ligaments that support the uterus include the (4), (j) *uterosacral* and (5), (b) *transverse cervical*.

**1.2** b, e

See pp. 9–10. The granulosa cells secrete oestradiol. Once the oocyte is released they become luteal cells and secrete oestradiol and progesterone. At menarche there are around 500000 oocytes in the ovary.

**1.3** a, d, e

See pp. 4, 10, 13. At the time of the luteinizing hormone (LH) surge the oocyte undergoes meiosis but with an unequal distribution of the cellular cytoplasm forming an oocyte ready for fertilization and the first polar body with 23 chromosomes in each. Glycogen is secreted in the luteal (secretory) phase of the cycle from the effects of progesterone on the endometrial glands. The endometrium is shed because the spiral arterioles go into spasm causing hypoxia and death of the endometrium. The follicular phase (from day one of the cycle to ovulation) can be very variable (cf. polycystic ovaries) whilst the luteal phase is of a fixed duration.

**1.4** a, c, d

Oestradiol exerts a negative feedback on follicle stimulating hormone (FSH) (i.e. when

**1.5**

Round ligament (j)

Ampulla of fallopian tube (e)
Infundibulopelvic ligament (f)

Uterine corpus (b)

Internal os of cervix (g)

oestradiol levels are low FSH levels rise). FSH and LH are controlled by the *hypo*thalamus which secretes gonadotrophin releasing hormone (GnRH). Testosterone is the major precursor of oestradiol and is secreted by the theca cells under the influence of LH, the testosterone passes to the granulosa cells and is converted to estradiol catalysed by FSH. Progesterone only starts to be secreted at the time of ovulation and reaches its peak seven days after ovulation in a non-conception cycle.

# Chapter 2

## Marking scheme

The marking schemes vary from medical school to medical school. Some mix marks for communication and details of the history together into one question. Some may group aspects of the question together and allow examiners to give a mark of 0, 1 or 2 depending on how well the candidate does in each section. The scheme outlined below gives a list of the things that may give you a mark (shown in parentheses) or that may be included in a group and is therefore only a guide to possible marks. It is wise to ask your medical school how their marking scheme is structured. You can then devise your own marking sheets and use the cases for practice.

## Communication

- Introduces themselves.  (1)
- Eye contact.  (1)
- Picks up on verbal clues. Patients often do not remember all the relevant details of their history immediately but may say something that implies you have an opportunity to ask another question to help them remember or feel comfortable answering the question. For example, the first patient may not be in a relationship because of dyspareunia and she may give a clue when answering the question about whether or not she has a boyfriend; the second patient may not remember the episode of being asked to take some tablets, or may know that she had had an infection causing her ectopic

pregnancy, but feels a bit stupid for not having followed medical advice.  (1)
- Picks up on non-verbal clues. Non-verbal clues include patients not looking at you, wriggling on their chair, not answering the question. You should notice this and re-ask the question in a different way or challenge the patient gently if she is looking very diffident or refusing to answer the question.  (1)
- Use of non-medical language.  (1)
- Listens.  (1)
- Allows questions.  (1)
- Structured history. This is marks for a logical order to the history which leads to a full assessment of the patient's problem. Do not get bogged down in irrelevant detail such as a long surgical history or detailed system questions as you will run out of time. Learn the list of headings and go through them quickly ignoring negative answers and going into further detail for a positive answer. (1/2)
- Accurate summary.  (1)

## History taking

- Identifies main complaint  (1)
- Explores main complaint appropriately  (1)
- Ascertains all details of main complaint  (1)
- Last menstrual period (LMP)/menstrual history  (1)
- Past gynaecological/sexual health history  (1)
- Past obstetric history  (1)
- Past medical and surgical history  (1)
- Family history  (1)
- Social history  (1)
- Medication/allergies  (1)
- Summary  (1)

The first three of these may be grouped together to give a score of 0–2.

In some medical schools the role-player may give marks for communication—did you trust this doctor, would you see him/her again, did you understand what they told you?—are questions that may be asked. Role-players have been shown to be very accurate in picking out the students who will do well and those that will not.

# Chapter 3

The relevant information for each scenario is given below.

**1** Turner's syndrome is associated with short stature in 100% of cases. Her ovaries are dysgenetic so they do not ovulate giving her a low oestrogen with a high LH and FSH. They should receive oestrogen replacement in the form of the pill or hormone replacement therapy (HRT). Egg donation is their only means of becoming pregnant.

**2** This young girl has a low body mass index (BMI) and does a lot of exercise. Both of these predispose young women to hypogonadotrophic hypogonadism. They have a low oestrogen and low LH and FSH. The most appropriate treatment is weight gain and a reduction in exercise (unlikely to be accepted in a talented athlete, but they can still gain weight). Treatment for fertility should not be started until weight gain has been achieved.

**3** This young girl has the stigmata of polycystic ovary syndrome—secondary oligoamenorrhoea, acne and hirsutism. Her family history of type 2 diabetes makes her more likely to be insulin resistant leading to anovulation and hirsutism. Her LH may be raised, FSH and oestradiol will be normal whilst her testosterone will be raised. First line treatment should be the pill with a non-androgenic progestogen (cyproterone acetate, desorgestrol, gestinone). To achieve fertility clomiphene is the first line of treatment.

**4** Galactorrhoea is diagnostic of hyperprolactinaemia. Her LH, FSH and oestradiol will be low and her prolactin raised. First line treatment is with a dopamine agonist. This is usually all that is required to restore menses and fertility.

**5** This is a classic presentation of cryptomenorrhoea—imperforate hymen. All her hormone profile will be normal. First line of treatment is surgery—a cruciate incision in the hymen. Menses will continue normally and fertility will be unaffected.

## Answers

    **3.1** (1) f, (2) j, (3) d, (4) h, (5) b
    **3.2** (1) d, (2) f, (3) b, (4) c, (5) a
    **3.3** (1) h, (2) a, (3) f, (4) e, (5) c

# Chapter 4

## Answers

**4.1** a, d, f, i, j

Women with premature ovarian failure (POF) do not respond to FSH, their only recourse to achieve pregnancy is through egg donation. The risk of multiple pregnancy is 10%. A sperm count of >20 million per ml with >50% motility and >10% normal forms is considered normal.

**4.2** b, c, e

**4.3** (a) 5, (b) 8, (c) 2, (d) 10, (e) 1

Tubal surgery is less successful than *in vitro* fertilization (IVF) in achieving an intrauterine pregnancy in women with tubal damage. The first line treatment for ovulation induction in women with polycystic ovary syndrome (PCOS) is clomiphene. FSH is successful for women with hypogonadotrophic hypogonadism. Klinefelter's syndrome men should not be offered intracytoplasmic sperm injection (ICSI) because of the high risk of triploidy in the offspring.

# Chapter 5

## Answers

**5.1** Marking scheme as for communication in Chapter 2 and:

- History of menarche and cycle length    (1)
- Nature of relationship with boyfriend including his age    (1)
- Implications of starting sex at this age    (1)
- Relationships within the family    (1)
- Telling her that she is below the legal age for sex    (1)
- Trying to persuade her to tell her parents    (1)
- Agreeing that this consultation is confidential    (1)
- Discussing the pros and cons of the oral contraceptive pill    (1)
- Explaining how to take the pill and the 7 day rule    (1)
- Bringing the consultation to a close    (1)

Following the Gillick case doctors are able to prescribe contraception for under-age girls and are bound to keep it confidential from her parents if the girl so wishes. This does not, however, remove the responsibility of the doctor to act in the best interests of the girl. She should be encouraged to tell her parents/guardian. She should be aware of the risks of entering into a sexual relationship—increased risk of PID, finding it unsatisfactory/ painful, need for cervical smears and of pregnancy even if on the pill. When you have agreed to give her the pill it is important to give her the advice on how to take it (see pp. 49–50).

5.2 Marking scheme:
- Establishes age and size of family (1)
- Establishes stability of relationship (1)
- Discusses male sterilization (1)
- Discusses alternative methods including Mirena (1)
- Agrees to sterilization (1)
- Explains operation/day case (1)
- Explains failure rate (1:300) (1)
- Explains that sterilization is irreversible and permanent (1)
- Explains need for mini-lap if necessary (unlikely) (1)
- Reassures about weight gain and periods (1)

Vasectomy (male sterilization) should always be discussed as there are fewer risks of the operation compared to laparoscopy. The stability of the relationship is very important although difficult to assess as divorce followed by a new partnership is a common reason for women to request reversal of sterilization. Couples sometimes feel that removing the threat of further pregnancies will solve their relationship difficulties—seldom the case. There is no evidence that contraceptive pills in any form increase weight gain but it is a commonly held belief amongst women.

5.3 b, d
The combined oral contraceptive pill (COCP) should be started on the first day of a period. By missing the first two pills in a packet the pill free interval has been lengthened beyond 7 days significantly increasing the risk that ovu-lation will occur. The COCP does not need to be taken at the same time each day, although the progestogen only pill does because the mechanism for pregnancy prevention is not by suppression of ovulation. Antiepileptic medication interferes with the metabolism of the COCP so a higher dose of oestrogen is required to suppress ovulation (50 µg vs 35 µg).

5.4 a, e
Intrauterine contraceptive devices (IUCDs) do not increase the risk of a sickle cell crisis but a careful sexual history should be taken. An IUCD does not increase the risk of cervical cancer.

5.5 b, c, e
Oestrogen alone does not reduce the risk of implantation. High dose progestogen alone is now the recommended form of oral emergency contraception. Oral emergency contraception is only effective up to 72 hours after unprotected intercourse whilst an IUCD can be used up to 5 days after intercourse. Endometrial curettage does not prevent implantation.

# Chapter 6

## Answers

6.1 None of these statements is correct.
Gonorrhoea is best diagnosed by endocervical culture on specialized media. High diagnostic yields occur if multiple sites are cultured, i.e. endocervix, urethra and anorectum. Erythromycin is used to treat penicillin-allergic pregnant women but has poor transplacental distribution. In addition, it is not as reliable as penicillin or doxycycline in the treatment of syphilis. Therefore, it is recommended that the mother is re-treated with doxycycline after breastfeeding has stopped. Consideration should be given to treating the baby with procaine penicillin at birth. First attack genital herpes can occur months or years after initial infection with the herpes virus, so contact tracing has limited value. Bacterial vaginosis is best diagnosed by Gram stain of high vaginal

swab (HVS) material and culture for *Garnerella vaginalis* is no longer recommended. Endocervical specimens should be used to test for *Chlamydia trachomatis* but this is usually done by DNA amplification or enzyme linked immunoassay (ELISA) techniques, as culture requires specialist laboratories.

**6.2** c, e

Human immunodeficiency virus (HIV) is a retrovirus and contains RNA and the reverse transcriptase enzyme which allows a DNA copy of the single RNA strand to be made. HIV uses the CD4 receptor to enter cells. Most seroconversions are asymptomatic. Patients with CD4 counts between 200 and $350 \times 10^6$/L will also be encouraged to start anti-HIV drugs if they have severe HIV-related symptoms, have had an opportunistic infection or have a rapidly falling CD4 count in the presence of a high viral load. Antiretroviral resistance testing may give false reassurance about susceptibility to anti-HIV drugs used in the past as resistant virus may be archived in the body and re-emerge under selective pressure should the drug be introduced. Tenofovir belongs to a new class of nucleotide reverse transcriptase inhibitors.

**6.3** Marking scheme:

- Communication
  - Introduces themselves (1)
  - Eye contact (1)
  - Pick up anxiety over sexually transmitted infection (STI) (1)
- History-taking
  - Asked about extramarital partners (1)
  - Asked about condoms (1)
  - Took a drug history (1)
  - Asked about nature of discharge (1)
  - Asked about past STIs (1)
- Investigations
  - Offered full STI screen* (2)
  - Offered HIV test (1)
  - Discussed 3 month window period for HIV (1)

*Half mark for each of chlamydial infection, trichomoniasis, gonorrhoea and syphilis.

**6.4** c

Vulvovaginal candidiasis is not usually associated with an offensive smell, which suggests either bacterial vaginosis or trichomoniasis. Condylomata lata are lesions seen in secondary syphilis and do not respond to podophyllotoxin although condylomata acuminata (warts) respond well to this therapy. Women who have been raped before are more often victims of rape again. For this reason, it is important to offer hepatitis B vaccination to all women who have been raped. The forensic examination should be done as soon as possible after the rape to collect evidence for the police. The STI screen is best done at 7–10 days after the assault, when STI pathogens are more likely to be detected. The sexual history should not be taken by the same doctor who did the forensic examination (who will likely attend court) as juries and judges sometimes view women with a past history of STIs in 'bad light'. It is best for this 'sensitive' information to be given to another doctor unlikely to be called to court. The best diagnostic method for trichomoniasis uses DNA amplification technology, although this is not widely available at the present time.

**6.5** a, c

Ejaculation is under sympathetic control mediated by adrenoreceptors. Psychosexual problems usually involve conflicts, often between couples. Psychosexual medicine works best when both members of the couple participate in the therapeutic intervention and understand the rationale. Vaginismus can be observed during the clinical examination on insertion of a speculum or fingers during a bimanual examination. Anorgasmia occurs more commonly in women than men and has both psychological and physical causes.

# Chapter 7

## Answers

**7.1** (1) c, (2) f, (3) h, (4) e, (5) a

In pregnancy the maternal cardiac output increases principally because of a greater (1), (c) *stroke volume*. Haemoglobin concentrations decrease because of an increased (2), (f) *plasma volume* despite an increased (3), (h) *red cell mass*. The uterus grows by (4), (e) *hypertrophy* with a blood flow at term of (5), (a) *100–150ml/kg/min*.

If you got any of these wrong please reread the text pp. 83–85.

**7.2** b, e

Fetal haemoglobin has a higher oxygen affinity than haemoglobin A and shifts the dissociation curve to the left as it becomes saturated with oxygen at lower oxygen concentrations. In fetal life oxygenated blood flows in the umbilical vein and deoxygenated blood in the umbilical arteries. In fetal life the lungs are filled with fluid produced by the pneumocytes which has a different chemical composition to amniotic fluid. This is confusing as the lungs do not develop properly in the absence of amniotic fluid (anhydramnios) presumably because growth factors in amniotic fluid are absorbed from the fetal mouth and gut as the fetus drinks the amniotic fluid although we do not have direct evidence for this. Fetal organogenesis is complete by 12 weeks of gestation although growth and maturation of all tissues continue throughout pregnancy. Exposure to infections in the second trimester (e.g. rubella, toxoplasmosis, cytomegalovirus (CMV), listeriosis) can lead to mental retardation, blindness, deafness, etc., because of failure of maturation rather than congenital abnormality.

**7.3** a, c, e

The placenta acts as a filter so that nutrients, oxygen and hormones pass from the mother to the fetus whilst waste products pass from the fetus to the mother. Human placental lactogen regulates the metabolism of insulin and glucose. Progesterone from the placenta relaxes the uterine muscle helping to maintain the pregnancy.

**7.4** b, c, d

- b = face presentation
- c = vertex presentation
- d = dimension used in ultrasound and is one of the diameters of a vertex presentation

All of these have an average diameter of 10 cm. The largest diameter is the mentovertical with an average diameter of 13 cm.

# Chapter 8

## Answers

**8.1** a, c, d, e

After two miscarriages the chances of a successful pregnancy next time are 75%. The majority of miscarriages are due to chromosomal abnormalities in the baby which are not inherited and occur by chance. In giving this piece of information many parents assume that there is something wrong with them and it is important to present this with sensitivity and emphasise that it is a chance occurrence in the majority of miscarriages. Women should also be advised to take folic acid to reduce the risk of neural tube defects.

**8.2** b, d

Subserosal fibroids are not associated with an increased risk of ectopic pregnancy. A corpus luteal cyst is a normal finding in pregnancy. For other risk factors see Box 8.2, p. 100.

**8.3** a, d, e

Hydatidiform mole is commoner in the Far East than in the UK. It is associated with hyperemesis and early onset pre-eclamptic toxaemia (PET). Because of the risk of developing choriocarcinoma, regular follow-up with serial human chorionic gonadatrophin (hCG) estimations is essential. Surgical evacuation is the treatment of choice with chemotherapy used for those with persistently raised hCG concentrations.

**8.4** c, e

Choriocarcinoma spreads to the lungs. 40% of cases of choriocarcinoma follow a hydatidiform mole whilst the risk of developing choriocarcinoma after a hydatidiform mole is 4%.

## Chapter 9

### Answers

9.1 Checklist (see pp. 109–110).
  - Introduction and verbal consent to examine.
  - Check with woman for areas of tenderness.
  - Inspection: the abdomen is distended compatible with pregnancy. Check for scars, rashes, linea nigra, (pigmented midline), anaemia, fetal movements.
  - Palpation: measure symphysiofundal height (SFH), lie, presentation, engagement, fetal movements, liquor volume.
  - Auscultation of fetal heart with a Pinard or Doppler.
  - Some stations also require you to take the blood pressure and check the urine. It is common in exams for albumin or glucose to be added to the urine to catch out the unwary student.

9.2 b, d
  Toxoplasmosis and CMV are not routinely screened in the UK although in regions with a high prevalence they may be. Syphilis is easily treated with penicillin and prevents transmission to the fetus. For rubella, whilst vaccination cannot be given in pregnancy, knowing the immunity status allows the non-immune woman to avoid contact with children or adults with rubella and to be immunized in the postnatal period. Hepatitis B is screened but not Hepatitis A, as Hepatitis A usually resolves with no risk of transmission to the baby whilst Hepatitis B may affect the baby postnatally and immunization can be offered at birth to the neonate.

9.3 a, c, e
  A reduced liquor volume has been shown to be one of the most sensitive indicators for fetal distress. Polyhydramnios may be associated with gestational diabetes or fetal abnormality, e.g. tracheoesophageal fistula. Fetal movements are a good indicator of well-being. Umbilical artery dopplers are reassuring if the pressure index and flow are normal. Uterine artery dopplers are used as identifiers of women at

increased risk of developing PET if notches are present at 20 and 24 weeks. An abnormal fetal lie may be associated with congenital abnormalities but is not a predictor of fetal distress.

9.4 b
  This woman is in her sixth pregnancy so she is Gravida 6. She has had three babies born after 24 weeks of pregnancy although one died — Para 3. She has had two pregnancy losses below 24 weeks — Para 3 + 2. Even though the 21 week gestation baby was born alive it is still classified as a miscarriage because the gestation is less than the legal definition of viability — 24 completed weeks of pregnancy.

## Chapter 10

### Answers

10.1 c, d
  Raised blood pressure without proteinuria is called pregnancy-induced hypertension and is rarely associated with increased risks for the mother or fetus. Women with gestational diabetes are at increased risk of developing PET rather than the other way round. An eclamptic fit secondary to cerebral oedema can be fatal to both the mother and baby whilst HELLP syndrome is usually more insidious in onset and resolves spontaneously after delivery of the baby.

10.2 b
  This woman is at high risk of developing eclampsia and requires immediate treatment for her blood pressure and cerebral irritation (fulminating pre-eclampsia). Magnesium sulphate has been shown to be the most effective prophylactic treatment for pre-eclampsia. It does have an effect on hypertension but is quite slow-acting. This woman's blood pressure is at a level which predisposes her to cerebral haemorrhage. Hydrallazine given in bolus doses every 15 minutes until the diastolic blood pressure is between 90–100 acts more rapidly. Once the blood pressure is controlled, the baby should

be delivered by whichever method is most appropriate (see p. 125).

**10.3** a, c, d, e

All pregnant women should have their blood group checked regardless of gestation or site of the pregnancy. Anti-D should be given when there is any bleeding in pregnancy. The commonest cause of rhesus iso-immunization is now the failure to give anti-D following a miscarriage, therapeutic abortion or ectopic pregnancy.

**10.4** d

Placenta praevia, cervical cancer and cervical polyp/ectropion can present with an antepartum haemorrhage but are usually painless. Von-Willebrand's disease predisposes a woman to bleeding but the diagnosis is usually known prior to pregnancy. Placental abruption can be concealed so the uterus may be large for dates due to haemorrhage behind the placenta. The uterus is classically tender and hard (woody). The maternal tachycardia suggests haemorrhage. Young women can maintain their blood pressure despite a large loss of blood so it is easy to underestimate the degree of haemorrhage.

**10.5** a, e

Renal agenesis is associated with anhydramnios because the fetus does not excrete any urine. PET is associated with oligohydramnios particularly if there is intrauterine growth restriction. Obstetric cholestasis does not alter the liquor volume. In a fetus with tracheoesophageal fistula, the fetus is unable to ingest the amniotic fluid and so liquor volume increases.

## Chapter 11

## Answers

**11.1** c, d

Ketoacidosis is never seen in gestational diabetes and is very rare even in women with type 1 diabetes. Women with a first degree relative with type 2 diabetes (non-insulin dependent/ late onset) are at increased risk of

developing gestational diabetes. It is most commonly controlled by diet alone. All women with diabetes whether pre-existing or gestational are at increased risk of developing PET.

**11.2** a, b, c, e

Congenital abnormalities are rare in gestational diabetes but three times more common in poorly controlled pre-existing diabetes.

**11.3** c, e

Iron and folate deficiency are the two most important common causes of anaemia in pregnancy. Supplements should be given particularly if the diet is not balanced (e.g. strict vegetarians).

**11.4** a, c, d

β-haemolytic streptococcus is a vaginal commensal that cannot be eradicated with penicillin as it will return, so there is no point in treating it prior to labour. The main risk to the neonate is of pneumonia and/or septicaemia which is associated with a high perinatal mortality. Treatment of the mother with penicillin during labour reduces the risk to the baby.

## Chapter 12

## Answers

**12.1** c, a, e, b, d

See pp. 165–166. If possible find a doll and a pelvis and rehearse the stages of rotation and delivery of the fetal head.

**12.2** c, d

See pp. 115, 167–70.

**12.3** a, c, e

Meconium may be a sign of fetal hypoxia and so all fetuses should be electronically monitored. Electronic fetal heart rate monitoring (EFM) is indicated if a deceleration is heard on intermittent monitoring. An alteration in the fetal heart rate is often the first sign of impending scar dehiscence in labour after a Caesarean section. Spontaneous rupture of membranes with clear liquor is not an indication for EFM provided the onset of labour is spontaneous.

**12.4** b, c, d

Uterine contractions are generated in the fundus of the uterus and pass down the uterus to the lower segment. In a woman using epidural anaesthesia who is fully dilated the normal practice is to allow the head to descend for 1 hour and for the woman to push for 1 hour. If the baby is not delivered then she should be assessed by an obstetrician and decision made with regard to delivery. Women with an epidural should be continuously electronically monitored.

## Chapter 13

## Answers

**13.1** b, c, e

The WHO definition of the active phase of labour is when the cervix is 3 cm or more dilated. To revise the Bishop's score see p. 184. In early labour women should be encouraged to mobilize as this encourages the fetal head to descend and put pressure on the cervix, helping it to dilate.

**13.2** a, d, e

Brow presentation cannot deliver spontaneously as the presenting diameter is the largest (13 cm). Occipitotransverse diameter is also large and the baby requires rotation to occipitoanterior (vertex position) before delivery. Occipitoposterior positions can deliver spontaneously although they commonly require operative intervention with forceps.

**13.3** a, b, d

Most babies that are breech before 34 weeks turn to become cephalic so that the incidence at term is 3% compared to 10% in preterm babies. The more preterm the infant the higher the likelihood of a breech presentation. Offering external cephalic version (ECV) prior to 37 weeks is often a waste of time, firstly the baby may spontaneously turn to cephalic and secondly the baby is more likely to revert to breech if turned before 37 weeks but

highly unlikely to do so beyond 37 weeks. Breech presentation is associated with an increased prevalence of congenital abnormalities and at term the perinatal morbidity and mortality are higher even if the baby is delivered by Caesarean section. There is no evidence that the outcome for the second twin is improved by elective Caesarean section if the first twin is cephalic, since the first twin will have dilated up the vaginal passage and the second twin is usually smaller than the first twin.

**13.4** 1 Adequate analgesia

2 Head not palpable per abdomen

3 Empty bladder

4 Full dilatation

5 Head at spines or below

**13.5** a, c, d

Syntometrine is a combination of syntocinon and ergometrine, both effective uterotonics which reduce the incidence of postpartum haemorrhage (PPH) significantly. Neither spontaneous vaginal delivery nor pre-eclampsia (in the absence of HELLP syndrome) increase the risk of PPH.

## Chapter 14

## Answers

**14.1** c, d, e

Bottle feeding does not predispose a woman to develop postnatal depression (PND) unless she wanted to breastfeed and is unable to — this would be rare at only 48 hours after birth. Sleeplessness, a strong family history and a recent life event all predispose a woman to PND. Rejection of the infant is more likely to be an early sign of postnatal psychosis.

**14.2** (1) f, (2) c, (3) j, (4) d, (5) h

A high temperature in a woman passing clots is most likely to indicate retained products of conception with endometritis. Salpingitis is usually a late sequelae. The left loin tenderness would indicate pyelonephritis rather than cystitis. The fluctuant mass in her breast makes the diagnosis one of breast abscess rather than simple engorgement. Pulmonary emboli rarely present with a temperature over 38°C or a productive cough although pleuritic pain is common. Deep vein thrombosis usually gives a low grade pyrexia or none at all with deep pain in the muscle of the calf rather than tenderness and erythema.

**14.3** (1) i, (2) a, (3) h, (4) b, (5) f

Flucloxacillin is a broad spectrum antibiotic which is particularly effective against *Staphylococcus aureus* and is used for any infection near the skin. A breast abscess will not settle without surgical incision and drainage. All urinary tract infections require increased fluid intake and antibiotics. Bronchitis with a temperature as high as this may go on to develop pneumonia and so physiotherapy is very helpful to clear the infected tissue from the lungs. Retained products of conception are a focus for infection and should be removed after 24 hours of broad spectrum antibiotics to reduce the risk of uterine perforation and bleeding.

## Chapter 15

## Answers

**15.1**  1  Heart rate
2  Respiratory effort
3  Muscle tone
4  Reflex irritability
5  Colour

**15.2**  d
- Heart rate >100 = 2
- Respiratory effort, irregular = 1
- Muscle tone, flaccid = 0
- Reflex irritability, grimace = 1
- Colour, pink = 2

**15.3**  Marking scheme:
Breastfeeding
*For* (5 marks)
- Breast milk is designed for babies
- Contains right balance of nutrients

- Contains immunoglobulins
- Reduces infections in the baby particularly GI upset
- Cheap and always available on demand
- No bottles to make up or heat up
- No sterilising kit needed

*Against* (5 marks)
- Engorged breasts
- Cracked nipples
- May not be enough milk
- May leak but can get pads
- Exposed in public but more acceptable now, with special bras and clothes can be very discrete.
- Have to take baby with you
- Only one that can feed the baby

**15.4**  c, d

If the baby is rhesus negative and the mother positive fetal blood cells can not sensitize the mother. If the baby is positive and the mother negative then the fetal cells can sensitize the mother who makes anti-D antibodies which then cross the placenta and haemolyse the fetal red blood cells causing jaundice. At birth the antibodies persist in the babies circulation and combined with the normal breakdown of blood cells can lead to significant jaundice. A baby of blood group A born to a mother with blood group B may suffer from an ABO incompatibility because the antigens and antibodies on the surface of the baby's red blood cells are different from that of its mother. They commonly become severely jaundiced in the first 24 hours of life. It is rare if the mother is blood group O.

## Chapter 16

## Answers

**16.1**  Marking scheme:
- Introduction and getting basic details                                    (1)
- Menstrual history                                        (0–4)
  - Previous cycle
  - Change in nature of period

- Protection used
- Impact on life
- Past contraceptive history      (1)
- Last smear test      (1)
- Past obstetric history      (1)
- Social history      (1)
- Medication and allergies      (1)

**16.2** b, e, g

Hysteroscopy and endometrial biopsy are not routine in women under the age of 40 as endometrial cancer is rare in this age group. They are indicated if the ultrasound scan is abnormal (see p. 221). Cervical pathology is common and may not be visible to the naked eye so a smear is always indicated even if it has been done quite recently. A full blood count is a reasonably objective measure of blood loss since a Hb of less than 11 g/dl with a microcytic picture indicates anaemia secondary to menstrual blood loss. Thyroid function tests are rarely informative in an asymptomatic woman. It is rare for women to become menopausal below the age of 40 (3%) so a hormone profile is likely to be normal. PCOS usually presents much earlier

**16.3** c

First line treatment with non-hormonal medication has been shown to be the most effective first-line therapy with the least side-effects. Antifibrinolytics, antiprostaglandins and fenamates are the most effective. Paracetamol is ineffective. Norethisterone is only effective if taken continuously. Mirena IUS is a second or third line therapy whilst endometrial ablation is only indicated if all other treatments have failed.

**16.4** a, c, d

Penicillin V does not affect anaerobic organisms and so is not suitable for infection prophylaxis in gynaecology. Subcutaneous heparin is reserved for women at high risk of thrombosis. TED stockings and flowtron boots are recommended internationally for all women undergoing pelvic surgery.

**16.5** All are correct.

Although damage to the bladder and ureters are rare complications they are serious and so

women should be warned. The ovaries may need removal if they are very adherent to the uterus or are abnormal. Infection and haemorrhage are a risk for all operations however small.

# Chapter 17

## Answers

**17.1** Marking scheme:

*History*

- Nature of pain      (0–2)
  - Site, onset, cyclicity, radiation
- Dyspareunia      (0–2)
  - Nature, deep, relationship, sensitivity
- Menstrual history      (0–2)
  - Regular, normal flow, contraception, desire for fertility,
- Logical sequence      (0–2)
  - Past medical, surgical, gynaecological and obstetric history, SH, FH, medication, allergies
- Management      (0–2)
  - Endometriosis, pelvic examination, USS, laparoscopy

**17.2** b, d

Submucous fibroids protrude into the uterine cavity and are lined by endometrium. The increased surface area and the increased vascularity of the fibroid commonly leads to menorrhagia. The uterus recognizes the fibroid as being abnormal and tries to extrude it through the cervix commonly causing severe secondary dysmenorrhoea. Constant lower abdominal pain is usually associated with fibroid degeneration. Vomiting and ectopic pregnancy are rare associations.

**17.3** d

Pelvic inflammatory disease (PID) presents with a pyrexia of >38°C, bilateral pain and no vomiting. Bleeding into or rupture of a cyst can cause localized peritonism but rarely vomiting. A torted ovarian cyst is commonly associated with vomiting.

**17.4** b, c, d, e

Fibroids degenerate whilst ovarian cysts can rupture causing acute abdominal pain. Dermoid cysts contain well differentiated tissues such as teeth, hair, sebaceous glands, renal, neural and other tissues. Endometriomas or luteal cysts which have bled internally contain altered blood (chocolate cysts). Ovarian cysts can secrete androgens (sertoli-leydig cell tumours/androblastomas) or oestrogen (granulosa cell tumours).

**17.5** a

This is a classic presentation of appendicitis. Pyelonephritis usually presents with loin pain, a swinging pyrexia of >38°C, vomiting, frequency and dysuria. A torted ovarian cyst is not usually associated with pyrexia nor absence of bowel movements. Bowel obstruction presents with generalized abdominal pain and apyrexia and a ruptured ovarian cyst rarely causes GI symptoms.

# Chapter 18

## Answers

**18.1** 1 Mammography for all women aged 50–65
2 Clinical examination
3 Ultrasound +/– MRI
4 Needle cytology

**18.2** 1 *Genetic*: Mutations in either of the two recognized breast cancer genes (BRCA1 and BRCA2) Cowden's Syndrome and ataxia telangiectasia.

2 *Hormonal factors*: early menarche, late menopause, no full-term pregnancies, full-term pregnancy occurring after the age of 40. HRT of all types but particularly continuous combined HRT (see Chapter 21).

3 *Environmental factors*:
• Radiation.
• Alcohol increases the risk of breast cancer in a dose-dependent manner.
• Diet has a large effect on breast cancer risk. Diets rich in fresh fruit and vegetables are associated with a much lower risk of breast cancer (50% reduction).

**18.3** a, b, e

Cisplatin is commonly used in ovarian cancer but is not effective for breast cancer. Provera is used in endometrial cancer. Other adjuvant therapies include tamoxifen, cyclophosphamide, 5-fluorouracil and epirubicin.

**18.4** 1 Breast itself (breast primary)
2 Axillary lymph nodes
3 Micrometastases

# Chapter 19

## Answers

**19.1** Marking scheme (potential 15 marks)
• Introduces him/herself (1)
• Fills in the form correctly* (0–3)
  • Name and address of woman
  • Date of birth
  • Hospital/NHS number (if known)
  • GP's name and address
  • Clinical details
  • Last menstrual period
  • Hormone treatment/IUCD
• Fills in slide correctly (0–3)
  • Name of woman
  • Date of birth
  • Date of test
  • Hospital/NHS number (if known)
• Explains procedure and obtains verbal consent (0–2)
• Assembles and inserts speculum correctly (1)
• Uses Aylesbury spatula (not blunt ended) (0–2)
  • Rotates spatula through 360°
• Removes speculum correctly (1)
• Wipes both sides of spatula onto slide (1)
• Fixes slide with fixative (1)
*not always expected under exam conditions but vital in clinic.

It is difficult to remember that a model should be spoken to as if she were a real woman. Most OSCE questions award marks for the communication part of the vaginal examination. It is therefore vital that the student practices this acting technique with a model and a critical observer prior to the examination.

**19.2** a, c

All women with a single cervical smear showing mild/moderate/severe dyskaryosis should be referred to colposcopy. Colposcopy with a cervical biopsy is essential for an accurate diagnosis of the degree of cervical intraepithelial neoplasia (CIN). The correlation between the degree of dyskaryosis and CIN is not strong and so cervical screening does not give an accurate diagnosis. The guideline for the referral of mild dyskaryosis has recently been updated. The previous practice of repeating the smear after 6 months and referring to colposcopy if the smear is abnormal again has been changed such that all these women should be referred for colposcopy. Additionally if a woman has three abnormal smears in the preceding 5 years that may not have been consecutive then she should be referred for colposcopy if she has not already been seen. In pregnancy the cervical smear is more likely to give a false positive result rather than a negative result.

**19.3** d, b, e, a, c

It is important that 4% acetic acid is painted onto the cervix prior to staining with iodine since the density of the white staining and the rapidity of change give an idea of the degree of abnormality whilst iodine only shows the area of abnormality. A biopsy should be taken prior to undertaking treatment to give an accurate histological diagnosis. The loop diathermy can distort the histology result due to heat artefact.

**19.4** 1 Not all women attend for cervical screening.
2 There will be false negatives (inadequate sampling/misinterpretation of the slide by a cytopathologist/glandular abnormality).
3 The infrequency of screening may miss a rapidly progressive case.
4 Treatment may be incorrectly given.
5 Treatment may not be adequate (full excision may not be achieved/reported on histology).

6 Recurrences may occur even if treatment was initially effective (see p. 262).

**19.5** 1 GPs keep a computerized register of all patients by age and sex.
2 The computer generates automatic letters of recall every 3 years for all women between the ages of 20–64.
3 Results are sent to the woman and her GP regardless of where the test was taken.
4 GPs are rewarded financially for achieving a >85% uptake of the programme.
5 Smear tests are offered in a variety of community and hospital based clinics.

# Chapter 20

# Answers

**20.1** b, d

Ovarian cancer is now the most common gynaecological malignancy (breast cancer is not classified as a gynaecological malignancy) and carries the poorest prognosis because the majority of cases present with Stage 3. Cervical carcinoma most commonly presents with postcoital bleeding whilst endometrial cancer presents with postmenopausal bleeding. Ovarian cancer remains asymptomatic until late in the disease when women usually present with a pelvic mass and/or ascites.

**20.2** a, c, d

This woman has carcinoma of the cervix until proved otherwise. Staging for cervical carcinoma includes:
• Examination under anaesthetic (including rectovaginal examination to assess the size of the tumour, parametrial spread, extension into the rectovagina; septum).
• Cystoscopy and sigmoidoscopy to assess bladder and bowel involvement.
• Biopsy of the suspicious area.
• Chest X-ray.
• IVU.
CT or MRI may be offered if available to give further information on tumour size, nodal involvement but does not alter the

FIGO staging which is determined by the above investigations.

**20.3** a

Carcinoma of the uterus and cervix nearly always present with vaginal bleeding. Stage 1 cancer of the ovary usually presents with a mobile mass which is rarely palpable per abdomen since ovarian cancer often spreads beyond the ovary at diameters of less than 10 cm. Stage 4 ovarian cancer can only be diagnosed clinically if there are palpable supraclavicular glands, a pleural effusion or a palpable liver edge—all of these are rare. The most common stage of ovarian carcinoma at presentation is stage 3.

**20.4** b, c, d

A hysteroscopy and curettage is not helpful in ovarian carcinoma but essential in the staging and diagnosis of uterine and cervical carcinoma. Whilst urea and electrolytes are essential pre-operative tests they are not useful in the staging of ovarian cancer. Imaging of the chest abdomen and pelvis should confirm the stage of the disease prior to operation giving the surgeon and the patient useful information about the nature of the proposed operation and its likely success. Together with the medical oncologists a plan for postoperative chemotherapy can be drawn up and the patient made fully aware of what is in store prior to major surgery.

**20.5** a, c

This woman has vulval carcinoma until proven otherwise. A careful examination of her vulva will reveal an ulcerated area which is probably secondarily infected. A swab and a biopsy should be taken from the ulcerated area. A high vaginal swab, cervical smear and hysteroscopy are unlikely to be informative. Abdominal palpation is indicated to detect enlarged inguinal nodes.

# Chapter 21

## Answers

**21.1** Marking scheme:

| | |
|---|---|
| 1 Oestrogen only | (1) |
| 2 Ideally till the age of 55 or a minimum of two years | (1) |
| 3 Minimal side effects, transient breast tenderness and abdominal bloating | (1) |
| 4 Can take orally, transdermally or by implant every 6 months | (1) |
| 5 Main benefit is longterm reduction in risk of osteoporosis | (1) |
| 6 Longterm increased risk of breast cancer particularly after 5 years | (1) |
| General ability to discuss with the patient, ability to give accurate information, reassures the patient, appreciates her concerns and helps her make a decision | (0–4) |

**21.2** a, e

Endometrial polyps are a common cause of postmenopausal vaginal bleeding. Atrophic vaginitis may spontaneously bleed but this is more common following sexual intercourse. It is also rare in women who are on HRT as they do not get vaginal dryness. Subserosal fibroids usually become inactive following the menopause even in women on HRT. Ovarian cancer virtually never presents with vaginal bleeding whilst cervical cancer often does.

**21.3**

• Inspection of vulva and vagina to check for vulval ulceration. Urethral caruncle, atrophic vaginitis (unlikely in this woman).

• Speculum examination of the cervix; to exclude cervical polyp, ectropion or frank carcinoma.

• Cervical smear; to detect carcinoma *in situ* or cervical dysplasia.

• Bimanual vaginal examination; to exclude uterine enlargement.

• Transvaginal ultrasound scan; to check for endometrial abnormalities including polyps.

• Endometrial biopsy; to ensure that the histology of the endometrium is normal.

• Hysteroscopy and biopsy if transvaginal scan is abnormal or equivocal.

## Chapter 22

### Answers

22.1 Marking scheme:
  • Introduction, name and age of patient (1)
  • Identifying main complaint accurately (1)
  • History taking
  • Leaking when coughing/exercising
  • Nocturia
  • Symptoms of prolapse } (0–4)
  • Disruption to life
  • Past obstetric history
  • Past gynae history
  • Family history } (0–4)
  • Social history

22.2
  • Abdominal palpation to check for masses.
  • Vaginal examination — dorsal initially to check for descent and the size of the uterus and presence of any pelvic masses.
  • Place her in the Sims position. Ask her to cough. Note presence or absence of cystourethrocoele and uterine descent. Note any urinary leaking.
  • Management — her symptoms are suggestive of genuine stress incontinence. She requires urodynamic assessment with video cystourethrography before deciding on treatment. Whilst awaiting this she should be referred to the physiotherapists for pelvic floor exercises including voluntary retention of vaginal cones. If urodynamics confirm a diagnosis of GSI then a retropubic or vaginal sling operation will give her the best chance of cure rather than a vaginal colporrhaphy.

22.3 Any five of the following:
  1 Urinary tract infection.
  2 Local infection.
  3 Primary or secondary haemorrhage.
  4 Urinary retention.
  5 Dyspareunia/vaginal stenosis.
  6 Venous thrombosis.
  7 Vaginal discharge.
  8 Chest infection.
  9 Fistula formation.

22.4 An involuntary loss of urine from the urethra when the transmitted intra-abdominal pressure causes a rise in the intravesical pressure which exceeds the intraurethral pressure in the absence of a detrusor contraction.

22.5 a, d, e

Incomplete emptying and a slow urinary stream are more often associated with overflow incontinence. Frequency and urgency are the commonest symptoms of detrusor instability but are not specific enough to establish the diagnosis without urodynamic investigation.

## Chapter 23

### Answers

23.1 1 Total birth rate = births per year × 1000/midyear population.
  2 General fertility rate = births per year × 1000/ women aged 15–45.
  3 Maternal mortality: deaths of women while pregnant or within 42 days of delivery, miscarriage, termination of pregnancy, from any cause related to or aggravated by the pregnancy or its management but not from accidental or incidental causes.
  4 Maternal mortality rate = no. of maternal deaths/ 1000 births or 100 000 maternities.
  5 Perinatal mortality rate = total of stillbirths + deaths in the first 7 days of life over 24 weeks of gestation/ 1000 births.

23.2 Hypertensive disease of pregnancy, thromboembolism, haemorrhage.

23.3 Introduction of evidence based guidelines, incident reporting and investigation, regular audit.

23.4 Place of residence, past nutrition and diseases, education, social class, age and parity.

**23.5** Full blood count, fasting blood sugar and HbA1C, Kleihauer test, clotting studies, lupus anticoagulant and anticardiolipin antibodies, Liver function tests, post-mortem examination, fetal karyotyping, X-ray or MRI of the baby if post-mortem declined.

## Additional reading

Meadow R. & Newell S. (2001) *Lecture Notes on Paediatrics*, 6th edn. Blackwell Publishing, Oxford.
Confidential enquiry into Maternal deaths 1997–1999—Why Mothers die
Confidential enquiry into Stillbirth and Death in Infancy (CESDI)

## Web sites and relevant published guidelines

NICE guidelines *www.nice.org.uk*
Caesarean section
Osteoporosis
Assessment and treatment of fertility
Electronic fetal monitoring
Induction of labour
Anti-D immunoglobulin for Rh prophylaxis
Confidential enquiry into maternal and child health

RCOG guidelines 1999–2002 *www.rcog.org/guidelines*
Male and female sterilization
Antenatal corticosteroids
Gestational trophoblastic disease
Alcohol consumption in pregnancy
Amniocentesis
Anti-D immunoglobulin for Rh prophylaxis
Breast cancer (pregnancy after)
Breech presentation (management)
Chickenpox in pregnancy
Early pregnancy loss—management
Eclampsia (management)
Endometriosis (investigation and management)
Genital herpes in pregnancy
HRT and venous thromboembolism
Instrumental vaginal delivery
Pelvimetry—clinical indications
Perineal repair
Peritoneal closure
Placenta praevia: diagnosis and management
Recurrent miscarriage—management
Small for gestational age fetus—investigation and management
Third and fourth degree perineal tears following vaginal delivery—management
Thromboembolic disease in pregnancy and the puerperium
Tocolytic drugs for women in pre-term labour.
Tubal pregnancies

# Index

Page numbers in *italics* represent figures, those in bold represent tables